Brow and Upper Eyelid Surgery: Multispecialty Approach

Editors

BABAK AZIZZADEH
GUY G. MASSRY

CLINICS IN PLASTIC SURGERY

www.plasticsurgery.theclinics.com

January 2013 • Volume 40 • Number 1

ELSEVIER

1600 John F. Kennedy Boulevard • Suite 1800 • Philadelphia, Pennsylvania 19103-2899

http://www.theclinics.com

CLINICS IN PLASTIC SURGERY Volume 40, Number 1
January 2013 ISSN 0094-1298, ISBN-13: 978-1-4557-5844-9

Editor: Joanne Husovski

Clinics in Plastic Surgery (ISSN 0094-1298) is published quarterly by Elsevier Inc., 360 Park Avenue South, New York, NY 10010-1710. Months of issue are January, April, July, and October. Business and Editorial Offices: 1600 John F. Kennedy Blvd., Suite 1800, Philadelphia, PA 19103-2899. Periodicals postage paid at New York, NY and additional mailing offices. Subscription prices are $448.00 per year for US individuals, $666.00 per year for US institutions, $221.00 per year for US students and residents, $509.00 per year for Canadian individuals, $779.00 per year for Canadian institutions, $578.00 per year for international individuals, $779.00 per year for international institutions, and $279.00 per year for Canadian and foreign students/residents. To receive student/resident rate, orders must be accompanied by name of affiliated institution, date of term, and the *signature* of program/residency coordinator on institution letterhead. Orders will be billed at individual rate until proof of status is received. Foreign air speed delivery is included in all *Clinics* subscription prices. All prices are subject to change without notice. **POSTMASTER:** Send address changes to *Clinics in Plastic Surgery*, Elsevier Health Sciences Division, Subscription Customer Service, 3251 Riverport Lane, Maryland Heights, MO 63043. **Customer Service: 1-800-654-2452 (US and Canada). From outside of the United States and Canada, call 314-447-8871. Fax: 314-447-8029. E-mail: JournalsCustomerService-usa@elsevier.com (for print support); JournalsOnlineSupport-usa@ elsevier.com (for online support).**

Reprints. For copies of 100 or more of articles in this publication, please contact the Commercial Reprints Department, Elsevier Inc., 360 Park Avenue South, New York, New York 10010-1710. Tel.: (+1) 212-633-3812; Fax: (+1) 212-462-1935; E-mail: reprints@elsevier.com.

Clinics in Plastic Surgery is covered in *Current Contents, EMBASE/Excerpta Medica, Science Citation Index, MEDLINE/ PubMed (Index Medicus), ASCA,* and *ISI/BIOMED.*

Printed and bound by CPI Group (UK) Ltd, Croydon, CR0 4YY

Transferred to digital print 2012

Contributors

CONSULTING EDITORS

MACK L. CHENEY, MD
Professor of Otology and Laryngology, Harvard
Medical School, Massachusetts Eye and Ear
Infirmary, Boston, Massachusetts

ROGER A. DAILEY, MD, FACS
Chief, Division of Oculofacial Plastic Surgery,
Casey Aesthetic Facial Surgery Center, Oregon
Health and Sciences University, Portland,
Oregon

MITCHEL P. GOLDMAN, MD
Volunteer Clinical Professor of Dermatology,
University of California, San Diego, San Diego,
California

FOAD NAHAI, MD, FACS
Paces Plastic Surgery, Atlanta, Georgia

GUEST EDITORS

BABAK AZIZZADEH, MD
Center for Advanced Facial Plastic Surgery,
Beverly Hills, California

GUY G. MASSRY, MD
Spalding Drive Cosmetic Surgery and
Dermatology, Beverly Hills, California

SECTION EDITORS

DORIS DAY, MD, Dermatology
Day Dermatology and Aesthetics, New York,
New York, www.DrDorisDay.com

JENNIFER C. KIM, MD, Facial Plastic Surgery
Center for Facial Cosmetic Surgery, University
of Michigan Health System Livonia, Michigan,
www.MichiganFacialPlasticSurgery.com/
Our_Doctors3.htm

FARZAD R. NAHAI, MD, Plastic Surgery
PACES Plastic Surgery, Atlanta, Georgia,
www.PacesPlasticSurgery.com/the-practice/
Meet-the-Doctors/Farzad-r-Nahai-md

**JULIE ANN WOODWARD, MD, Oculoplastic
Surgery**
Oculoplastic and Reconstructive Surgery
Service, Duke University Health System,
Durham, North Carolina, www.DukeHealth.
org/Physicians/Julie_Ann_Woodward

AUTHORS

SANG TAE AHN, MD
Professor of Plastic Surgery, Seoul St. Mary's
Hospital, The Catholic University of Korea,
Seocho-gu, Seoul, South Korea

SHAN R. BAKER, MD
Professor, Center for Facial Cosmetic Surgery,
University of Michigan, Livonia, Michigan

KOFI D. BOAHENE, MD
Assistant Professor, Division of Facial Plastic
and Reconstructive Surgery, Johns Hopkins
School of Medicine, Baltimore, Maryland

JEREMY A. BRAUER, MD
Laser & Skin Surgery Center of New York,
New York, New York

VIVIAN W. BUCAY, MD, FAAD
Private Practice; Department of Physician Assistant Studies, Clinical Assistant Professor, University of Texas Health Science Center, San Antonio, Texas

PATRICK J. BYRNE, MD
Associate Professor, Division of Facial Plastic and Reconstructive Surgery, Johns Hopkins School of Medicine, Baltimore, Maryland

RYAN M. COLLAR, MD
Clinical Instructor, Division of Facial Plastic and Reconstructive Surgery, Johns Hopkins School of Medicine, Baltimore, Maryland

CRAIG N. CZYZ, DO, FACOS
Chair, Division of Ophthalmology, Section Head, Section Oculofacial Plastic and Reconstructive Surgery, Ohio University/Ohio Health Doctors Hospital; Assistant Professor, Department of Ophthalmology, Ohio University College of Osteopathic Medicine, Columbus, Ohio

DORIS DAY, MD, MA
The Ronald O. Perelman Department of Dermatology, New York University Langone Medical Center; Day Dermatology and Aesthetics, New York, New York

REBECCA FITZGERALD, MD
Dermatology Private Practice, Assistant Clinical Instructor, Department of Medicine, David Geffen School of Medicine, University of California, Los Angeles, California

JILL A. FOSTER, MD, FACS
Division of Ophthalmology, Section Oculofacial Plastic and Reconstructive Surgery, Ohio Health Doctors Hospital; Associate Clinical Professor, Division of Oculofacial Plastic and Reconstructive Surgery, Department of Ophthalmology, The Ohio State University; Medical Director, Plastic Surgery Ohio, Columbus, Ohio

GARRETT R. GRIFFIN, MD
Fellow, Division of Facial Plastic & Reconstructive Surgery, Keck School of Medicine at USC, Los Angeles, California

ELIZABETH K. HALE, MD
Laser & Skin Surgery Center of New York, New York, New York; The Ronald O. Perelman Department of Dermatology, New York University Langone Medical Center, New York, New York

ROBERT H. HILL, MD
Division of Ophthalmology, Section Oculofacial Plastic and Reconstructive Surgery, Ohio Health Doctors Hospital; Division of Oculofacial Plastic and Reconstructive Surgery, Department of Ophthalmology, The Ohio State University, Columbus, Ohio

DON O. KIKKAWA, MD
Professor and Chief, Division of Oculofacial Plastic and Reconstructive Surgery, Department of Ophthalmology, University of California - San Diego, Shiley Eye Center, La Jolla, California

MONIKA KIRIPOLSKY, MD, FAAD
Scripps Health, Encinitas, California

JENNIFER C. KIM, MD
Division of Facial Plastic and Reconstructive Surgery, Department of Otolaryngology–Head and Neck Surgery, University of Michigan Health System, Ann Arbor, Michigan

NAKYUNG KIM, MD
L Plastic Surgery – Form & Function, San Francisco, California

BOBBY S. KORN, MD, PhD
Associate Professor, Division of Oculofacial Plastic and Reconstructive Surgery, Department of Ophthalmology, Shiley Eye Center, University of California - San Diego, La Jolla, California

VINCENT B. LAM, MD
Department of Ophthalmology, Drexel University College of Medicine, Philadelphia, Pennsylvania

PHILLIP R. LANGSDON, MD, FACS
Professor, Division of Facial Plastic and Reconstructive Surgery, Department of Otolaryngology–Head and Neck Surgery; University of Tennessee Health Science Center, Memphis, Tennessee; Chief of Facial Plastic Surgery and Director, The Langsdon Clinic, Germantown, Tennessee

CHARLES K. LEE, MD
Chief of Plastic Surgery, St. Mary's Medical Center; Assistant Clinical Professor of Plastic and Reconstructive Surgery, University of California, San Francisco (UCSF), San Francisco, California

JUDY W. LEE, MD
Assistant Professor, Department of
Otolaryngology, Center for Facial Cosmetic
Surgery, University of Michigan, Livonia,
Michigan

DAVID M. LIEBERMAN, MD
Facial Plastic and Reconstructive Surgery,
The Redwood Center for Facial Plastic
Surgery, Palo Alto, California

LEE HOOI LIM, MBBS
International Clinical Fellow, Division of
Oculofacial Plastic and Reconstructive
Surgery, Department of Ophthalmology, Shiley
Eye Center, University of California - San
Diego, La Jolla, California; Consultant,
Oculoplastic Department, Singapore National
Eye Center, Singapore

JOHN J. MARTIN Jr, MD
Facial Plastic and Cosmetic Surgery, Coral
Gables, Florida

CLINTON D. McCORD, MD
Paces Plastic Surgery, Atlanta, Georgia

JEFFREY S. MOYER, MD, FACS
Division of Facial Plastic and Reconstructive
Surgery, Department of Otolaryngology–Head
and Neck Surgery, Center for Facial Cosmetic
Surgery, University of Michigan, Livonia,
Michigan

FARZAD R. NAHAI, MD
Private Practice, Paces Plastic Surgery,
Assistant Clinical Professor of Plastic Surgery,
Emory University, Atlanta, Georgia

TANUJ NAKRA, MD
Texas Oculoplastic Consultants, Austin, Texas

UTPAL PATEL, MD, PhD
The Ronald O. Perelman Department of
Dermatology, New York University Langone
Medical Center, New York, New York

JON-PAUL PEPPER, MD
Division of Facial Plastic and Reconstructive
Surgery, Department of Otolaryngology–Head
and Neck Surgery, Center for Facial
Cosmetic Surgery, University of Michigan,
Livonia, Michigan

VITO C. QUATELA, MD
Facial Plastic and Reconstructive Surgery,
Lindsay House Center for Cosmetic and
Reconstructive Surgery, Rochester, New York

DAVID W. RODWELL III, MD
Resident, Division of Facial Plastic and
Reconstructive Surgery, Department of
Otolaryngology–Head and Neck Surgery,
University of Tennessee Health Science
Center, Memphis, Tennessee

AMY E. ROSE, MD
The Ronald O. Perelman Department of
Dermatology, New York University Langone
Medical Center, New York, New York

NATALIE A. STANCIU, MD
Texas Oculoplastic Consultants, Austin, Texas

HEMA SUNDARAM, MD, FAAD
Sundaram Dermatology, Cosmetic & Laser
Surgery Center, Rockville, Maryland

ADAM M. TERELLA, MD
Instructor/Fellow, Division of Facial Plastic and
Reconstructive Surgery, Department of
Otolaryngology–Head and Neck Surgery,
Oregon Health and Science University,
Portland, Oregon

PARKER A. VELARGO, MD
Resident, Division of Facial Plastic and
Reconstructive Surgery, Department of
Otolaryngology–Head and Neck Surgery,
University of Tennessee Health Science
Center, Memphis, Tennessee

JOSEPH D. WALRATH, MD
Paces Plastic Surgery, Atlanta, Georgia

TOM D. WANG, MD
Professor, Division of Facial Plastic and
Reconstructive Surgery, Department of
Otolaryngology–Head and Neck Surgery,
Oregon Health and Science University,
Portland, Oregon

KATHERINE M. WHIPPLE, MD
Instructor, Division of Oculofacial Plastic
and Reconstructive Surgery, Department
of Ophthalmology, Shiley Eye Center,
University of California-San Diego,
La Jolla, California

ALLAN E. WULC, MD, FACS
Department of Ophthalmology
and Otolaryngology, Drexel University
College of Medicine; Department of
Ophthalmology, Scheie Eye Institute,
University of Pennsylvania, Philadelphia,
Pennsylvania

Contents

The Brow-Eyelid Continuum: An Anatomic Perspective　　　　1

Vincent B. Lam, Craig N. Czyz, and Allan E. Wulc

> Surgical rejuvenation of the upper eyelids cannot be performed without taking into consideration the complex aesthetic and anatomic relationships that exist in the upper third of the face. This article discusses the concept of evaluating this facial area as a unit, the brow-eyelid continuum. In addition, the ideal aesthetic goal, the clinical and surgical anatomy, and aging changes relevant to this region are discussed.

Contemporary Concepts in Brow and Eyelid Aging　　　　21

Rebecca Fitzgerald

> This article outlines current concepts in aging brows and lids, and focuses on the current "evolution" to the 3-dimensional construct. Relevant anatomy is reviewed in detail because thoughtful analysis of the underlying anatomy, ethnicity, gender, and goals of each patient will greatly enhance our ability to address site-specific corrections to achieve optimal and natural-looking results.

Preoperative Evaluation of the Brow-Lid Continuum　　　　43

Craig N. Czyz, Robert H. Hill, and Jill A. Foster

> This article presents a thorough review for evaluation of the upper eyelid and brow preceding rejuvenation surgery. It is emphasized that surgical and nonsurgical rejuvenation is directed toward modifying the anatomic causes of facial aging. Relevant anatomy of the lid and brow area is delineated. The discussion includes surgical notes that highlight cautions or tips related to the anatomic area concerned.

patients about outcomes of this surgery. Detailed steps of the endoscopic brow-lift technique are presented. Complications are discussed and the authors conclude with a summarization of what the ideal brow-lift procedure would accomplish.

The open brow lift procedure is discussed in terms of relevant surgical anatomy, preoperative evaluation, and detailed surgical technique for pretrichial coronal forehead lift with hair-bearing temporal lift, direct incisional brow lift, and coronal brow lift. Complications are discussed, and information is presented on patient evaluation and expectations, with a discussion of what patients can expect before and after brow lift surgery.

This article presents a review of the contribution of the periorbital musculature and brow depressors to the overall brow aesthetics. Special focus is given to the role of transblepharoplasty brow lift as well as myotomy of the corrugator and procerus muscles. The authors' preferred surgical technique and patient results are reviewed in detail.

Upper lid blepharoplasty is a procedure associated with a high level of patient and surgeon satisfaction. New insights into the anatomic underpinnings of the periorbital aging process have enabled more successful and reproducible surgical results. The authors provide a detailed discussion of the relevant anatomy and integrate this into their surgical philosophy for upper lid blepharoplasty. Special focus is given to presurgical planning.

Traditional upper blepharoplasty typically involves resection of excess upper eyelid skin and muscle with or without fat excision. Well-established concepts in periorbital aging have been challenged by newer morphologic and histologic studies that have characterized the changes that occur in the various periorbital soft tissue components. Several modified or adjunctive techniques have recently emerged to improve esthetic outcomes in upper blepharoplasty. The authors review surgical technique in detail: nasal fat repositioning, orbicularis oculi preservation, increasing lateral upper eyelid fullness, lacrimal gland resuspension, internal brow elevation, and glabellar myectomy, along with complications and aftercare involved with procedures.

The concept of the ideal female eyebrow has changed over time. Modern studies examining youthful brow aesthetics are reviewed. An analysis of ideal female brow characteristics as depicted in the Western print media between 1945 and 2011 was performed. This analysis provided objective evidence that the ideal youthful brow peak has migrated laterally over time to lie at the lateral canthus. There has been a nonstatistically significant trend toward lower and flatter brows. These findings are discussed in relation to current concepts of female brow aging, with re-percussions regarding endoscopic brow lift and aesthetic forehead surgery.

Upper eyelid blepharoplasty is one of the most common facial plastic surgeries per-formed in the United States. Understanding how brow position contributes to the up-per eyelid appearance is essential. Consistent and desirable surgical outcomes are best achieved with a detailed knowledge of periorbital anatomy. The surgeon must understand patients' expectations and ensure that surgical goals are realistic. The potential complications and their management are discussed. The goal of upper eyelid blepharoplasty is to create a sculpted upper lid with a visible pretarsal strip and subtle fullness along the lateral upper lid–brow complex. The trend toward vol-ume preservation is discussed.

Upper lid blepharoplasty is the most common plastic surgery procedure in Asia and has consistently maintained its position as cultural acceptance and techniques have evolved. Asian upper lid blepharoplasty is a complex procedure that requires com-prehensive understanding of the anatomy and precise surgical technique. The cre-ation of the supratarsal crease has gone through many evolutions in technique but the principles and goals remain the same: a functional, natural-appearing eyelid crease that brings out the beauty of the Asian eye. Recent advances have improved functional and aesthetic outcomes of Asian upper lid blepharoplasty.

This article is designed to offer a deeper understanding of complications that can occur with blepharoplasty and to highlight the realm of surgical and nonsurgical ther-apeutic interventions for revision.

This discussion focuses primarily on lipoatrophy and periorbital deflation in relation to adjunctive fat grafting of the brow and upper eyelid. Like with all clinical informa-tion for cosmetic and reconstructive surgeons in this multidisciplinary review of reju-venation of the brow and upper lid, the authors present anatomy, evaluation, patient expectations, technique, and complications – here, specifically in terms of fat graft-ing and its associated aspects of fat transfer and relocation and autologous fat, along with hyaluronic acid fillers. Fat harvest and preparation are also described in detail.

A straightforward approach to ptosis in a patient interested in aesthetic blepharo-plasty is presented. Beginning with an explanation of how ptosis often becomes apparent after an aesthetic surgery of the upper lid, this article describes functional anatomy of the eyelid relevant to ptosis, and discusses the various causes of ptosis, examination of the patient presenting with a drooping lid, aspects the surgeon should be aware of from the patient's perspective of this problem, and surgical options and techniques. The author describes in step-by-step detail external levator aponeurosis resection, pretarsal aponeurosis resection, Müller muscle–conjunctival resection, the complications that can arise with these procedures, and aftercare required.

CLINICS IN PLASTIC SURGERY

> This issue is the first of several volumes presenting topics from cosmetic specialists with training and practices in Plastic Surgery, Facial Plastic Surgery, Oculoplastic Surgery, and Dermatology. Upcoming are topics from specialists in MultispecialtyApproach to Midface, Perioral, Rhinoplasty, publishing in 2013–2014.

DOWNLOAD
Free App!

Review Articles
THE CLINICS

NOW AVAILABLE FOR YOUR iPhone and iPad

Foreword
Advances in Esthetic Surgery from Four Specialties

I commend guest editors Babak Azizzadeh, Guy Massry, and the four section editors for their vision in bringing together experts from four specialties in this issue of *Clinics in Plastic Surgery*. The topic, "The Multidisciplinary Approach to Brow and Upper Eyelid," is very timely given the dramatic and rapid changes in our approach to the brow and upper eyelid rejuvenation over the past few years. This is an up-to-date, state-of-the-art review. We have come a long way since the early 1990s where all we had to offer were coronal browlifts and perhaps collagen injections.

The development and popularity of the endoscopic approach to browlifting in the early 1990s were seen as a "disruptive technology" that changed our approach to browlifting and significantly reduced the number of open coronal browlifts. Later in the mid-1990s the emergence of toxins and their role in forehead rejuvenation and brow shaping was an even more impactful "disruptive technology." So effective was the impact of toxins that, in the years between 1997 and 2007, the number of browlifts performed dropped by a dramatic 51% according to the statistics reported in 2008 by the American Society for Aesthetic Plastic Surgery. Soon after, the rapid popularity of toxins for brow rejuvenation and the role of fillers emerged for brow, the temporal area, and the upper and lower eyelids. The injectables have proven to be efficacious, safe, and, at least in the short term, economical, with minimal down time or risk.

Parallel with the developing role of injectables, other approaches for brow rejuvenation emerged, the lateral or temporal browlift in isolation or in combination with a transpalpebral approach to modification of the corrugator and procerus muscles.

Currently, we have so many safe and effective options for brow and eyelid rejuvenation. In the right patient and in the right hands, each has a role and each may be considered the best option.

These recent advances were made possible through the efforts of all four core specialties of plastic surgery, facial plastic surgery, oculoplastic surgery, and dermatology. The willingness to share and to learn from each other has benefited us as physicians, and most of all, our patients benefit most from this shared information. Each of the authors in this volume is recognized as a contributor in his own field and we are indebted to them for sharing their expertise with the rest of us.

This volume, reviewing the current state of the art, belongs in the library of each of us who are involved in periorbital rejuvenation.

Foad Nahai, MD, FACS
3200 Downwood Circle
Paces Plastic Surgery
Atlanta, GA 30327, USA

E-mail address:
nahaimd@aol.com

Clin Plastic Surg 40 (2013) xiii
http://dx.doi.org/10.1016/j.cps.2012.11.001
0094-1298/13/$ – see front matter © 2013 Elsevier Inc. All rights reserved.

Foreword
Cross-Specialty Discussion Enables Educational Enlightenment

It is indeed a pleasure to contribute a foreword to this timely issue of *Clinics in Plastic Surgery*, dedicated to approaches to the brow and upper eyelid. It is refreshing to see a contribution to this series that emphasizes input from a wide variety of surgical specialties. Cross-specialty discussion and input uniformly lead to improved surgical outcomes and patient satisfaction. Unfortunately, this type of effective cross-talk has not always been the reality. Reflecting back several decades ago, a spirit of collaboration was the exception rather than the rule. Each specialty guarded its clinical knowledge very closely, and attempts to enter the gray zones of disparate surgical fields were met with vigorous resistance.

As reflected in this issue of *Clinics in Plastic Surgery*, this practice has changed. This shift is likely to have occurred because each specialty now acknowledges the positive impact of educational collaboration. It is now uniformly recognized that the tools employed by plastic surgeons, combined with those employed by facial plastic surgeons, oculoplastic surgeons, and dermatologists together, provide a stronger armamentarium with which to achieve superior clinical results. Also contributing to the openness of ideas across surgical specialties is the fact that gifted surgical teachers have emerged who have been willing to teach not only physicians within their discipline but also new generations of physicians from collaborating specialties. The combination of teaching excellence and surgical expertise embodied in our strongest thought leaders in facial surgery is inspiring and permits learners to seek cross-specialty guidance in their quest for improved results.

Specialty collaboration is a concept whose time has arrived, and with that it is each of our individual obligations to accurately assess our individual skill sets and experience. Collaboration should not lead to expansion of surgical "turf," but should be synergistic in its educational impact.

I applaud the gifted teachers represented in this publication for their dedication to this concept born of educational enlightenment.

Mack L. Cheney, MD
Massachusetts Eye and Ear Infirmary
Boston, MA, USA

E-mail address:
Mack_Cheney@meei.harvard.edu

Clin Plastic Surg 40 (2013) xv
http://dx.doi.org/10.1016/j.cps.2012.11.002
0094-1298/13/$ – see front matter © 2013 Published by Elsevier Inc.

plasticsurgery.theclinics.com

Foreword

The Core Four Subspecialties in Esthetic Surgery

It is my great pleasure to be asked to write the foreword for this excellent *Clinics in Plastic Surgery* issue that represents the collaborative efforts of "The Core Four Subspecialties" in facial esthetic surgery.

Obtaining the best surgical outcomes for our patients requires a detailed and thorough comprehension of surgical anatomy, preoperative evaluation techniques, and the varied surgical procedures we perform. There is no better way to assure precision and expertise in these areas than combining the education and experience of oculofacial plastic surgeons, general plastic surgeons, facial plastic surgeons, and dermatologic surgeons. The editors and section editors of this project have thus created a comprehensive and contemporary reference and shown the foresight to engage the core specialties to attain their goals.

I personally began my medical training at the Mayo Clinic Medical School in Rochester, Minnesota in 1978. During my anatomy course in the first year, our professor, Dr Don Cahill, mentioned to our class that there was a "turf" battle that existed among surgeons who operated on structures of the head and neck. I didn't really comprehend what he was saying at that time; it was only later that I was to come to understand this concept more fully.

While a student at Mayo, I was offered a residency in General and Plastic Surgery by Chairman of Surgery, Dr Donald McIlrath. As chance had it, though, a random elective with Dr Robert Waller (Chairman of Ophthalmology at the time) changed my plans. Dr Waller introduced and guided me toward a career in oculofacial plastic surgery. Since entering practice in 1988, I have occasionally witnessed the barriers present between the core specialties and the negative effects those conflicts created for the advancement of patient care, education, and safety.

In 2006, I was fortunate to serve as President of The American Society of Ophthalmic Plastic and Reconstructive Surgeons (ASOPRS). During my tenure, I had the great pleasure to be involved with Dr Mark Jewell (President of the American Society of Aesthetic Plastic Surgeons), Dr Alastair Carruthers (President of the American Society for Dermatologic Surgery, ASDS), and Dr Ira Papel (President of the American Academy of Facial Plastic and Reconstructive Surgeons, AAFPRS) in the creation of the Physicians Coalition for Injectable Safety**. Although ASOPRS, ASDS, and the AAFPRS had been working together through a loose-knit Federation for about 20 years to promote education and safety, it was not until Dr Jewell conceptualized the "core four" specialties that the organization was formed to unite our various specialties at least on the topic of patient safety. Twenty-five years after I finished medical school, my former student peers and I were working together again as concerned physicians to increase the quality of patient care and safety.

This issue is but one of many positive outcomes that continue to evolve from the collaborative efforts of our physicians and surgeons practicing facial esthetic surgery.

My thanks to the decision-makers who pushed this project forward and my congratulations to the outstanding editors and authors for the excellent product that they have created.

Roger A. Dailey, MD, FACS
Division of Oculofacial Plastic Surgery
Casey Aesthetic Facial Surgery Center
Oregon Health and Sciences University
Portland, OR 97221, USA

E-mail address:
daileyr@ohsu.edu

Clin Plastic Surg 40 (2013) xvii
http://dx.doi.org/10.1016/j.cps.2012.11.003
0094-1298/13/$ – see front matter © 2013 Elsevier Inc. All rights reserved.

Foreword

Engaging All Specialties for Advancement of Patient Care

As the baby boomer generation ages and the general public strives toward an ageless beauty, an increasing number of "noncore" medical providers are becoming "cosmetic surgeons." In addition, specialists including dermatologists, plastic surgeons, ophthalmologists, and otolaryngologists, whose primary training includes cosmetic procedures, are expanding their cosmetic practices to meet the increasing public demand for these services and to buffer the economic downturn of third-party reimbursement. The expansion of cosmetic surgery is not limited to private medical clinics. Academic centers have begun creating multidisciplinary cosmetic centers (MCCs) in response to increasing public demand for these services. The organization of multiple medical specialties under one roof is logical since there are multiple components in aging. Epidermal aging and photodamage require the expertise of a dermatologist. Resorption of bone and muscle and displacement of subdermal fat require the expertise of plastic, ophthalmologic surgeons as well as otolaryngologists and oromaxillofacial surgeons. No one specialty can claim to be expert in the vast variety of techniques and procedures required to reverse the aging process. It is therefore perfect timing that an edition of *Clinics in Plastic Surgery* provides a multidisciplinary approach to this growing field.

A survey of academic physicians from the departments of dermatology, plastic surgery, otolaryngology, and ophthalmology on their attitudes regarding MCCs and toward other specialties providing cosmetic services was recently conducted at Wake Forest University School of Medicine, Winston-Salem, North Carolina.[1] Among survey respondents, the overall opinion on MCCs was positive. Perceived benefits included improved patient care, resource sharing, increased opportunity for multidisciplinary research, improved resident education, and increased cross-referrals. Concerns included fear of competition, jealousy, and ego. Some specialists may feel that their field is self-reliant, that their field can do anything that other subspecialties can without needing to

collaborate, and that the other subspecialties will not bring anything to the table. A valid concern would be the difficulty to agree on the scope of practice for each subspecialty in areas where procedures can be performed by multiple disciplines. These attitudes could certainly impede cooperative care, leading to feelings of contempt across disciplines.

Employing a multidisciplinary approach has been successful in various aspects of medicine. Transplant surgery could not have evolved without the cooperation of multiple medical specialties, including immunologists and surgeons. The optimal management of a variety of cancers is aided by cooperation among surgeons, oncologists, and radiologists who meet in tumor boards. The first widespread use of a dermal filler, Zyderm collagen, was developed and tested by both dermatologic and plastic surgeons at Stanford University over 30 years ago. Liposuction was perfected with the advent of tumescent anesthesia by dermatologic surgeons with the surgical expertise of plastic surgeons. Vein surgery was revolutionized with the use of intravascular laser and radiofrequency catheters and tumescent anesthesia developed by dermatologic surgeons combined with ultrasound technology from radiologists and an understanding of the venous system by vascular surgeons. Laser resurfacing and the treatment of vascular and pigmented lesions, developed by dermatologic surgeons along with the surgical expertise of plastic, occuloplastic, otolaryngologist, and oromaxiofacial surgeons, has revolutionized the rejuvenation of photoaged skin as well as congenital birthmarks and traumatic scarring. This is just a short list of advancements in medicine and patient care from multidisciplinary teamwork. Future advancements will continue.

To be sure, one medical specialty alone can improve a patient's appearance, but how much more fun is it to collaborate and learn from one's colleagues? Medical technology has become so complex that one would be hard pressed to know it all. It is therefore optimal to integrate the

Clin Plastic Surg 40 (2013) xix–xx
http://dx.doi.org/10.1016/j.cps.2012.11.004

plasticsurgery.theclinics.com

knowledge of other specialties to accelerate advancements in patient care.

The concept of combining a variety of specialties together to enhance patient care has been adopted in academic centers with proven success. The University of Pennsylvania has been successful creating "incentives for a culture of collaboration rather than competition, a culture that stresses the success of the program, the team, and the institution, over that of the more traditional department."[2] This collection of articles from leaders in Facial Plastic Surgery, Occuloplastic Surgery, Plastic Surgery, and Dermatologic Surgery is an outstanding continuing attempt to engage all specialties toward the advancement of patient care. The editors and authors should all be congratulated for their joint efforts.

Mitchel P. Goldman, MD
University of California, San Diego
9339 Genesee Avenue, Suite 300
San Diego, CA 92121, USA

E-mail address:
MGoldman@GBKderm.com

REFERENCES

1. Schroeder RE, Levender MM, Feldman SR. Academic physicians' attitudes towards implementation of multi-disciplinary cosmetic centers and the challenges of subspecialties working together. Cosmetic Dermatol 2012;25:327–32.
2. Rodin J. A revisionist view of the integrated academic health center. Acad Med 2004;79:171–8.

Preface
Brow and Upper Lid Aesthetics and Rejuvenation: Views from Four Disciplines

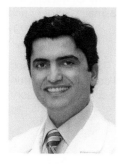 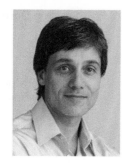

Babak Azizzadeh, MD   Guy G. Massry, MD
Guest Editors

Aesthetic surgery of the eyelids and periorbita is a unique component of plastic surgery. This is because the development and refinement of surgical and nonsurgical rejuvenative procedures inherent to this area of the face are founded on the contributions of specialists from various disciplines—primarily plastic surgery, facial plastic surgery, oculoplastic surgery, and dermatology. As such, a comprehensive reference on cosmetic interventions tailored to enhance the appearance of the eyelids and adjacent structures can only be complete with a multidisciplinary approach constructed with contributions from of each these core specialties. From this thinking, this volume of *Clinics in Plastic Surgery*, "Brow and Upper Eyelid Surgery: Multidisciplinary Insights," was born. A second volume dedicated to the lower lids and midface with a similar format and authorship will follow soon.

The forehead/eyebrows and upper lids act as an aesthetic unit. They intimately interact to convey expression, mood, demeanor, and thought. In addition, their function is critical to protecting the eyes and maintaining our most important sense—vision. Clearly, an in-depth understanding of the form and function of these dynamic structures is essential for all practitioners involved in their cosmetic enhancement.

In this text we sought out the expertise of leaders in each of the 4 core specialties mentioned above so that we could present a truly comprehensive, diverse, and multidisciplinary view of aesthetic forehead/eyebrow lifting, upper blepharoplasty, and pertinent associated noninvasive cosmetic refinements. This project was an invaluable and enjoyable experience that allowed us the opportunity to unite, debate, compare, and contrast different views on the same basic principles and procedures. From the experience, we feel we are better practitioners and surgeons. In addition the experience reinforced our strong belief that only through sharing ideas from varied backgrounds and ranges of experience can we develop the most contemporary and forward thinking reference on this ever-evolving area of facial cosmetic surgery.

We would like to thank all the contributing physicians for their time, which we know is limited to start with. We are only the gatekeepers and without their valued efforts there is no project.

Clin Plastic Surg 40 (2013) xxi–xxii
http://dx.doi.org/10.1016/j.cps.2012.09.002
0094-1298/13/$ – see front matter © 2013 Published by Elsevier Inc.

Also, we had the good fortune of working with Elsevier, a great publisher, with a wonderful staff, who never said no to anything we asked for. We are especially thankful to Joanne Husovski, our Senior Editor at *Clinics in Plastic Surgery*, who was by far the most invaluable resource and point person anyone could ask for. To our 4 contributing section editors, Jennifer Kim, MD, Farzad Nahai, MD, Julie Woodward, MD, and Doris Day, MD, we are indebted beyond words. You all did the real work, while our job was to smile at how easy it was to put together such an already finished product. Finally, we are both fortunate to have families and friends who support us in our varied professional endeavors. This is the greatest gift of all as their sacrifices are what allow us to grow and enhance our love for what we do.

Babak Azizzadeh, MD
Center for Advanced Facial Plastic Surgery
Beverly Hills, CA

Guy G. Massry, MD
Spalding Drive Cosmetic Surgery and
Dermatology
Beverly Hills, CA

E-mail addresses:
drazizzadeh@gmail.com (B. Azizzadeh)
gmassry@drmassry.com (G.G. Massry)

The Brow-Eyelid Continuum
An Anatomic Perspective

Vincent B. Lam, MD[a], Craig N. Czyz, DO[b,c],
Allan E. Wulc, MD[d,e],*

KEYWORDS

- Anatomy • Brow • Eyelid • Brow-lid continuum • Aging face • Plastic surgery

KEY POINTS

- Upper eyelid issues cannot always be addressed in isolation with upper blepharoplasty.
- Brow position and contour are integral components of eyelid appearance.
- Brows and eyelids should be considered as 1 aesthetic unit: the brow-eyelid continuum.
- The ideal distance from the eyelid crease to the central upper brow approximated at 2 times the vertical height of the eyelid crease is subjective, and should be based on the patient's and surgeon's aesthetic preferences.
- Ocular dominance and Hering law play a role in eyelid and brow position, and manipulation of one component often affects the position of other components.
- A multiprocedure approach involving ptosis repair, volumetric supplementation, and brow lifting in conjunction with conventional upper blepharoplasty is often necessary for ideal aesthetic improvement of the brow-eyelid continuum.

INTRODUCTION

Surgical rejuvenation of the upper eyelids cannot be performed without taking into consideration the complex aesthetic and anatomic relationships that exist in the upper third of the face. A surgeon who aims for successful eyelid rejuvenation with upper blepharoplasty in isolation may have difficulty attaining a personally satisfactory outcome, and, most importantly, may not meet the patient's expectations. When evaluating a patient, the upper eyelids should be viewed in contiguity with the other structures forming the upper third of the face, including the eyebrows, forehead, and the location of the frontal hairline. The term brow-eyelid continuum may help guide the patient's understanding that any or all of these structures may require treatment to obtain a harmonious and aesthetically pleasing rejuvenation.

CLINICAL SIGNIFICANCE OF THE BROW-EYELID CONTINUUM

The forehead-eyebrow complex is a critical aesthetic component of the upper facial third. The position and contour of the eyebrows play a role in the appearance of the eyelids. A ptotic brow, whether caused by gravitational changes

Funding sources: None.
Conflict of interest: None.
[a] Department of Ophthalmology, Drexel University College of Medicine, Philadelphia, PA, USA; [b] Section of Oculofacial Plastic and Reconstructive Surgery, Division of Ophthalmology, Ohio University/OhioHealth Doctor's Hospital, 5100 West Broad Street, Columbus, OH 43228, USA; [c] Department of Ophthalmology, Ohio University College of Osteopathic Medicine, Athens, OH, USA; [d] Department of Ophthalmology and Otolaryngology, Drexel University College of Medicine, 2900 West Queen Lane, Philadelphia, PA 19129, USA; [e] Department of Ophthalmology, Scheie Eye Institute, 51 N 39th Street #501, University of Pennsylvania, Philadelphia, PA 19104, USA
* Corresponding author. 610 West Germantown Pike, Suite 161, Plymouth Meeting, PA 19462.
E-mail address: awulcmd@gmail.com

or loss of three-dimensional volume in the brows and temples, can cause apparent increased skin redundancy and fullness in the upper sulcus and the temporal eyelid. These changes exacerbate the appearance of temporal eyelid hooding. The frontalis muscle, the prime elevator of the brow, contributes 2 mm of elevation to the upper eyelid, and thus overall resting frontalis tone can affect the position of the upper eyelid margin relative to the pupil.[1] When assessing the upper eyelids, the brows should be placed in a position consistent with the patient's appearance in youth. Old photographs are invaluable in customizing brow position to the patient.

Aging changes evidenced in the brow-eyelid continuum are related to complex alterations in the orbital rim (bone), fat compartments of the brow and lids, and skin. The traditional subtractive upper eyelid blepharoplasty addresses redundant skin, muscle, and fat, but usually does not fully address these complex alterations. Most patients benefit from additional procedures to address these associated periocular aging issues, such as volume augmentation, brow lifting, and skin resurfacing. When these senescent changes are addressed as a whole, a conservative blepharoplasty, often with only skin removal with minimal fat excision or preservation, can be performed to attain a more pleasing aesthetic result.

Excess Upper Eyelid Skin and Ptosis

Dermatochalasis, defined as the appearance of excess skin in the upper eyelids, is a chronic condition that produces compensatory frontalis muscle overaction as the eyebrows raise to elevate excess skin off the eyelashes. Upper eyelid ptosis also produces similar compensatory frontalis contraction.[1] Patients with these conditions often appear to have excellent brow position, but with significant horizontal forehead rhytids; however, when the frontalis is put at rest by the examiner's finger, with gentle pressure downwards to eliminate the forehead rhytids, these patients often manifest significant brow ptosis.

Isolated blepharoplasty in these patients unmasks this latent brow ptosis because the patient no longer needs to compensate for mechanical ptosis by contracting the frontalis (**Fig. 1**).[2] This procedure often leads to a poor aesthetic result. Bilateral ptosis repair also eliminates the drive for frontalis activation, and also unmasks brow ptosis and can compromise the aesthetic result when performed as an isolated procedure (**Fig. 2**). In both of these clinical situations, it is important to discuss the need for brow lifting surgery to prevent patient disappointment with the postoperative result. Many patients either opt for simultaneous brow lift or are prepared to deal with the aesthetic consequences if eyelid surgery alone is chosen.

Hering's Law Applied to Blepharoplasty and Ptosis Repair

In 1868, Ewald Hering described what is now known as the Hering law, stating that there is equal and simultaneous innervation to synergistic ocular yoke muscles.[3] Afferent innervation to the brainstem from the visual system drives a bilateral symmetrically mediated motor response that aligns the eyes. This phenomenon was first described to explain how, when fixating on a moving visual target, the eyes move symmetrically while maintaining fusion.[4–6] The Hering law also applies to the frontalis and levator muscles, and is the principle underlying the drop in the brows seen when blepharoplasty or ptosis repair is performed (as described previously). According to this principle,

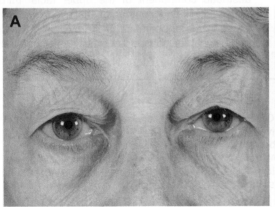 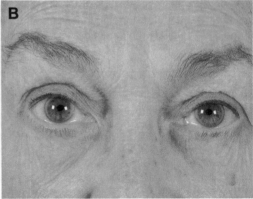

Fig. 1. (*A*) Preoperative photograph of patient showing bilateral upper eyelid dermatochalasis. (*B*) Postoperative photograph of the same patient after blepharoplasty showing unmasking of brow ptosis left greater than the right.

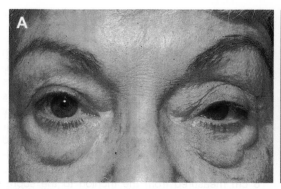
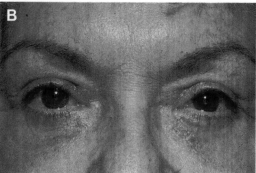

Fig. 2. (*A*) Preoperative photograph of patient showing bilateral upper eyelid dermatochalasis and left upper eyelid ptosis. (*B*) Postoperative photograph of the same patient after bilateral upper eyelid blepharoplasty and left upper eyelid ptosis repair resulting in bilateral brow ptosis, left greater than right.

the paired levator and frontalis muscles are symmetrically innervated from a motor standpoint, and correction of upper eyelid ptosis or dermatochalasis diminishes afferent input to the frontalis muscles, causing the brows to drop.

In cases of upper eyelid position asymmetry, such as in unilateral ptosis, the Hering law is equally important. In these cases, ocular dominance (preferred eye) must be determined. The dominant eye is the preferred afferent input that drives symmetric bilateral motor innervations to the levator muscle.[7] In cases of asymmetry, it can be assumed that alteration in the dominant eye's eyelid position may have an effect on the contralateral eye's lid position. This assumption can not be made when the nondominant eye is ptotic, and unilateral ptosis repair may be performed without alteration of the contralateral lid position. However, in cases in which unilateral ptosis occurs in the dominant eyelid, compensatory elevation of the contralateral (nonptotic) eyelid can occur. Once the unilateral ptosis is surgically corrected and the increased tone of the levator muscles is diminished bilaterally, latent ptosis

may become evident in the contralateral (nondominant) eyelid, either at the time of surgery or afterward. Thus, in cases of asymmetric bilateral ptosis or unilateral ptosis in the dominant eye, it is best to anticipate the potential to perform bilateral ptosis surgery.

Unilateral eyelid asymmetries can also have an effect on brow position because the impetus for frontalis muscle contraction is also not always symmetric. Asymmetric brow elevation can therefore be seen in patients with unilateral ptosis, with the ptotic eyelid appearing symmetric to the contralateral side (**Fig. 3**). An association between involuntary asymmetric eyebrow elevation and ocular dominance has been described, with ocular dominance matching the side of unilateral eyebrow elevation 77% of the time.[7] Unilateral brow asymmetries are also commonly seen in patients with preexisting conditions such as Bell palsy, previous trauma to the VII nerve, and scar tissue in the forehead from trauma or surgery. Thus, when evaluating the patient, it is important in all these instances to elevate the ptotic brow and depress the elevated brow to rule out unilateral

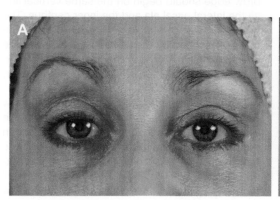
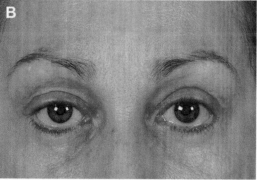

Fig. 3. (*A*) Patient with right brow overaction with no apparent eyelid ptosis. Note the higher eyelid crease in the right upper eyelid. (*B*) The same patient on another day with a relaxed right brow and unmasking of a right upper eyelid ptosis. Note the lowered right upper eyelid crease with frontalis relaxed.

compensatory frontalis overaction that could be concealing an eyelid ptosis.

Neurotoxin Effect on Brow-Eyelid Continuum

Now that the use of neurotoxins has become commonplace for the treatment of glabellar and transverse forehead wrinkles, their effect on the brow-eyelid continuum must be considered. It is common to evaluate patients for brow or upper eyelid ptosis who have exacerbated a preexisting condition such as upper eyelid skin excess or brow ptosis with neurotoxin placement. Depending on the placement and quantity of the neurotoxin injections, brow and eyelid contour can be significantly altered. It is common in our practices to see patients in consultation for blepharoplasty who have undergone recent injections and have not made the connection between their sudden skin excess or brow ptosis and their neurotoxin treatment.

Brow-Eyelid Continuum Evaluation

The upper eyelids must not be considered in isolation in evaluating patients for upper eyelid aesthetic surgery. Asymmetries of the upper eyelid or brow position must be carefully assessed before surgery, and often the solution to a unilateral problem involves bilateral surgery. Because of the integration of the brow-eyelid continuum, the region must be evaluated as a whole, even when the presenting issue seems obvious.

AESTHETIC ANATOMY OF THE FACE

Since the Renaissance, scholars and artists have developed guidelines for ideal facial proportions that continue to be studied, modified, and debated.[8,9] A wide variation exists in the ideal aesthetic of the upper third of the face and is influenced by age, sex, culture, and ethnicity. Alterations in what is considered aesthetically desirable also vary based on fashion and the epoch. The widespread use of Botox (Allergan, Inc., Irvine, CA) and its congeners may have altered perceptions of what is attractive in the periorbital region, because fashion models and celebrities often are photographed with brow ptosis or peaked brows from selective paresis of muscles. Although there is no universally applicable ideal eyebrow position and contour, certain principles must be followed to maintain harmony within the periorbital region. Following is a summary of the current guidelines of ideal aesthetics in the upper third of the face based on published anatomic guidelines.

Hairline, Forehead, and Temporal Fossa

Understanding the aesthetic anatomy of the hairline, forehead, and temporal fossa is important in achieving a balanced and harmonious rejuvenation of the upper third of the face.[10] This area is often overlooked when rejuvenating the eyebrows and upper eyelids, because certain techniques of brow lifting elevate the hairline, leading to a disproportionately long forehead with a receded hairline.[11,12] The hairline is variable between individuals. The average male hairline height is 6.5 to 8 cm measured from the trichion to the supraeyebrow line. The female hairline is lower, between 5 and 6 cm.[13,14] The forehead is delineated by the hairline superiorly, the glabella inferiorly, the frontonasal groove centrally, and laterally by the lateral brow. The forehead should transition smoothly to the temple. In general, the diagonal distance between the lateral brow and the temporal tuft should be less than 3.5 cm.

Eyebrows

The brow frames the appearance of the upper eyelid. Subtle alterations in brow position convey an array of emotions, from anger to surprise.[15] Best described by Laorwong and colleagues,[16] the brow is shaped like a curved sword. The superior brow edge is arched and tapered laterally. The horizontal length of the brows can measure 5.0 to 5.5 cm with a width of 1.3 to 1.5 cm. Men in general have thicker brows than women. The cilia in the medial brows are finer and directed upward. As the brow tapers laterally, the superior and inferior cilia are more transversely oriented and direct toward each other at approximately a 30° angle.[16]

The basis of the modern ideal female brow was described by Westmore[17] in 1974. The ideal brow is gently curved, with its apex aligned approximately above the lateral corneal limbus. The medial brow edge should begin on the same vertical line as the lateral nasal ala and the inner canthus. The lateral brow edge should end at the oblique line that is described by the lateral nasal alae and the lateral canthus (**Fig. 4**). The male brow should have similar medial to lateral alignment; however, it is usually lower and straighter.[18]

Additional aesthetic determinants of ideal brow position and contour have been reported since Westmore's[17] description; many of these are in conflict. Ellenbogen[15] thought that the brow was most aesthetically pleasing 1 cm above the supraorbital ridge, whereas Whitaker and colleagues[18] thought the ideal brow should be slightly below the supraorbital ridge. The greatest point of curvature of the brow has also been debated. Cook and colleagues,[19] Ellenbogen,[15] and Whitaker

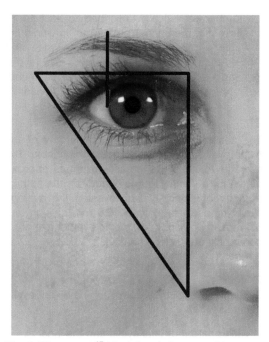

Fig. 4. Westmore's[17] ideal female brow position.

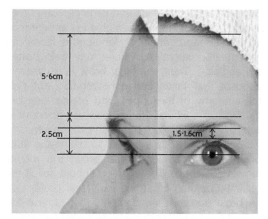

Fig. 5. Numeric guidelines that aid in defining the ideal brow position and hairline.

and colleagues[18] thought that the greatest curvature of the brow is positioned more laterally. Pham and colleagues[15,18,20,21] reported that the apex of the temporal curve correlates best with the temporal fusion line, and occurs more laterally. These contradictions arise because the aesthetic ideal is subjective.

The preference of brow position and contour can also depend on the age of the beholder. In one study, individuals younger than age 30 years preferred lower positioned brows, whereas those more than age 50 years preferred higher, more centrally arched brows.[22] An explanation of this phenomenon could be that individuals conceptualize beauty during their youth. The appearance of the youthful brow shape and position has changed through the years. Early in the 1930s and until the 1970s, the high arched eyebrow with the apex in the middle was the most popular brow shape.[23–25] The projected youthful brow in most fashion magazines is currently characterized by thick, full, and low-set eyebrows.[26,27]

Objective guidelines for determining ideal brow position

To make the subjective nature of brow position and contour more objective, investigators have proposed numeric guidelines for ideal brow position (**Fig. 5**).

- Connell and colleagues estimated the distance between the upper eyelid crease to the lower eyebrow edge at 1.5 cm.[28]

- Matarasso and Terino[29] estimated the distance from the upper edge of the eyebrow to the hairline as 5 to 6 cm, the lower edge of the middle eyebrow to the eyelid crease as 1.6 cm, the lower edge of the eyebrow to the midpupil as 2.5 cm, and the lower edge of the middle eyebrow to the superior orbital rim as 1 cm.
- McKinney and colleagues[30] described the distance from the midpupil to the upper edge of the eyebrow as 2.5 cm and the distance from the upper edge of the eyebrow to the hairline as 5 cm, on average.
- Numeric guidelines such as these provide a useful starting point, but cannot be applied universally because of variations among individuals.

Variables in determining ideal brow position

The racial composition of the patient is a variable that makes numeric determinations of ideal brow position universally challenging. Inter-racial anthropometric analyses of the eyebrows and eyelids were conducted by Kunjur and colleagues,[31] in which 3 different racial groups, white, Indian, and Chinese, were compared. The investigators found that the eyebrow was arched and bow shaped in all subjects and that the apex of the brow was between the lateral canthus and the lateral limbus, except in Indian men, in whom it was about 1 to 2 mm lateral to the lateral canthus. Price and colleagues,[32] in their study comparing eyelids and brows between African Americans and white people, found that African Americans had an overall higher brow position than white people. No significant racial differences were found in regard to the shape and apex of the brow.

Facial shape is an important factor in the determination of an individualized ideal brow position.[33]

Some investigators think that vertically long faces should have a flatter brow to give the appearance of a fuller face, whereas, for square faces, an accentuated lateral curvature may help soften the angles.[34] Thus, the ideal brow is a dynamic concept that takes into consideration not only the anatomy of the upper third of the face but the face as a whole. This precept is important in achieving a balanced, natural surgical result.

Despite numerous attempts to define the ideal position and contour of the brow, the results remain subjective. The surgeon should solicit the patient's opinion regarding individual preference on brow position and contour, then advise the patient as to whether these preferences can realistically be attained. The surgeon should also be honest about the aesthetic merits of the patient's chosen position.

Upper Eyelids

Ideal eyelid appearance varies with gender, race, and age. In general:

- The upper eyelid should rest approximately 1 to 2 mm below the superior corneal limbus.
- The lower eyelid should rest on or 1 mm above the inferior corneal limbus.
- The opening between the eyelid margins, the vertical palpebral fissure, measures 9 to 10 mm, whereas the horizontal aperture measures 28 to 30 mm.[35]
- Normal eyelid levator function is 14 to 16 mm and is defined as the excursion of the upper eyelid margin from downgaze to upgaze with the frontalis immobilized.[36]
- The greatest curve of the upper eyelid is observed slightly medial to the pupil, whereas the lower eyelid's greatest curve is seen lateral to the midpupillary line.
- The horizontal palpebral fissure is inclined with a slight upward tilt with the lateral canthus positioned about 2 mm above the medial canthus.[35–37] In a comparative inter-racial study, Kunjur and colleagues[31] found that canthal tilt varied among races. The author found that canthal tilt was greatest in Chinese subjects (5.7°), then white people (4.0°) and then Indians (1.2°).
- The eyelid crease, a significant component of eyelid aesthetics, is formed by the subcutaneous insertion of the levator aponeurosis onto the anterior lamella and varies in position with age, sex, and race. Eyelid crease height is generally higher in women than in men. The eyelid crease, as measured from the lid margin, is

characteristically described to be 8 to 10 mm in men and 10 to 12 mm in women.[36] In a recent study comparing white and African American eyebrow and eyelid dimensions, African Americans were found, in general, to have higher eyelid creases.[32]

Asian eyelid crease

The aesthetic appearance and anatomy of the Asian eyelid crease are unique and variable. The average Asian eyelid crease height is approximately 5 to 7 mm. Park's[38] study of the anthropometry of Asian eyelids revealed the average eyelid crease height to be 6.6 mm in men and 6.5 mm in women. In the Asian eyelid there are 3 commonly described variations:

1. Apparent double eyelid
2. Inner eyelid fold with a low-lying crease
3. Single eyelid that does not have an eyelid crease

The apparent double eyelid and the inner eyelid fold with a low-lying crease make up most of the Asian eyelids observed (**Fig. 6**).[39,40] Compared with the white eyelid, the Asian eyelid has been described to have a lower insertion point of the orbital septum onto the levator aponeurosis.[40,41] This anatomic difference results in an inferior extension of the preaponeurotic fat pad creating a thicker and lower eyelid crease. Kakizaki and colleagues,[42] using cadaveric Asian eyelids, recently showed that the distal end of the levator aponeurosis insertion site was located above the superior tarsal border, similar to its insertion site in white eyelids. This study suggests that the anatomic differences observed between Asian and white people are caused by inherent differences in upper eyelid fat volume rather than the attachment site of the orbital septum to the levator.

SURGICAL ANATOMY OF THE FACE
Forehead and Brows

Bony landmarks

The frontal and nasal bones are the primary bony landmarks encountered in aesthetic brow and upper eyelid surgery.

- In most patients, the supraorbital nerve originates from a notch over the superior orbital rim.
- In approximately 20% of patients, the nerve exits through a foramen.
- In 10% of patients, a lateral branch of the nerve exits the frontal bone approximately 2 cm above the rim.[43]

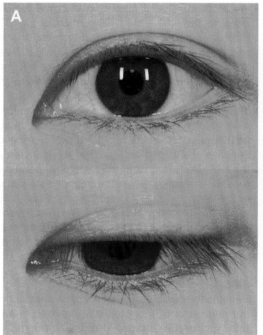 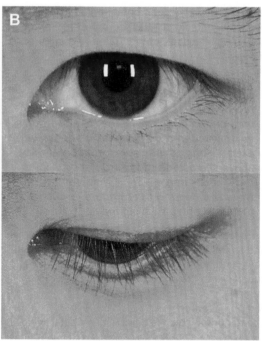

Fig. 6. (A) An Asian eyelid with an apparent double eyelid fold. (B) An Asian eyelid with an inner eyelid fold and low-lying crease.

Surgical note: The surgeon should be familiar with the location of these nerves to avoid injury, especially during dissection.

Muscles

The main elevator of the eyebrow and forehead is the frontalis muscle. The paired frontalis muscles join the occipitalis muscles posteriorly, the galea aponeurotica anteriorly, and the temporal fascias laterally. Frontalis fibers interdigitate with the orbital portion of the orbicularis muscle near the supraorbital rim and insert into the dermis beneath the eyebrow. The activation of the frontalis produces horizontal rhytids of the forehead skin.

The procerus and corrugator supercilii muscles are the primary brow depressors, along with the orbicularis to a lesser extent. Their origins, insertions, and primary actions are described later.

Soft tissue and suspensory ligaments

The forehead is usually described in layers from the skin to the periosteum[44]:

- Skin
- Connective tissue
- Aponeurosis, which fuses with the frontalis muscle
- Loose connective tissue
- Galea
- Periosteum

Surgical note: Adhesion zones have been described for the frontal periosteum by Moss and colleagues.[45] They are strongest along the frontal bone in the vicinity of the superior temporal crest ligament, and extend to the origin of the corrugator muscle.

- The inferior border of this adhesion zone is located 6 mm above the deep attachment of the periorbital septum.
- The upper border extends 20 to 40 mm above the orbital rim.

The galea aponeurotica descends laterally into the temporal fossa as the superficial temporal fascia. The galea aponeurotica splits anteriorly into a superficial and deep layer to include the frontalis and the orbicularis muscle. At the level of the brow, the deep layer of the galea also splits into an anterior and posterior facial layer to enclose the retro-orbicularis oculi fat (ROOF).[46] The posterior facial layer continues as the orbital septum of the eyelid, eventually fusing with the levator aponeurosis.

The conjoined tendon is an area of fusion between the soft tissues of the forehead and the fascias of the temple and is an important landmark in endoscopic brow surgery. The deep temporal fascia (DTF), superficial temporal fascia (STF), and frontal periosteum fuse forming the conjoint tendon. The inferior temporal septum, described by Moss and colleagues,[45] represents another area of confluence between deep and superficial tissues.

> *Surgical note: At this location, the DTF splits into its superficial and deep layers to envelope the superficial temporal fat pad, and is a landmark that is important in brow surgery. This zone of adhesion exists along a line approximately 1 cm above the course of the frontal branch of the facial nerve. This area must be traversed deep to the temporal branch of the facial nerve to avoid injury.[44]*

Perforating veins and sensory nerves (the medial and lateral zygomaticotemporal nerves) are pertinent landmarks that indicate that the nerve is superficial to the plane of dissection.[43,45]

Temporal region

The temporal region is complex and multilayered.

> *Surgical note: The frontal branch of the facial nerve is vulnerable at several locations in this dissection. It is important for the surgeon to become well acquainted with the anatomy of this region before embarking on surgery.*

The superficial musculoaponeurotic system (SMAS) of the temple is composed of the temporoparietal fascia (TPF; also known as the STF),

the most superficial fascial layer in the temple. Deep to this, the superficial portion of the DTF is observed; a white glistening fascia that is easily separated from the TPF above. This loose areolar layer between the TPF and the DTF has been referred to as the subaponeurotic plane (Fig. 7).[47,48]

The DTF splits into a superficial and a deep layer as it further descends toward the zygomatic arch. The superficial temporal fat pad is encased between the superficial and the deep layers of the DTF. In this location, the superficial portion of the DTF is also known as the intermediate fascia, or the innominate fascia, and the fat pad is known as the intermediate fat pad.[47,48] The deep layer of the deep temporalis fascia covers the temporalis muscle and blends inferiorly with the parotidomasseteric fascia of the face.[45,49]

ROOF

Beneath the ciliary portion of the brow and accompanying orbicularis is a fat pad encased in septated connective tissue. This fat compartment, the ROOF pad, continues into the upper eyelid as the postorbicularis fascia (POF).[50]

> *Surgical note: Although some investigators have advocated resection of the ROOF to improve the contour of the lateral eyelid,[51] deformities related to resection can ensue and this can add to normal involutional eyebrow/eyelid deficits.[52] Instead, vertical elevation of the ROOF via a brow*

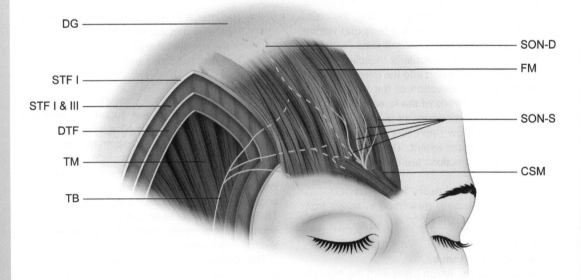

Fig. 7. Fascial layers of the temporal region. CSM, corrugators supercilii muscle; DG, deep galea plane; DTF, Deep temporal fascia; FM, frontalis muscle; SON-D, deep division of the supraorbital nerve; SON-S, superficial division of the supraorbital nerve; STF I, outer layer of STF; STF II and STF III, deep STF layers; TB, temporal branch of frontal nerve; TM, temporalis muscle.

lifting procedure is often necessary to achieve the desired contour of the brow-eyelid continuum.

In Asian people, the ROOF continues into the lid proper as a fatty layer called the preseptal fat, located between the orbicularis muscle and orbital septum. This layer contributes to the apparent fullness of the Asian upper eyelid.[53]

Eyelids

Upper eyelids

The upper eyelid skin is the thinnest skin in the body because of its lack of subcutaneous fat.[54] It is thinnest near the ciliary margin and becomes thicker approaching the eyebrows. The eyebrow skin is significantly thicker, containing sebaceous glands, sweat glands, and hair follicles.

The eyelid margin is approximately 2 mm in width. From anterior to posterior, the eyelid margin consists of the skin, the eyelashes, the gray line (terminal orbicularis muscle), the tarsus with associated meibomian gland orifices, and the mucocutaneous junction.

Surgical note: The gray line serves as an important surgical anatomic landmark and represents the muscle of Riolan, which is the most anterior and superficial portion of the pretarsal orbicularis muscle.[55] The gray line is useful to the surgeon in aligning the eyelid margin.

The eyelid can be divided through the gray line into 2 segments:

1. Anterior lamellae
2. Posterior lamellae

Throughout the eyelid, the anterior lamella is composed of skin and orbicularis muscle. Above the tarsus, the posterior lamella is composed of the eyelid retractors and palpebral conjunctiva. Below the tarsus, the posterior lamella consists of the tarsus and conjunctiva. Connective tissue attachments of the levator aponeurosis traverse anteriorly and attach to the pretarsal orbicularis muscle and skin, forming the upper eyelid crease.

Tarsus

The tarsal plates are rigid structures formed from connective tissue (collagen type I, III, VI, and multiple glycosaminoglycans) and serve as the supporting framework of the eyelids.[56] Within the tarsus are meibomian glands that secrete mebum, the oily external component of the 3-layered tear film. The tarsal plates measure approximately 29 mm horizontally, with a thickness

of 1 mm. The superior tarsus has a vertical height of 8 to 12 mm.[57] Asian people have a smaller superior tarsal plate, with a vertical height measuring 8 mm.[58]

Orbital septum

The orbital septum is a fibrous multilayered connective tissue that originates at the arcus marginalis, a circumferential thickening of periosteum at the orbital rim. The orbital septum defines the separation of the orbit proper from the eyelid, and can be thought of as a physical barrier that encloses the orbital fat and internal orbital structures. The septum fuses with the levator aponeurosis in the upper eyelid and the capsulopalpebral fascia in the lower eyelid.[36,59]

Surgical note: It is imperative the orbital septum never be sutured when closing a blepharoplasty incision or lid motility dysfunction can result.

Eyelid/orbital fat

The eyelid fat compartments or pads lie posterior the orbital septum. The upper eyelid has 2 distinct fat compartments, nasal and central, separated by a connective tissue septum. The nasal fat is in continuity with deeper orbital fat because it is not separated from extraconal and intraconal fat by the levator aponeurosis. The central fat compartment is an important landmark in upper eyelid surgery because it lies directly anterior to the levator aponeurosis.[36] The potential space between the orbital septum and the levator aponeurosis is greatest immediately inferior to the superior orbital rim over the central fat pad, and therefore is an ideal location for dividing the orbital septum to expose the fat without injury to the levator and other deep structures. This preaponeurotic fat pad can be differentiated from the nasal fat pad by its color. The central fat pad has a yellow appearance, whereas the nasal fat pad has a whiter appearance. This color difference has been attributed to a higher carotenoid and retinol content in the central fat pad.[60] Korn and colleagues[61] suggest that this difference relates to differing embryologic origins, with the central fat pad derived from mesodermal cells and the nasal fat pad from neural crest cells.

Lacrimal gland

The lacrimal gland is a bilobed structure composed of orbital and palpebral segments divided by the lateral horn of the levator aponeurosis. The orbital lobe lies in the lacrimal fossa located in the superior lateral orbit and is connected to the palpebral lobe posterior to the lateral horn of the levator. With aging, the lacrimal gland can prolapse, adding to brow/sulcus fullness. Lacrimal gland prolapse has been reported to occur in 15% of patients and may be associated with normal aging of the orbit.[62] The dehiscence of the fibrous interlobular septae that connect the gland to the orbital rim fossa, along with thinning of septal connective tissue, contribute to prolapse of the lacrimal gland.[63]

Eyelid Muscles

Protractors

The circular orbicularis oculi muscle, the main protractor of the eyelid, lies directly beneath the eyelid skin. The orbicularis oculi muscle, innervated by the facial nerve (cranial nerve [CN] VII), encircles the orbit and eyelids, extending beyond the orbital rim. The orbicularis is divided into 3 segments, all named for the structures they overlie:

1. Pretarsal segment
2. Preseptal segment
3. Orbital segment

The pretarsal portion rests over the upper and lower tarsal plates, the preseptal portion over the orbital septum, and the orbital portion over the orbital rim.[64] The orbicularis acts both voluntarily to close the eyes and involuntary with the blink mechanism. The action of the pretarsal and preseptal orbicularis contribute to lacrimal drainage via the lacrimal pump mechanism.[36]

The pretarsal orbicularis fibers insert at the canthal tendon laterally and originate from 2 locations medially: the posterior lacrimal crest (deep head) and the anterior limb of the medial canthal tendon (superficial head). The superficial and deep heads of the upper and lower pretarsal orbicularis collectively form the Horner muscle, located posterior to the medial canthal tendon. Preseptal orbicularis fibers originate medially from the superficial and deep heads. The preseptal superficial head originates from the medial canthal tendon and the deep head originates from the fascia of the lacrimal sac and medial orbital wall above and below the Horner muscle. The orbicularis laterally inserts into the lateral palpebral raphe. The superior portion of the orbital orbicularis muscle is formed from fibers originating from the anterior limb of the orbital portion of the frontal bone. The orbicularis fibers interdigitate with the frontalis muscle superiorly, procerus and corrugators supercilii muscle medially, and anterior temporalis fascia laterally.[35]

Three muscles (brow depressors) work in conjunction with the orbicularis to aid in upper eyelid closure:

1. Procerus
2. Corrugator supercilii
3. Depressor supercilii

The procerus muscle originates on the nasal bone, inserting into the skin of the nasal bridge and lower forehead. Contraction results in an inferior-directed force that causes medial brow descent and the formation of horizontal glabellar rhytids.

The paired corrugator superciliaris muscles originate in the medial superciliary ridge and extend obliquely superolaterally where they blend with the frontalis and orbicularis oculi muscle, and insert onto the skin of the middle eyebrow. Activation of the muscle results in inferomedial depression of the medial brow and the development of vertical glabellar furrows.

The depressor supercilii originates from the frontal process of the maxilla about 1 cm superior to the medial canthal tendon and ascends superiorly to insert in the skin about 14 to 15 mm superior to the medical canthal tendon.[64] Activation of the muscle also depresses the medial brow and contributes to the formation of oblique glabellar frown lines.

Retractors

There are 2 upper eyelid elevating muscles:

1. Levator palpebrae superioris
2. Müller muscle

Levator muscle The levator is the primary retractor of the upper eyelid. It is innervated by the superior division of CN III, which enters the muscle approximately 12 mm from the orbital apex. The levator muscle originates from the lesser wing of the sphenoid at the orbital apex. It extends anteriorly above the superior rectus muscle until the Whitnall ligament (the superior transverse ligament), where it transitions into the levator aponeurosis and inserts onto the anterior surface of the tarsus. The orbital (muscular) portion of the levator has a horizontal vector of action, whereas the aponeurotic portion has a vertical vector (**Fig. 8**). The levator muscle with its aponeurosis measures 54 to 60 mm in length from origin to insertion, with the aponeurotic portion of the levator complex being 14 to 20 mm.[65]

The levator aponeurosis is composed of an anterior and posterior layer. The anterior layer is robust and ends in a junction with the orbital septum and submuscular fibroadipose tissue. The posterior layer extends over the anterior surface of the Müller muscle and attaches to the anterior lamella of the upper eyelid and the anterior one-third of the tarsus. Together, the anterior and posterior layers

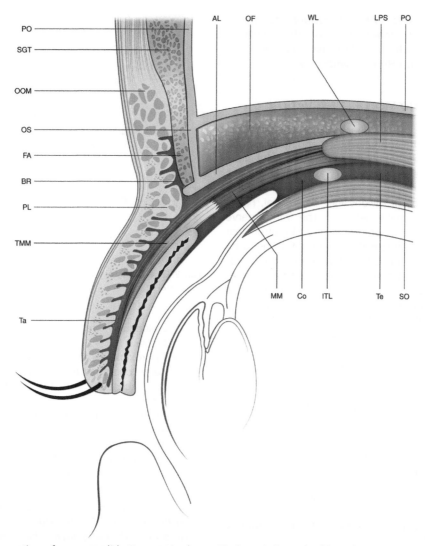

Fig. 8. Cross section of upper eyelid. AL, anterior layer; BR, branch from the fibroadipose layer; Co, connective tissue; FA, fibroadipose layer; ITL, intermuscular transverse ligament; LPS, levator palpebrae superioris muscle; MM, Müller muscle; OF, orbital fat; OOM, orbicularis oculi muscle; OS, orbital septum; PL, posterior layer; PO, periorbita; SGT, subgaleal tissue; Ta, tarsus; Te, Tenon capsule; TMM, tendon of Müller muscle; SR, superior rectus muscle; WL, Whitnall ligament.

exert a posterosuperior pull on the preaponeurotic fat pad, skin, muscle, and tarsus to elevate the eyelid (see **Fig. 8**).[66]

The levator complex is suspended by a transverse band of fibrous condensation, the superior transverse ligament of Whitnall. The Whitnall ligament attaches medially to connective tissue surrounding the trochlea and the superior oblique tendon. It passes through the stroma of the lacrimal gland laterally and attaches to the inner aspect of the lateral orbital wall approximately 10 mm above the lateral orbital tubercle.[67] The Whitnall ligament functions as a fulcrum for the levator, converting the anterior-posterior pulling force of the levator muscle to a superior-inferior pulling force. It also acts as a suspensory ligament, supporting the upper eyelid.

Müller muscle Posterior to the levator aponeurosis lies the Müller muscle, a sympathetically innervated smooth muscle that originates at the level of the Whitnall ligament, and inserts along the superior tarsal margin (see **Fig. 8**).[68] The posterior surface of the Müller muscle is intimately adherent to the palpebral conjunctiva. The Müller muscle measures 15 to 20 mm in width and 15 to 20 mm in length. Contraction of this muscle is involuntary, and related to resting sympathetic tone. The Müller muscle contributes approximately 2 mm to eyelid elevation.[36]

Surgical note: Any disruption to the sympathetic innervation of the Müller muscle results in mild ptosis, as seen in patients with Horner syndrome.

SENSORY AND MOTOR INNERVATION

Sensory innervation to the upper third of the face is supplied by the ophthalmic (V1) and maxillary (V2) divisions of the trigeminal nerve. The ophthalmic division courses in the lateral wall of the cavernous sinus and through the superior orbital fissure to enter the orbit. It divides into the frontal, naso-ciliary, and lacrimal nerves.[69] The frontal nerve divides into the supraorbital and supratrochlear nerves. The supraorbital nerve exits the orbit through the supraorbital notch or foramen to provide sensory innervation to the upper eyelid, forehead, and scalp (see **Fig. 7**).[70] A medial and a lateral branch are usually seen and occasionally arise separately. The lateral branch courses deep supplying the temporal scalp, compared with the more superficial medial branch, which supplies the forehead and central scalp. The supratrochlear nerve courses above the trochlea and innervates the skin of the glabella, and the medial forehead, upper eyelid, and medial conjunctiva.

Facial Nerve

Motor innervation of the brows and upper lids is supplied by the facial nerve (CN VII).

- The facial nerve divides into 3 to 5 major branches deep to the parotid gland.
- One of these branches is the temporofacial trunk of the nerve.
- Approximately 1 to 2 cm after leaving the parotid gland, the trunk divides into the zygomatic and frontal (temporal) terminal nerve branches (**Fig. 9**).

The temporofacial branch of the facial nerve follows a regular course described by Pitanguy and Ramos.[71]

- The nerve can be traced along a line from approximately 0.5 cm below the tragus to 1.5 cm above the tail of the brow (see **Fig. 9**).
- After exiting the parotid gland, the temporal branch travels in an anterosuperior direction.[45]
- At the level of the zygomatic arch and to about 1 cm above the arch, the nerve travels below the SMAS in a layer of fat above the zygomatic periosteum and underneath a fascia that Trussler and

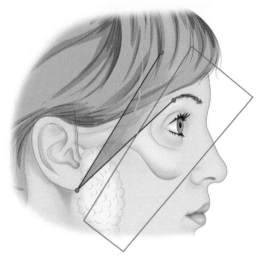

Fig. 9. The trajectory of the temporal branch of the facial nerve.

colleagues[72] termed the parotid temporal fascia.[47]
- Approximately 2 cm above the arch, the nerve becomes more superficial, abutting the back surface of the parotid temporal fascia.
- Eventually the nerve becomes encased within the parotid temporal fascia (**Fig. 10**).[72]
- The nerve then continues to course parallel and caudal to the inferior temporal fusion line (inferior temporal septum).

Surgical note: Here the nerve is no longer within the parotid temporal fascia and runs in a fibrofatty layer above the deep surface of the STF (Fig. 11).[45] In this location, the unprotected frontal branch is vulnerable to injury.

Surgical note: The sentinel veins and the branches of the zygomaticotemporal nerve penetrate radially through the fascias from deep to superficial, roughly approximating the course of the nerve, and are important surgical landmarks during forehead dissection.

The temporal branch of the facial nerve commonly branches into 3 rami:

1. Anterior
2. Middle
3. Posterior

The anterior and middle rami supply the upper orbicularis oculi and frontalis muscle through their deep surfaces.[73] The middle ramus supplies the

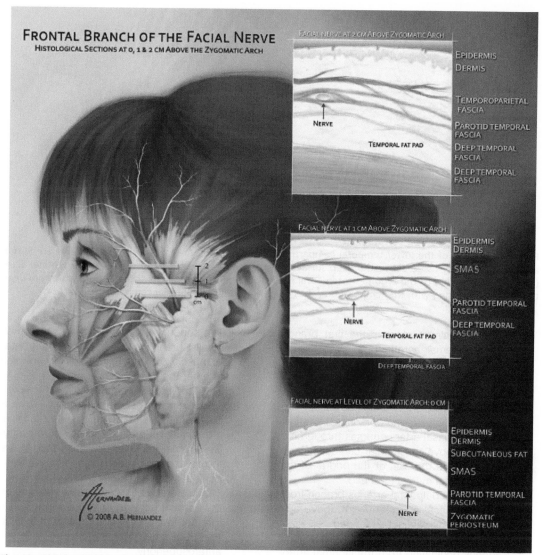

Fig. 10. Histologic tissue sections harvested at 1-cm intervals over the zygomatic arch. (© 2008 A.B. Hernandez "Alexandra Hernandez, M.A. of Gory Details Illustration.")

corrugator muscle and courses deep to the frontalis, bounded superiorly by the supraorbital adhesion and inferiorly by the periorbital septum.[45,74]

The brow and forehead muscles along with the orbicularis oculi are innervated by the branches of the facial nerve (CN VII). Innervation of the orbicularis oculi is supplied by the temporal and zygomatic branches, whereas the frontalis and corrugator supercilii are supplied by the temporal branch (see **Fig. 7**). The procerus receives innervation via the branch of the facial nerve.[57]

VASCULATURE

The complex vascular supply of the upper facial third is derived from the internal and external carotid arteries. The branches of the external carotid artery that supply the eyelid, temporal region, and scalp include the superficial temporal artery and tributaries of the facial artery.

- In the vicinity of the eyelids, the facial artery gives off the angular artery, which anastomoses with branches of the dorsal nasal artery.

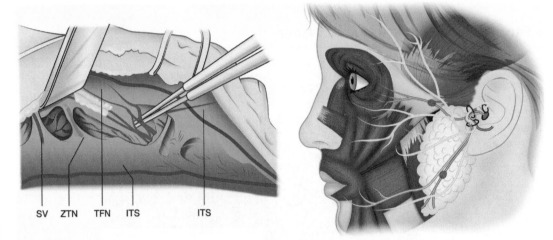

SV   ZTN   TFN   ITS   ITS

Fig. 11. Dissection of the lower temporal compartment. The temporal branches of the facial nerve are within a layer of fibrofatty tissue above the deep surface of the superficial temporal fascia (STF). The sentinel veins (SV) and the branches of the zygomaticotemporal nerve (ZTN) penetrate radially through the fascia from deep to superficial, crossing with the temporal branches perpendicularly. ITS, inferior temporal septum.

- The ophthalmic artery is the first branch of the internal carotid and gives rise to multiple tributaries, including the lacrimal and supraorbital arteries, supplying the sinuses and orbit.
- The ophthalmic artery branches distally into the supratrochlear and dorsonasal arteries.
- The dorsonasal artery courses through the septum above the medial canthal tendon and supplies the skin at the bridge of the nose and the medial forehead.
- Two medial palpebral arteries branch from the dorsonasal artery and exit above and below the medial canthal tendon.
- The medial palpebral and lateral palpebral arteries originating from the lacrimal artery join to form the marginal arcades supplying the upper and lower eyelids. The marginal arcade lies approximately 2 mm superior to the lid margin in the upper eyelid, whereas the single lower eyelid arcade lies at its inferior tarsal border.
- The peripheral arcade of the upper eyelid also originates from the medial and lateral palpebral arteries. It lies superior to the superior tarsal border between the levator aponeurosis and the Müller muscle.[75]
- The supraorbital artery joins the supraorbital nerve along the roof of the orbit and exits the supraorbital foramen or notch to supply the brow, forehead, scalp, and upper eyelids.
- After exiting the supraorbital rim, the supraorbital artery immediately divides into superficial and deep branches.

- The superficial branch further divides into smaller branches that penetrate the frontalis muscle and continue to extend cephalad to enter the frontal scalp.
- The deep branch courses between the periosteum and the galea aponeurotica, extending laterally toward the temporal fusion line.
- It then follows the superior temporal fusion line, forming smaller branches that pierce the galea aponeurotica to supply the frontoparietal scalp.[76,77]
- The midforehead and scalp are supplied by the supratrochlear artery, which exits through the orbital septum, accompanying the supratrochlear nerve, and courses anterosuperiorly.

The upper third of the face is unique in that the venous supply does not precisely follow arterial supply, varies between individuals, and is valveless. The venous drainage of the forehead comprises a plexus of veins referred to as the frontal vein.

- The frontal vein communicates laterally with the superficial temporal vein and inferiorly with the supraorbital vein at the level of the medial canthus.
- The supraorbital vein supplies the forehead above the brows, communicating with the superficial temporal vein.
- The converged veins then continue as the angular vein in an oblique, inferior direction and become the anterior facial vein as it passes the inferior orbital rim.
- Before merging with the frontal vein, a branch of the supraorbital vein often

transverses the supraorbital notch into the orbit and communicates with the superior ophthalmic vein.

Surgical note: This communication is significant because the superior and inferior orbital (ophthalmic) veins drain into the cavernous sinus. This valveless venous communication from the skin to the cavernous sinus creates a potential route for intracranial spread of orbital infection.[78]

LYMPHATICS

The lymphatic system of the upper facial third primarily involves the preauricular, deep cervical, and submandibular lymph nodes.

- The central forehead, medial brow, medial third of the upper eyelid, and medial two-thirds of the lower eyelid drain into the submandibular lymph nodes.
- The lateral forehead and brow, lateral two-thirds of the upper eyelid, and lateral third of the lower eyelid drain into the preauricular lymph nodes, then into deep cervical lymph nodes.[75]

Surgical note: Lymphatics can play a role in postoperative edema, but surgical avoidance is rare.

THE AGING UPPER THIRD OF THE FACE
Multifactorial Process

Facial aging is a multifactorial process that results from bony changes, soft tissue deflation (volume loss), tissue descent, and skin changes. Dermatochalasis, upper eyelid and brow ptosis, lacrimal gland prolapse, obliteration of the upper eyelid crease, and steatoblepharon can all occur as part of the aging process (**Fig. 12**). Cutaneous aging occurs globally throughout the face, but may first become evident in the periorbital region. The skin loses collagen structure (elasticity), dermal appendages, and becomes thinner, which may lead to the development of folds and rhytids.[79] These changes are associated with ultraviolet radiation, smoking, and intrinsic aging, and have been described extensively elsewhere.[80]

Bony Remodeling in Aging

Bony remodeling occurs with aging and has been shown to result in skull enlargement.[81,82]

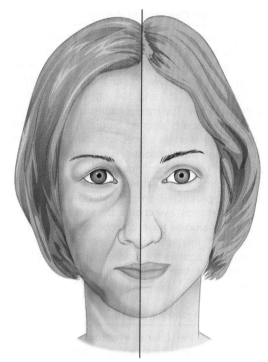

Fig. 12. The left panel shows the characteristics of a youthful face. The right side shows changes that occur from aging.

The supraorbital bar of the frontal sinus appears to increase in size, particularly in men, perhaps because of an apparent enlargement of the frontal sinus.[83] The orbital aperture increases in size, with vertical lengthening and scalloping of the superomedial and inferolateral orbit, described as curve distortion by Pessa.[84] Bony remodeling in the superomedial orbit may contribute to the apparent enlargement of the medial upper eyelid fat pad. These orbital changes may also lead to the eyebrow soft tissues descending into the orbital aperture, causing the appearance of brow ptosis and lateral orbital hooding.[85] The expanding remodeled orbit may give rise to the deepened sulci, the enophthalmos, and the ptosis often observed with aging.

Brow Changes in Aging

The forehead may increase in apparent size because of recession of the hairline in both men and women. Brow hairs are equally susceptible to the aging process. With age, brow hair can decrease in density, particularly in women, in the temporal third. The color of the brow hairs may become lighter over time and gray. In men, eyebrow hairs can become longer and coarser.

Morphologic Changes in Aging

Using carefully photographed comparisons of patients over a period of years, Lambros[86] described the morphologic changes that occur in the aging upper face. He found that the eyebrows descended slightly and the upper eyelid peak shifted laterally. The medial canthus was observed to stay in place or migrate medially, whereas the lateral canthal angle moved medially, decreasing the size of the horizontal palpebral aperture.[86] Lambros[86] also confirmed other age-related changes, including hollowing of the temples and adjacent periorbital areas, the development of forehead rhytids, eyelid ptosis, and dermatochalasis. Other studies have corroborated these findings.[79,87,88] Inspection and observation of these changes in aging patients compared with photographs from their past further confirms these findings.

Periorbital Aging

Descent of the lateral eyebrow is commonly observed in periorbital aging.[52] Knize[46] posited that the soft tissues lateral to the temporal fusion line lacked the support necessary to counteract the effects of gravity, leading to lateral eyebrow descent. Contrasting studies have found that the eyebrow paradoxically elevates with age and does not descend.[89,90] This elevation causes the horizontal forehead rhytids and is related to frontalis overaction.[32,89] Proposed mechanisms include chronically activated frontalis muscle as compensation for a primary acquired subclinical upper eyelid ptosis, aponeurotic dehiscence, and/or chronic elevation of the brows to reduce visual obstruction from dermatochalasis.[89,91]

Eyelid Skin in Aging

Redundant and lax upper eyelid skin, dermatochalasis, develops with aging and may interfere with vision. Dermatochalasis has been attributed to gravitational effect, volume loss, loss of tissue elasticity, and connective tissue degeneration, although no exact causes have been determined. A recent histologic study postulated that lymphedema contributes to the development of dermatochalasis, although its role is not clearly understood.[92] Despite these involutional changes in upper eyelid skin, the orbicularis remains intact with no discernable change in the bulk of muscle fibers.[93–95]

In the presence of dermatochalasis, the lid crease tends to diminish, and redundant skin can hang over the lashes, often resulting in lash ptosis. In the setting of aponeurotic ptosis, the upper eyelid skin becomes stretched over the ptotic eyelid. In conjunction with this, the lid crease elevates and the upper eyelid sulcus deepens as the central (preaponeurotic) fat pad recesses into the orbit with the dehiscent aponeurosis, which gives the appearance of a hollow superior orbit.

As mentioned earlier, aging can lead to the dehiscence of the levator aponeurosis, resulting in involutional blepharoptosis. Age-related changes contributing to aponeurotic dehiscence include[96,97]:

- Attenuation of the medial aponeurosis
- Lateral displacement of the upper eyelid tarsal plate
- Fatty degeneration of the levator muscle

It is important to determine the degree of ptosis that is solely attributable to levator aponeurosis dehiscence rather than other involutional processes of the brow-eyelid continuum.

The fat pads of the brows, temple, and midface, as described by Rohrich and colleagues,[98] seem to lose volume and descend with aging. The ROOF may diminish in quantity, leading to apparent redundancy of skin, or may descend. Temporal hooding caused by brow ptosis must be distinguished from lacrimal gland prolapse, another age-associated change that causes temporal bulging in the lateral upper eyelid.[62]

Orbital Fat in Aging

Within the orbit, there is an apparent paradoxic increase in upper eyelid nasal fad pad volume and a decrease in the upper eyelid central fat pad.[99] In the lower eyelid, Darcy and colleagues[100] showed with magnetic resonance imaging studies that orbital fat seems to increase with aging. Whether orbital fat increases in amount or simply becomes more apparent because of weakness of the septum is debatable but, in either situation, orbital fat becomes more visible in the upper eyelid. Fat atrophy may also occur, causing relative enophthalmos and hollowing of the upper sulcus.

SUMMARY

Surgery involving the upper eyelids must take into account all aspects of the brow-eyelid continuum. Eyelid surgery alone may not improve the aesthetics of the periorbital area, and has the potential to worsen them. It is important that the surgeon performing procedures in this area understands the complex interactions that may occur when eyelid surgery alone is performed, understands the anatomic and morphologic alterations that occur with aging, and be able to create a surgical plan that involves management of the brows and forehead to obtain optimal results.

REFERENCES

1. Karacalar A. Compensatory brow asymmetry: anatomic study and clinical experience. Aesthetic Plast Surg 2005;29(2):119–23.
2. Frankel AS, Kamer FM. The effect of blepharoplasty on eyebrow position. Arch Otolaryngol Head Neck Surg 1997;123(4):393–6.
3. Teske SA. Hering's law and eyebrow position. Ophthal Plast Reconstr Surg 1998;14(2):105–6.
4. Mehta HK. The contralateral upper eyelid in ptosis: some observations pertinent to ptosis corrective surgery. Br J Ophthalmol 1979;63(2):120–4.
5. Gay AJ, Salmon ML, Windsor CE. Hering's law, the levators, and their relationship in disease states. Arch Ophthalmol 1967;77(2):157–60.
6. Kersten RC, de Conciliis C, Kulwin DR. Acquired ptosis in the young and middle-aged adult population. Ophthalmology 1995;102(6):924–8.
7. Shah CT, Nguyen EV, Hassan AS. Asymmetric eyebrow elevation and its association with ocular dominance. Ophthal Plast Reconstr Surg 2012;28(1):50–3.
8. Le TT. Proportionality in Asian and North American Caucasian faces using neoclassical facial canons as criteria. Aesthetic Plast Surg 2002;26(1):64–9.
9. Farkas LG. Vertical and horizontal proportions of the face in young adult North American Caucasians: revision of neoclassical canons. Plast Reconstr Surg 1985;75(3):328–38.
10. Ramirez AL, Ende KH, Kabaker SS. Correction of the high female hairline. Arch Facial Plast Surg 2009;11(2):84–90.
11. Holcomb JD, McCollough EG. Trichophytic incisional approaches to upper facial rejuvenation. Arch Facial Plast Surg 2001;3(1):48–53.
12. Owsley TG. Subcutaneous trichophytic forehead browlift: the case for an "open" approach. J Oral Maxillofac Surg 2006;64(7):1133–6.
13. Camirand A. Hairline incisions. Plast Reconstr Surg 1999;103(2):736–7.
14. Beehner M. Hairline design in hair replacement surgery. Facial Plast Surg 2008;24(4):389–403.
15. Ellenbogen R. Transcoronal eyebrow lift with concomitant upper blepharoplasty. Plast Reconstr Surg 1983;71(4):490–9.
16. Laorwong K, Pathomvanich D, Bunagan K. Eyebrow transplantation in Asians. Dermatol Surg 2009;35(3):496–503 [discussion: 503–4].
17. Westmore M. Facial cosmetics in conjunction with surgery. In: Aesthetic Plastic Surgical Society Meeting. Vancouver, May 1974.
18. Whitaker LA, Morales L Jr, Farkas LG. Aesthetic surgery of the supraorbital ridge and forehead structures. Plast Reconstr Surg 1986;78(1):23–32.
19. Cook BE Jr, Lucarelli MJ, Lemke BN. Depressor supercilii muscle: anatomy, histology, and cosmetic implications. Ophthal Plast Reconstr Surg 2001;17(6):404–11.
20. Cook TA. The versatile midforehead browlift. Arch Otolaryngol Head Neck Surg 1989;115(2):163–8.
21. Pham S, Wilhelmi B, Mowlavi A. Eyebrow peak position redefined. Aesthet Surg J 2010;30(3):297–300.
22. Feser DK. Attractiveness of eyebrow position and shape in females depends on the age of the beholder. Aesthetic Plast Surg 2007;31(2):154–60.
23. Romm S. The changing face of beauty. Aesthetic Plast Surg 1989;13(2):91–8.
24. Oestreicher JH, Hurwitz JJ. The position of the eyebrow. Ophthalmic Surg 1990;21(4):245–9.
25. Volpe CR, Ramirez OM. The beautiful eye. Facial Plast Surg Clin North Am 2005;13(4):493–504.
26. Fagien S. Advanced rejuvenative upper blepharoplasty: enhancing aesthetics of the upper periorbita. Plast Reconstr Surg 2002;110(1):278–91 [discussion: 292].
27. Rohrich RJ. Current concepts in aesthetic upper blepharoplasty. Plast Reconstr Surg 2004;113(3):32e–42e.
28. Connell BF, Lambros VS, Neurohr GH. The forehead lift: techniques to avoid complications and produce optimal results. Aesthetic Plast Surg 1989;13(4):217–37.
29. Matarasso A, Terino EO. Forehead-brow rhytidoplasty: reassessing the goals. Plast Reconstr Surg 1994;93(7):1378–89 [discussion: 1390–1].
30. McKinney P, Mossie RD, Zukowski ML. Criteria for the forehead lift. Aesthetic Plast Surg 1991;15(2):141–7.
31. Kunjur J, Sabesan T, Ilankovan V. Anthropometric analysis of eyebrows and eyelids: an inter-racial study. Br J Oral Maxillofac Surg 2006;44(2):89–93.
32. Price KM. Eyebrow and eyelid dimensions: an anthropometric analysis of African Americans and Caucasians. Plast Reconstr Surg 2009;124(2):615–23.
33. Alex JC. Aesthetic considerations in the elevation of the eyebrow. Facial Plast Surg 2004;20(3):193–8.
34. Baker SB. The influence of brow shape on the perception of facial form and brow aesthetics. Plast Reconstr Surg 2007;119(7):2240–7.
35. McCord CD, Codner MA. Eyelid and periorbital surgery. St Louis (MO): Quality Medical Publishing; 2008. p. xiv, 784.
36. American Academy of Ophthalmology. Orbit, eyelids, and lacrimal system, 1992-1993. Basic and clinical science course. San Francisco (CA): American Academy of Ophthalmology; 1992. p. 254.

37. Most SP, Mobley SR, Larrabee WF Jr. Anatomy of the eyelids. Facial Plast Surg Clin North Am 2005; 13(4):487–92, v.

38. Park DH. Anthropometry of Asian eyelids by age. Plast Reconstr Surg 2008;121(4):1405–13.

39. Cho M, Glavas IP. Anatomic properties of the upper eyelid in Asian Americans. Dermatol Surg 2009; 35(11):1736–40.

40. Jeong S. The Asian upper eyelid: an anatomical study with comparison to the Caucasian eyelid. Arch Ophthalmol 1999;117(7):907–12.

41. Doxanas MT, Anderson RL. Oriental eyelids. An anatomic study. Arch Ophthalmol 1984;102(8): 1232–5.

42. Kakizaki H. Orbital septum attachment sites on the levator aponeurosis in Asians and whites. Ophthal Plast Reconstr Surg 2010;26(4):265–8.

43. Beer GM. Variations of the frontal exit of the supra-orbital nerve: an anatomic study. Plast Reconstr Surg 1998;102(2):334–41.

44. Mendelson BC, Jacobson SR. Surgical anatomy of the midcheek: facial layers, spaces, and the midcheek segments. Clin Plast Surg 2008;35(3): 395–404 [discussion: 393].

45. Moss CJ, Mendelson BC, Taylor GI. Surgical anatomy of the ligamentous attachments in the temple and periorbital regions. Plast Reconstr Surg 2000;105(4):1475–90 [discussion: 1491–8].

46. Knize DM. An anatomically based study of the mechanism of eyebrow ptosis. Plast Reconstr Surg 1996;97(7):1321–33.

47. Stuzin JM. Anatomy of the frontal branch of the facial nerve: the significance of the temporal fat pad. Plast Reconstr Surg 1989;83(2):265–71.

48. Stuzin JM, Baker TJ, Gordon HL. The relationship of the superficial and deep facial fascias: relevance to rhytidectomy and aging. Plast Reconstr Surg 1992;89(3):441–9 [discussion: 450–1].

49. Babakurban ST. Temporal branch of the facial nerve and its relationship to fascial layers. Arch Facial Plast Surg 2010;12(1):16–23.

50. Chen WP. Oculoplastic surgery: the essentials. New York: Thieme; 2001. p. xi, 499.

51. May JW Jr, Fearon J, Zingarelli P. Retro-orbicularis oculus fat (ROOF) resection in aesthetic blepharoplasty: a 6-year study in 63 patients. Plast Reconstr Surg 1990;86(4):682–9.

52. Boo-Chai K. In Orientals, be careful when you're on the ROOF. Plast Reconstr Surg 1991;88(1):178.

53. Ichinose A, Tahara S. Extended preseptal fat resection in Asian blepharoplasty. Ann Plast Surg 2008;60(2):121–6.

54. Southwood WF. The thickness of the skin. Plast Reconstr Surg (1946) 1955;15(5):423–9.

55. Wulc AE, Dryden RM, Khatchaturian T. Where is the gray line? Arch Ophthalmol 1987;105(8): 1092–8.

56. Milz S. An immunohistochemical study of the extra-cellular matrix of the tarsal plate in the upper eyelid in human beings. J Anat 2005;206(1):37–45.

57. Ridgway JM, Larrabee WF. Anatomy for blepharo-plasty and brow-lift. Facial Plast Surg 2010;26(3): 177–85.

58. Goold LA. Tarsal height. Ophthalmology 2009; 116(9):1831–1831.e2.

59. Meyer DR. Anatomy of the orbital septum and associated eyelid connective tissues. Implications for ptosis surgery. Ophthal Plast Reconstr Surg 1991;7(2):104–13.

60. Sires BS. The color difference in orbital fat. Arch Ophthalmol 2001;119(6):868–71.

61. Korn BS, Kikkawa DO, Hicok KC. Identification and characterization of adult stem cells from human orbital adipose tissue. Ophthal Plast Reconstr Surg 2009;25(1):27–32.

62. Massry GG. Prevalence of lacrimal gland prolapse in the functional blepharoplasty population. Oph-thal Plast Reconstr Surg 2011;27(6):410–3.

63. Petrelli RL. The treatment of lacrimal gland prolapse in blepharoplasty. Ophthal Plast Reconstr Surg 1988;4(3):139–42.

64. Dutton JJ. Atlas of clinical and surgical orbital anatomy. 2nd edition. Philadelphia: Elsevier Saunders; 2011. p. xiii, 262.

65. Stasior GO. Levator aponeurosis elastic fiber network. Ophthal Plast Reconstr Surg 1993;9(1):1–10.

66. Kakizaki H. The levator aponeurosis consists of two layers that include smooth muscle. Ophthal Plast Reconstr Surg 2005;21(5):379–82.

67. Codere F, Tucker NA, Renaldi B. The anatomy of Whitnall ligament. Ophthalmology 1995;102(12): 2016–9.

68. Kuwabara T, Cogan DG, Johnson CC. Structure of the muscles of the upper eyelid. Arch Ophthalmol 1975;93(11):1189–97.

69. Tyers AG, Collin JRO. Colour atlas of ophthalmic plastic surgery. Oxford (United Kingdom); Boston: Butterworth-Heinemann/Elsevier; 2008.

70. Janis JE. The anatomy of the corrugator supercilii muscle: part II. Supraorbital nerve branching patterns. Plast Reconstr Surg 2008;121(1):233–40.

71. Pitanguy I, Ramos AS. The frontal branch of the facial nerve: the importance of its variations in face lifting. Plast Reconstr Surg 1966;38(4):352–6.

72. Trussler AP. The frontal branch of the facial nerve across the zygomatic arch: anatomical relevance of the high-SMAS technique. Plast Reconstr Surg 2010;125(4):1221–9.

73. Ishikawa Y. An anatomical study on the distribution of the temporal branch of the facial nerve. J Craniomaxillofac Surg 1990;18(7):287–92.

74. Hwang K, Kim YJ, Chung IH. Innervation of the corrugator supercilii muscle. Ann Plast Surg 2004; 52(2):140–3.

75. American Academy of Ophthalmology. Fundamentals and principles of ophthalmology, 2005-2006. Basic and clinical science course. San Francisco (CA): American Academy of Ophthalmology; 2005. p. xvi, 520.

76. Kleintjes WG. Forehead anatomy: arterial variations and venous link of the midline forehead flap. J Plast Reconstr Aesthet Surg 2007;60(6):593–606.

77. Knize DM. A study of the supraorbital nerve. Plast Reconstr Surg 1995;96(3):564–9.

78. Larrabee WF, Makielski KH, Henderson JL. Surgical anatomy of the face. 2nd edition. Philadelphia: Lippincott Williams & Wilkins; 2004. p. xii, 195.

79. Warren RJ, Aston SJ, Mendelson BC. Face lift. Plast Reconstr Surg 2011;128(6):747e–64e.

80. Fan GB, Wu PL, Wang XM. Changes of oxygen content in facial skin before and after cigarette smoking. Skin Res Technol 2011. [Epub ahead of print].

81. Bartlett SP, Grossman R, Whitaker LA. Age-related changes of the craniofacial skeleton: an anthropometric and histologic analysis. Plast Reconstr Surg 1992;90(4):592–600.

82. Pessa JE. Aging and the shape of the mandible. Plast Reconstr Surg 2008;121(1):196–200.

83. Israel H. The dichotomous pattern of craniofacial expansion during aging. Am J Phys Anthropol 1977;47(1):47–51.

84. Pessa JE, Chen Y. Curve analysis of the aging orbital aperture. Plast Reconstr Surg 2002;109(2):751–5 [discussion: 756–60].

85. Kahn DM, Shaw RB. Overview of current thoughts on facial volume and aging. Facial Plast Surg 2010;26(5):350–5.

86. Lambros V. Observations on periorbital and midface aging. Plast Reconstr Surg 2007;120(5):1367–76 [discussion: 1377].

87. Yeh CC, Williams EF 3rd. Fat management in lower lid blepharoplasty. Facial Plast Surg 2009;25(4):234–44.

88. Chen HH, Williams EF. Lipotransfer in the upper third of the face. Curr Opin Otolaryngol Head Neck Surg 2011;19(4):289–94.

89. Matros E, Garcia JA, Yaremchuk MJ. Changes in eyebrow position and shape with aging. Plast Reconstr Surg 2009;124(4):1296–301.

90. van den Bosch WA, Leenders I, Mulder P. Topographic anatomy of the eyelids, and the effects of sex and age. Br J Ophthalmol 1999;83(3):347–52.

91. Troilius C. Subperiosteal brow lifts without fixation. Plast Reconstr Surg 2004;114(6):1595–603 [discussion: 1604–5].

92. Nagi KS, Carlson JA, Wladis EJ. Histologic assessment of dermatochalasis: elastolysis and lymphostasis are fundamental and interrelated findings. Ophthalmology 2011;118(6):1205–10.

93. Pottier F, El-Shazly NZ, El-Shazly AE. Aging of orbicularis oculi: anatomophysiologic consideration in upper blepharoplasty. Arch Facial Plast Surg 2008;10(5):346–9.

94. Cheng NC. Fiber type and myosin heavy chain compositions of adult pretarsal orbicularis oculi muscle. J Mol Histol 2007;38(3):177–82.

95. Lee H. Histopathologic findings of the orbicularis oculi in upper eyelid aging: total or minimal excision of orbicularis oculi in upper blepharoplasty. Arch Facial Plast Surg 2012;14(4):253–7. [Epub ahead of print].

96. Shore JW, McCord CD Jr. Anatomic changes in involutional blepharoptosis. Am J Ophthalmol 1984;98(1):21–7.

97. Pereira LS. Levator superioris muscle function in involutional blepharoptosis. Am J Ophthalmol 2008;145(6):1095–8.

98. Rohrich RJ, Pessa JE. The fat compartments of the face: anatomy and clinical implications for cosmetic surgery. Plast Reconstr Surg 2007;119(7):2219–27 [discussion: 2228–31].

99. Oh SR. Analysis of eyelid fat pad changes with aging. Ophthal Plast Reconstr Surg 2011;27(5):348–51.

100. Darcy SJ. Magnetic resonance imaging characterization of orbital changes with age and associated contributions to lower eyelid prominence. Plast Reconstr Surg 2008;122(3):921–9 [discussion: 930–1].

Contemporary Concepts in Brow and Eyelid Aging

Rebecca Fitzgerald, MD

KEYWORDS

- Dermatology • Facial rejuvenation • Brow aging • Eye aging • Aging face

KEY POINTS

- Aging is a 3-dimensional process, with changes in multiple tissues contributing to the overall effect.
- Patients most commonly correlate aging changes with expressions of anger, sadness, and fatigue.
- The role of volume loss in the clinical changes observed in the aging face is becoming widely appreciated. Mastery of volume replacement has become essential to the successful practice of esthetic medicine.
- Lifting techniques alone, without addressing volume loss, can no longer adequately address the aging process in the upper third of the face. In fact, this approach may actually exacerbate, rather than ameliorate, the aging process.
- Rejuvenation of the eyelids and eyebrows requires an understanding of the interrelationships between these and other facial structures to ensure optimal outcomes.
- Anatomy informs concepts, concepts inform technique, and technique determines outcomes.

INTRODUCTION

Current literature suggests that the aging process is occurring in all tissue structures of the face and that a change in one area may greatly influence the neighboring tissues, leading to a cascade of secondary events. The central role of volume loss and deflation in the aging face, rather than ptosis alone, has been clearly illustrated by Lambros[1] in a longitudinal photographic analysis of more than 100 patients spanning an average period of 25 years. These studies have eloquently demonstrated that volume loss in fact mimics gravitational descent.

The age-related changes in the eyelid and eyebrow continuum, similar to other regions of the face, should be thought of as a 3-dimensional construct with deflation rather than ptosis being the primary factor in the aging process. Esthetic facial rejuvenation has traditionally focused on surgical procedures, which are based on a paradigm of removing and lifting "excess" tissues to counteract gravitational changes. Open and endoscopic browlifting techniques, as well as "nonsurgical" eyebrow lift with chemodenervation, have been widely used in clinical practice. Approaching the aging face from the standpoint of volume loss invokes an entirely different paradigm of rejuvenation. Instead of simply excising and lifting the tissues, the volume paradigm invokes the concept of "filling" the face. The focus of this article, outlining current concepts in the aging brows and lids, therefore focuses on this current "evolution" to the 3-dimensional construct. Although we often look for ideals, such as the perfect cheek, perfect lip, or perfect brow position, there is likely no singular esthetic that fits every individual face. Thoughtful analysis of the underlying anatomy, ethnicity, gender, and goals of each patient will greatly enhance our ability to address site-specific corrections to achieve optimal and natural-looking results. For this reason, relevant anatomy is reviewed in detail here.

Department of Medicine, David Geffen School of Medicine, University of California, Los Angeles, 321 North Larchmont Boulevard, Suite 906, Los Angeles, CA 90004, USA
E-mail address: fitzmd@earthlink.net

Clin Plastic Surg 40 (2013) 21–42
http://dx.doi.org/10.1016/j.cps.2012.08.005
0094-1298/13/$ – see front matter © 2013 Elsevier Inc. All rights reserved.

plasticsurgery.theclinics.com

YOUTHFUL AND AGING BROWS AND LIDS

In youth, the 3-dimensional surface contours of the face predominantly reflect light. Volume changes over time result in broken reflections with intervening shadows. This is beautifully illustrated in **Fig. 1**, which shows 2 pictures of the same woman, one from her high school years and the other 37 years later.[2] The profound global volume loss in the older photograph is easy to appreciate. The youthful oval face in the frontal view dramatically flattens with age. The young eye appears long and full, the bony orbit is not visible, the skin is elastic and thick, most of the upper lid is concealed by the full brow, with only a few millimeters of upper lid show. The upper lid sulcus lacks a shadow, and the eye has an overall "almond" configuration, with the lid margin, lid crease, and eyebrow all parallel.

All of these characteristics are affected by aging in predictable ways. In the older photograph, we see brow deflation that does not result in significant brow ptosis, but rather results in the brow laying flat against the orbital rim. Shadows develop below the brow and in the concave temple. As the upper lid deflates, a fold of skin develops where there was once fullness, and the shadow of the upper lid sulcus emerges. With increasing age, this fold of upper lid skin often droops and may encroach on the lash line, completely effacing

any visibility of the upper lid ("hooding"). The eyelid skin may also slip into the lid crease, revealing the upper lid veiled in youth by the full brow. Often this is initially most pronounced medially resulting in the so-called "A-frame" deformity.

More than 20 years ago, Van den Bosch and colleagues[3] collected and analyzed data on eyeball and eyelid position of 320 men and women, equally divided into 10-year age cohorts between the ages of 10 and 89 years, and found that aging mainly affects the size of the horizontal eyelid fissure, which lengthens by about 10% between the ages of 12 and 25, and then shortens by almost the same amount between middle age and old age. Additional findings from their study were a higher skin fold (meaning increased upper lid show), and higher eyebrow position in both sexes. Sagging of the lower eyelid was noted, especially in men. These changes seen with aging (an increased upper lid show, which makes the eye look taller vertically, in combination with a horizontal shortening) result in a perceived "rounding" of the eye.

These changes are extremely well illustrated in **Fig. 2**, taken from Lambros' article on volumizing the brows.[4] The top pair of pictures of the same woman at 21 and 64 years old demonstrate how the eyes have an almost "almond"-shaped appearance in youth and a more rounded configuration with aging. In the middle row, a photograph of

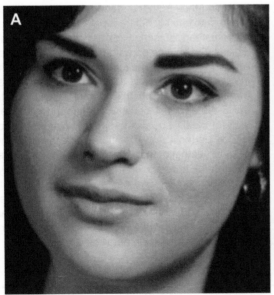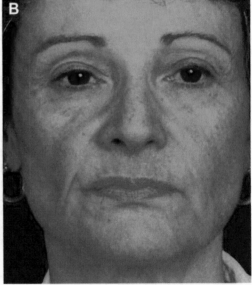

Fig. 1. The concept of aging is shifting from 2-dimensional to 3-dimensional, as illustrated by these photographs. (*A*) High school photograph exhibiting fullness and highlights. (*B*) The same person 37 years older. (*From* Glasgold M, Lam SM, Glasgold R. Volumetric rejuvenation of the periorbital region. Facial Plast Surg 2010;26:3; with permission.)

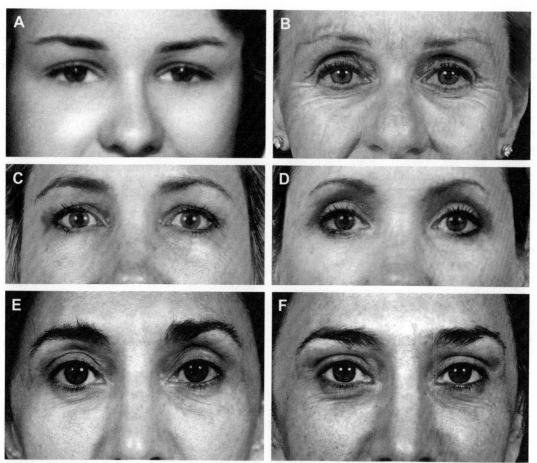

Fig. 2. (*Upper*) A typical pattern of upper lid aging. (*A*) View of a 21-year-old woman. Note that the young eye is long and full, without much upper lid showing. The bony orbital rim is not visible. (*B*) The same woman at 64 years of age. The older eye is rounder, shorter, and more hollow. The orbital rim is visible. (*Middle*): (*C*) Pretreatment view of a 45-year-old woman. (*D*) Posttreatment view 2 years after upper lid blepharoplasty. Although the eye is more defined, it retains many characteristics seen with aging, as it is rounder, shorter, and more hollow. Also note the superior orbital rim is visible. (*Lower*): (*E*) Pretreatment view of a 48-year-old woman. (*F*) Posttreatment view a few minutes after an ice cube was applied, and local anesthetic was infiltrated and massaged into place to form a new brow curve. Note that the patient's eyes look more youthful. (*Adapted from* Lambros V. Volumizing the brow with hyaluronic acid fillers. Aesthet Surg J 2009;29(3):174–9; with permission.)

a 45-year-old woman before and after blepharo-plasty illustrates that conventional excisional techniques involving removal of "excess" skin and fat may actually exacerbate the hollowing of the orbit, with the subsequent appearance of a rounder shortened eye (ie, an older-appearing eye). Finally, on the bottom row, we see an older woman with rounded eyes. As the upper lid deflates, a fold of skin develops where there once was fullness, and the shadow of the upper lid sulcus emerges (especially on her right). Volumizing the upper brow with local anesthesia in this patient results in a less-rounded, more almond-shaped eye, resulting in a more youthful-appearing periorbital area.

Aging of the upper third of the face, of course, affects much more than esthetics. The eyes and the periorbital structures convey a wide range of expressions, representing a critical nonverbal form of communication that is fundamental to all of our social interactions. The basic expressions of happiness, sadness, fear, anger, and surprise appear to cross cultural lines and may be considered a universal means of nonverbal communication. Facial interpretation is in fact considered to be among the most important acquisitions in our development.[5] Some forms of facial expressions, such as anger (glabellar furrows), sadness (downward angulation of the oral commissure), and fatigue (tear trough deformity), may be mimicked by the aging process. This generally leads to an unintended and undesirable misinterpretation of mood by others that is unwelcome to most all of us as we age and is one of the most common presenting complaints (**Fig. 3**).

In a study in 2008, Knoll and colleagues[6] had a set of images adjusted to only one variable reviewed by subjects and graded for of each of 7 expressions/emotions as follows: "surprise," "anger," "sadness," "disgust," "fear," "happiness," and "tiredness." They found statistically significant values for tiredness were achieved by changes of increasing and decreasing the pretarsal skin crease (to simulate a long upper lid show or "hooding" with no lid show) and by depressing the lateral brow. Elevation of the medial brow elicited a minimal increase for sadness. All of these changes may also be seen with aging. Interestingly, simulating the skin resection of an upper blepharoplasty resulted in an increase in the perception of tiredness, perhaps indicating that skin excision without regard to volume may exacerbate, rather than ameliorate, the appearance of aging.

RELEVANT ANATOMY
Skin

Over the past decade, substantial progress has been made toward understanding the underlying mechanisms of the aging process. A major feature of aged skin is fragmentation of the dermal collagen matrix that leads to the loss of structural integrity and impairment of fibroblast function. Fragmentation results from actions of specific enzymes (matrix metalloproteinases) observed in both intrinsic and extrinsic aging. Fibroblasts that produce and organize the collagen matrix cannot attach to fragmented collagen and subsequently collapse. Collapsed fibroblasts produce low levels of collagen and high levels of collagen-degrading enzymes. Once a critical amount of collagen has been lost, this imbalance advances the aging process in a self-perpetuating, never-ending deleterious cycle. This is well illustrated by the difference in skin elasticity seen on the driver's side and non–driver's side window of the truck driver pictured in **Fig. 4**. The production of new collagen demonstrated by electron microscopy after the

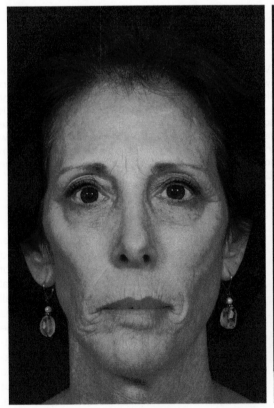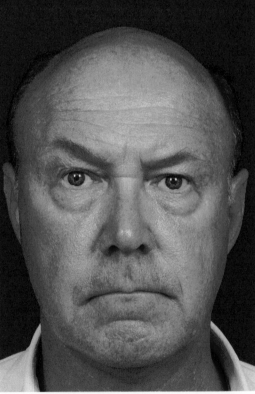

Fig. 3. Brow changes seen with aging may also communicate an unintended feeling of sadness, fatigue, or anger. (*Courtesy of* Rebecca Fitzgerald, MD.)

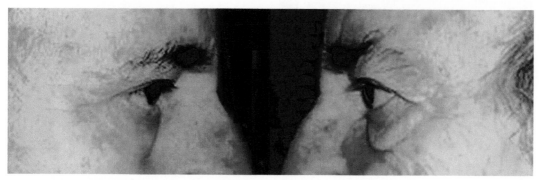

Fig. 4. Intrinsic and extrinsic aging in the skin affects its ability to adjust well to underlying volume loss. This patient looks older on his left side. He is a truck driver in the Mojave Desert and has more pronounced elastosis on the left side, which faces the driver's side window. (*Courtesy of* Rebecca Fitzgerald, MD.)

injection of hyaluronic acid is felt likely to be attributable to a mechanical stretch effect, serving to rebalance collagen production and degradation, and thereby slowing its loss.[7,8]

Bone

Craniofacial bony remodeling is increasingly being recognized as an important contributor to the facial aging process. More than a decade ago, Pessa and Chen[9] studied 30 male skulls in 3 age categories at the Smithsonian Institution and found that although there was no change in width or height of the orbit with increasing age, there was curve distortion of the superomedial and inferolateral orbit. They also noted that this change in shape as well as size reflected a selective pattern of resorption and renewal occurring with age.

Subsequently, drawing on the common observation that a change in the underlying bony support from facial trauma could lead to changes in the draping of the soft tissues of the face, Pessa[10] then hypothesized a corollary: it was logical that changes in the bony orbit could also be associated with changes in the overlying soft tissue. Specifically, that the redraping of soft tissue overlying the remodeled bony orbit may contribute to the development of a lateral suborbital tear trough and increased scleral show (**Figs. 5** and **6**). Multiple studies have now demonstrated these craniofacial skeletal changes with age, most notably the landmark study by Shaw and Kahn.[11–15]

Soft Tissue (Muscle and Fat)

Muscle dynamics play a central role in the changes seen in the aging forehead and brow.

Ellis and Masri studied 60 patients, age 20 to 74 years, who they split into 3 groups according to the dominant animation pattern: brow lifters, frowners, and squinters. They found that brow ptosis was accentuated laterally in the squinters and medially in the frowners, and that the brow lifter group showed more uniform displacement of the eyebrows.[16] Animation patterns acquired in childhood, therefore, may have a significant effect on patterns of brow ptosis.

What happens to muscles with aging is likely contingent on a number of variables. Traditional thought holds that muscles become more lax with time. Some researchers now believe the muscles of facial animation may adjust to shifts in underlying volume by adjusting (and increasing) their resting tone. This may have clinical relevance regarding the depth at which we choose to place our fillers, as there may be some advantage to deeper placement.[17,18]

The medial brow depressors are made up of the centrally located procerus, surrounded laterally by 2 pairs of muscles: the corrugator supercilli and the depressor supercilli. The procerus is often a bifid muscle. It originates over the nasal dorsum, inserts into the skin of the glabella, and contributes to the horizontal lines over the nasal dorsum. The corrugator supercilii is the largest of the depressor muscles. It has both a transverse and a medial head with an origin at the medial orbital bone and an insertion on the underside of the frontalis muscle over the midbrow. The corrugator pulls in and down, contributing to the formation of the vertical glabellar rhytides, commonly referred to as "the elevens." The depressor supercilii is a small muscle relative to the other depressors and runs almost vertically between the medial orbital bone and the medial head of the brow (**Fig. 7**).

The orbicularis oculi muscle is a concentric muscle originating at the medial orbital bone and consists of 3 parts:

1. Pretarsal: starting at the lid margin
2. Preseptal: between the distal edge of the tarsal plate and the orbital rim

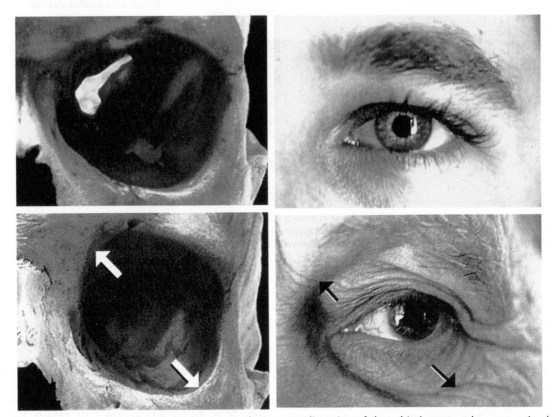

Fig. 5. Pessa's hypothesis that skeletal aging results in curve distortion of the orbital aperture has now gained support from numerous studies. These changes may have both cosmetic and functional consequences, as they are accompanied by secondary changes in the position of the facial soft tissues. This is illustrated here in a photograph of both a young and aged individual. (*From* Pessa JE, Chen Y. Curve analysis of the aging orbital aperture. Plast Reconstr Surg 2002;109:751; with permission; and Pessa JE. An algorithm of facial aging: verification of Lambros's theory by three-dimensional stereolithography, with reference to the pathogenesis of midfacial aging, scleral show, and the lateral suborbital trough deformity. Plast Reconstr Surg 2000;106(2):479–88; with permission.)

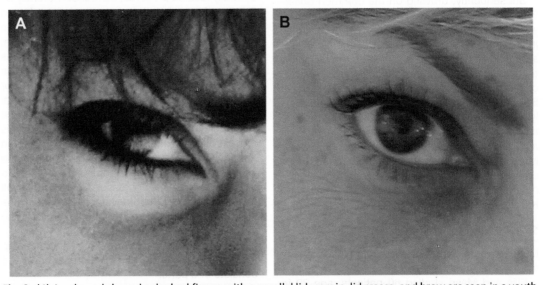

Fig. 6. (*A*) An almond-shaped palpebral fissure with a parallel lid margin, lid crease, and brow are seen in a youthful eye. (*B*) Corresponding changes in the soft tissues accompany the underlying bony remodeling in an aging eye. A linear example with similar changes in the same woman at ages 20 and 46. Note the distortion of the lower lateral lid and the slight scleral show. (*Courtesy of* Rebecca Fitzgerald, MD.)

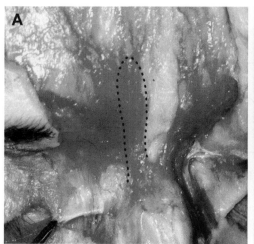
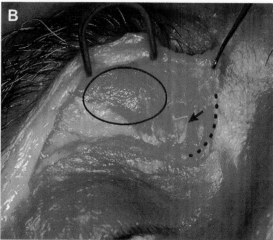

Fig. 7. (*A*) The dotted area denotes the right procerus. Note the fascial insertion over the nasal bones. (*B*) The cut edge of the orbicularis is dotted. The arrow shows a single-headed depressor supercilii that originates above the medial canthal tendon to insert into the medial brow. The black circle shows an obliquely oriented lower corrugator. (*From* Zide BM, Jelks G. Surgical anatomy around the orbit. The system of zones. Philadelphia: Lippincott, Williams and Wilkins; 2006. p. 67; with permission.)

3. Preorbicularis: covering the bony orbit distal to the rim

The medial portion of the orbicularis oculi is also a depressor of the medial brow. The lateral orbicularis oculi is a lateral brow depressor (which contributes to the formation of crow's feet).

The elevator of the brow is the frontalis muscle. It is also most often found as a bifid muscle in which the right and left halves do not usually meet in the middle of the forehead (**Fig. 8**). Using cadaveric dissections, Knize[19] noted that the lateral margin of frontalis muscle almost always ends or becomes markedly attenuated along or just lateral to the temporal fusion line of the skull and its continuation as the superior temporal line. Among cadaver specimens, the temporal line was found to intersect the eyebrow at variable points ranging from the middle third of the eyebrow to just lateral to the eyebrow. The more medially that the plane of the temporal line meets the eyebrow, the less frontalis muscle resting tone there is for suspensory support for the lateral eyebrow. Among different patients, then, the ability of the frontalis muscle to maintain lateral eyebrow position may be variable. Additionally, the presence of a lateral orbital retaining ligament between the superficial temporal fascia and the zygomaticofrontal suture fixes the lateral eyebrow, preventing movement to a degree equivalent to the medial brow. Additionally, Knize notes that the preseptal fat pad and galea fat pad may facilitate gravitational descent of the unsupported overlying lateral eyebrow (**Fig. 9**). The photos to the right of the schematic were chosen to illustrate how this may appear clinically. Details on medial brow anatomy are outlined in the schematic seen in **Fig. 10** and cadaveric dissections of this region are seen in **Figs. 11** and **12**.

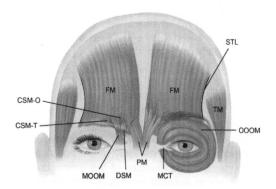

Fig. 8. Muscles of the forehead and temporal fossa. The characteristic appearance of the aged upper face is produced by the combination of bony remodeling, volume changes, and the action of the following muscles: frontalis (FM), oblique head of the corrugator supercilii (CSM-O), transverse head of the corrugator supercilii (CSM-T), depressor supercilii (DSM), procerus (PM), medial head of the orbicularis oculi (MOOM), and the orbital portion of the orbicularis oculi (OOOM). Also labeled are the superior temporal fusion line of the skull (STL), the medial canthal tendon (MCT), and the temporalis (TM) muscle. (*From* Knize D. Anatomic concepts for brow lift procedures. Plast Reconstr Surg 2009;124(6):2118–26; with permission.)

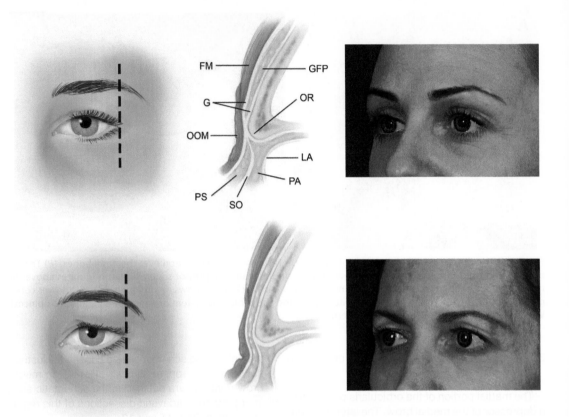

Fig. 9. When the layers of the galea (G) completely envelop the galea fat pad (GFP) by re-fusing along the entire superior orbital rim (OR), as shown above, lateral eyebrow position will be more stable during the aging process. If envelopment of the galea fat pad is incomplete laterally, as shown below, lateral eyebrow ptosis would be expected to appear earlier in the aging process as the fat pads slide down over the orbital rim. The photographs to the right of the schematic were chosen to illustrate how this may appear clinically. (*Courtesy of* Knize D. An anatomically based study of the mechanism of eyebrow ptosis. Plast Reconstr Surg 1996;97:1321–33, with permission; and Rebecca Fitzgerald, MD.)

Anatomy informs concepts, concepts inform technique, and technique determines outcomes. Treatment of the periorbital area, therefore, should theoretically include not only neuromodulation of the hyperdynamic muscles of the region but also volumizing to account for changes in the skeletal platform, as well as the fat pads seen with aging of the brow/lid continuum.

Facial Topography

Over the past several years, Rohrich and Pessa[20–22] have performed numerous cadaveric dissection studies revealing that the adipose tissues of the face exist as distinct regions and zones rather than as one confluent soft tissue mass.

Boundary zones between these anatomic regions can exist both superficial and deep to fascia and muscle. Deep fat pads impart a specific shape and contour to the overlying skin, and are a primary determinant of anterior projection. This can be easily appreciated in the cheek, brow, and upper and lower eyelids. In their new text, they present detailed dissections illustrating that the surface of the face is a roadmap for the underlying anatomy and a few important points are reviewed here.[23] The work of Pessa and Rohrich reveals that deep vascular arcades and regional differences in fat usually define topographic "creases," which are the indentations that occur in between folds. As nerves run with the arteries, creases indicate their position as well. "Wrinkles," on the other hand, may be predictors of the course of superficial vessels but differences in adipose tissue thickness are not typically seen.

These anatomic variations allow the practitioner to more carefully plan filler injection techniques, ie, fillers injected superficially directly beneath

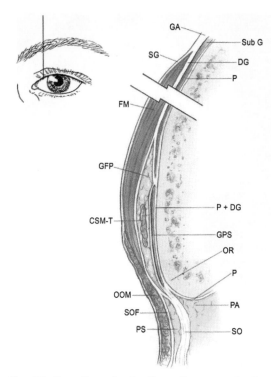

Fig. 10. Over the calvaria, the galea aponeurotica (GA) lies on the subgalea fascia plane (Sub G), which separates the galea aponeurotica from periosteum (P). As the galea aponeurotica approaches the upper forehead, it splits into the superficial galea plane (SG) and the deep galea plane (DG) to envelop the frontalis muscle (FM). The deep galea plane splits again to envelop the galea fat pad (GFP), which at the level indicated in this illustration, contains the transverse head of the corrugator supercilii muscle (CSM-T). Over the lower forehead, the deep galea plane splits a third time to form the glide plane space (GPS), a space deep to the corrugator supercilii muscle that contains only loose areolar tissue. Under the GPS "floor," the subgalea fascia plane, which separated the deep galea plane from periosteum over the upper forehead, is obliterated. The floor of the glide plane space is the deepest layer of the deep galea plane fused with periosteum (PDG) and is fixed to the underlying frontal bone. The multiple layers of the deep galea plane rejoin and fuse to the orbital rim (OR) before they enter the orbit to form the suborbicularis oculi muscle fascia (SOF) and the septum orbitale (SO). The preseptal fat pad (PS) lies superficial to the septum orbitale, whereas the preaponeurotic fat pad (PA) lies deep to it. The superficial galea plane that covers the surface of the frontalis muscle continues over the surface of the orbicularis oculi muscle (OOM). (*Adapted from* Knize D. The forehead and temporal fossa: anatomy and technique. Philadelphia: Williams & Wilkins; 2001. p. 46; with permission; and Knize D. The importance of the retaining ligamentous attachments of the forehead for selective eyebrow shaping and forehead rejuvenation. Plast Reconstr Surg 2007;119(3):1119–20; with permission.)

true creases should not be associated with a significant complication rate (as is seen in clinical practice), whereas superficial injections under wrinkles, on the other hand, may be more prone to inadvertent injury. Most importantly, this anatomic finding indicates that deeper injections into creases run the risk of injuring the regional blood supply.

Orbital Ligaments

Understanding the underlying ligamental structures of the periorbital region is crucial. The orbicularis retaining ligament (ORL) plays a key role in the topographic anatomy of the upper lids and eyebrows. It is a membrane that is created when the fascia beneath the orbicularis oculi muscle inserts into the periosteum of the supraorbital rim. It acts to tether the orbicularis oculi muscle and provides a point of stability. The ORL is the boundary between the forehead and the upper eyelid and extends onto the zygomatic arch as the lateral orbital thickening. The ORL inserts 2 to 3 mm above the inferior edge of the supraorbital rim and this point is of extreme clinical importance. Any injection performed below this insertion point places material into the upper eyelid, rendering the levator muscle and fat vulnerable to injury. This complication is avoidable if one palpates the supraorbital rim and always injects 2 to 3 mm above its inferior edge where the ORL inserts.

It should be emphasized that the ORL seal at the boundary between forehead and upper eyelid is imperfect where vessels and nerves traverse anatomic compartments. For example, if an injection is placed directly adjacent to the supraorbital foramen, product can migrate along the supraorbital artery and nerve into the upper eyelid. This is one suspected mechanism of eyelid ptosis that can occur as a result of chemodenervation of the levator palpebrae muscle when an extraorbital injection of a neuromodulater is performed.

Finally, we know that periorbital injections are most safely performed with small volumes and low pressure to decrease the risk of retrograde injection into the ophthalmic artery system. As discussed earlier, creases may serve as landmarks of where to avoid deep injections around the eyelid. They also serve as a warning that complications may arise from failure to recognize the imperfect seal between anatomic boundaries.

The aging anatomic changes in all of the previously mentioned structures are illustrated in **Fig. 13.**

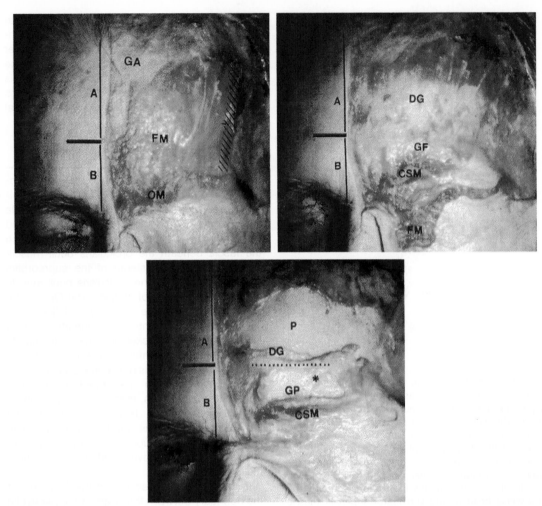

Fig. 11. Forehead anatomy. (*Left*) Cadaver specimen with left forehead skin and subcutaneous tissue removed. The frontalis muscle (FM) is enveloped by galea aponeurotica (GA). The glistening surface of the left frontalis muscle shown here is the thin superficial galea plane. The lateral margin of the frontalis muscle falls over the zone of fixation (*slanted lines*) just medial to the temporal fusion line of the skull and its continuation as the superior temporal line. The orbicularis oculi muscle (OM) overlaps the lower frontalis muscle. Zone A (A) and zone B (B) of the forehead are indicated. (*Right*) The frontalis muscle has been transected and its inferior half elevated off the underlying deep galea plane (DG). Frontalis muscle along with orbicularis oculi muscle is reflected over the orbital area to expose the lateral end of the corrugator supercilii muscle (CSM). Corrugator supercilii muscle, which passes through the galea fat pad (GF), was transected at the level of entrance into the plane of frontalis muscle and orbicularis oculi muscle. Galea fat pad is enveloped by deep galea plane, seen as a glistening film over the fat pad. The galea fat pad essentially covers zone B. (*Bottom*) The deep galea plane is shown raised off the periosteum (P) and reflected down to the level (*dotted line*) below which the deepest layer of deep galea plane and periosteum are fused and fixed to frontal bone over zone B. Deep to the galea fat pad is the subgalea fat pad glide plane (GP) space. The floor of the glide plane space is lined with smooth connective tissue, the deepest layer of the deep galea plane. Note the deep division of the supraorbital nerve (*asterisk*) running between the floor and the underlying periosteum. The roof of this space is the layer of deep galea plane that lines the undersurface of galea fat pad. Corrugator supercilii muscle rests on the medial roof of this space as corrugator supercilii muscle passes through the galea fat pad en route to the dermis. (*From* Knize D. An anatomically based study of the mechanism of eyebrow ptosis. Plast Reconstr Surg 1996;97:1321–33; with permission.)

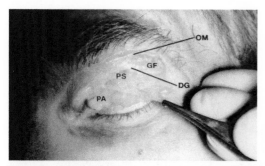

Fig. 12. Periorbital fat pads. Cadaveric photography showing how the septum orbitale (grasped by forceps) separates preaponeurotic fat pad (PA) from preseptal fat pad (PS). Deep to orbicularis oculi muscle (OM), the inferior edge of the lateral galea fat pad (GF) has been exposed by removing some of its overlying layer of the deep galea plane (DG). In this specimen, the preseptal fat pad and the galea fat pad were separated by the deep galeal fascial plane (DG). (*From* Knize D. An anatomically based study of the mechanism of eyebrow ptosis. Plast Reconstr Surg 1996;97:1321–33; with permission.)

EVALUATION OF BROW AND EYELIDS

Eyebrow position and shape determine not only the overall esthetic look of the face, but also serve as a key factor in facial recognition. Sadro and colleagues[24] performed a study that removed various key facial features of well-known historical figures and asked observers to identify the figures. They found a significantly greater decrement in facial recognition with the absence of eyebrows

as compared with absence of eyes (**Fig. 14**). As a result, to obtain "natural" brow rejuvenation results, it is important to avoid significant and dramatic changes to the region.

Brow Shape and Position

The definition of one ideal brow shape that can be used as a standard to predict and measure all outcomes has been elusive and perhaps counterproductive in obtaining optimal results. This may be, in part, because there is no one ideal brow shape. The traditional description by Westmore[25] in 1974 described characteristics of the ideal eyebrow as an arch where the brow apex terminates above the lateral limbus of the iris, with the medial and lateral ends of the brow at the same horizontal level. Brow shape and position have since been variably described in a number of ways, using various landmarks, and with differing esthetics over the past 30 years. Multiple studies reveal that descriptions of an "ideal brow" have varied, contingent on many factors, including the age of the subject or the observer, as well as race, gender, and even the shape of the face that the brow sits on.[25–33]

Studies have looked at the preferences of plastic surgeons, cosmetologists, lay public, and even the patients themselves. In their analysis of eyebrow shape and position of attractive models from popular fashion magazines, Gunter and Antrobus[34] found that although there were individual variations, the brows usually started low medially and were often flat as they ascended slightly to the midpupil. Freund and Nolan[35] tested the

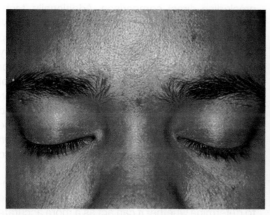 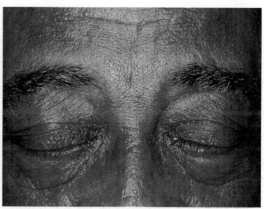

Fig. 13. Periorbital features are intimately related. The eyelids and eyebrows cannot be evaluated individually. The changes in skin elasticity, fat volume, resting muscle contraction, and progressive distortion of the orbital aperture, which affects the position of the overlying soft tissues, is well illustrated in this photograph of a younger and older African American man. Note the increased frontalis muscle action, even in relaxation, in the older subject on the right compared with the younger subject on the left. (*From* Price KM, Gupta PK, Woodward JA, et al. Eyebrow and eyelid dimensions: an anthropometric analysis of African Americans and Caucasians. Plast Reconstr Surg 2009;124:615–23; with permission.)

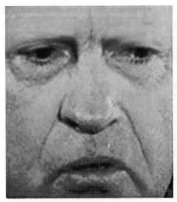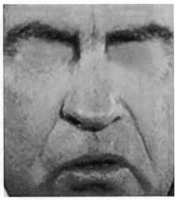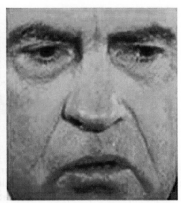

Fig. 14. Simulation of an experiment assessing the contribution of eyebrows to facial recognition: original images of President Richard Nixon along with modified versions lacking either eyebrows or eyes. (*Courtesy of Pawan Sinha, PhD, Cambridge, MA; with permission.*)

opinions of 11 cosmetic surgeons and 9 cosmetologists with computer graphics to isolate changes in brow shape or position as the only variables of appearance. They concluded that the medial brow should be located at or below the supraorbital rim, not above it, and that the brow should be shaped with its highest point located lateral to the pupil ("apex lateral slant").

Schreiber and colleagues[36] surveyed 100 randomly selected lay people who were asked to rank 27 photographs and found that most people preferred placement of the eyebrow in a lower position, including the arch, than had previously thought to be ideal by the classic "Westmore" ideals (**Fig. 15**).

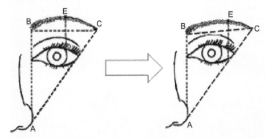

Fig. 15. Schreiber and colleagues' rendition of Westmore's classic illustration of periorbital esthetic ideals with the following changes: first, the overall position of the eyebrow is lower; second, the arch is more lateral in relation to its position over the lateral limbus; and third, the lateral eyebrow is higher than the medial eyebrow. The second and third changes have been previously described. (*From* Schreiber JE, Singh NK, Klatsky SA. Beauty lies in the eyebrow of the beholder: a public survey of eyebrow aesthetics. Aesthet Surg J 2005;25:348–52; with permission.)

Most recently, when Sclafani and Jung[37] had patients (n = 30) position their own "ideal" brow (photographs were taken of subjects in 5 poses: eyes open and eyes closed, maximum brow elevation and brow contraction, and brow positioned optimally by the subject), they found that most patients preferred brows with a shapely but comparatively unelevated brow. Most women in this study desired the medial brow head at or below the orbital rim.

Variance in Measurement Techniques for Brow Position

Unfortunately, data regarding brow position in women at different ages all use different landmarks and techniques for measurement, precluding direct comparison. Additionally, techniques used in the measurement of eyebrow height have often been based on the relationship of the eyebrow to structures that tend to vary with age (eg, eyelid margin or crease position) or are difficult to accurately measure because of landmark ambiguity (ie, central pupil to eyebrow height). Cole and colleagues[38] provide a detailed review of many previous studies and describe a new technique measuring eyebrow position form the inferior corneal limbus in an effort to provide an easily reproducible standard.

More recently, Pham and colleagues[39] examined the position of the deep temporal fusion line to determine whether it can act as a more accurate and functional landmark than prior anatomic landmarks for the eyebrow peak position.

Several articles in the literature conclude that brow lifts produce eyebrows with shape and position that are not esthetically pleasing, citing overelevation, hollowing, and sometimes a look of "perpetual

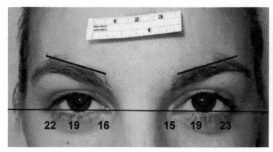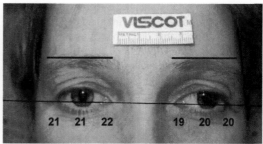

Fig. 16. Brow shape changes with aging were studied in 2 age cohorts by Matros and Garcia. They published this photograph to illustrate the typical results seen for patients from the 20-year-old to 30-year-old (*left*) and 50-year-old to 60-year-old (*right*) cohorts. They note that younger patients have a medial brow that is low, with an apex lateral configuration. Older patients have an elevated medial and middle brow, which contributes to a flattened appearance. Measurements to the top of the brow margin are shown for each point measured. Although this particular study was not designed to evaluate inflation or projection of the brow, this photograph does beautifully illustrate the striking differences in 3-dimensional contour between the youthful and aging brow. (*From* Matros E, Garcia JA. Change in eyebrow position and shape with ageing. Plast Reconstr Surg 2009;124:1296–301; with permission.)

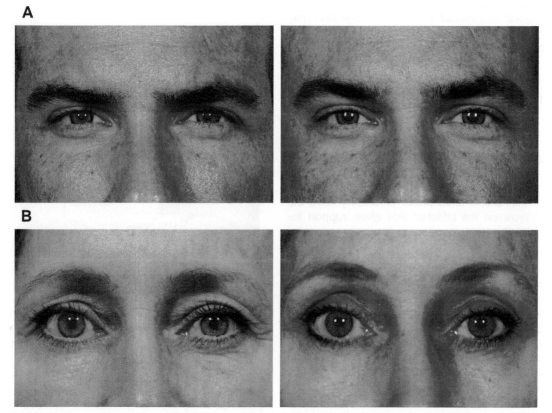

Fig. 17. (*A*) Chemodenervation with pleasing result in volumized male orbit. Lateral frontalis treated as well to prevent "spocking." (*B*) Chemodenervation with suboptimal result in "deflated" female orbit lifts brows and skin unmasking skeletonization of the orbital rim. (*Courtesy of* Rebecca Fitzgerald, MD.)

surprise." This is substantiated by the fact that some patients undergo brow lift reversal surgery.[40]

Whether or not this discrepancy is technical or conceptual is not yet clear. There are technical and perceptual complexities that are still being unraveled. Lambros[41] has commented that the best person for a brow lift is one with no eyebrows at all, as you can then lift enough to uncrumple redundant skin from the orbit and subsequently paint the brows where you want them.

Analysis of the Aging Brow

Patient selection and the particular surgical goal (raising the brow versus smoothing orbital skin) undoubtedly play a role. Some feel the confusion arises from lack of definitive studies showing what actually happens to our brow position as we age. Although traditional thinking is that aging brows fall, 1 old and 2 new studies cite that brows actually elevate with age. Matros and colleagues[42] recently studied 70 women from 2 age groups (20–30-year-olds and 50–60-year-olds) and found that, contrary to popular principles of forehead aging, the lateral brow position was similar in both groups, whereas the medial and midbrow were more elevated in the older group. The findings suggest why medial and midbrow elevation may result in esthetically unpleasing results for patients.[42]

They[42] suggest 2 different mechanisms that might explain this phenomenon:

1. First, the elevation may be attributable to a hyperactive frontalis muscle compensating for visual field obstruction secondary to upper lid dermatochalasia.
2. Second, the frontalis may be contracting to compensate for subclinical age-related lid ptosis. They note that the fact that patients with unilateral lid ptosis chronically raise the brow on the affected side gives support for this theory.

These authors[42] also note that most of the scientific literature on eyebrow height documents only postsurgical change and found only 2 reports describing changes in female brow height through time. The first was from the aforementioned study by Van den Bosch and colleagues,[3] who, using a fixed measurement at a single point above the pupil, found that the midbrow elevates with advancing age in a large cohort of men and women.

In the second study, Lambros[1] evaluated aging of the brow by comparing longitudinal photographs of individuals spanning 10 to 50 years. Using digital animation, he observed that brows

descended in 29% of patients, remained stable in 30%, and elevated in the remaining patients.

Patil and colleagues[43] recently used methodology similar to Matros and colleagues[42] to study brow position with aging in Indian women (20–30-year-olds and 50–60-year-olds, n = 160) and found similar results (that brows elevate with age).

Most would agree that overelevation of the brows creates a surprised look. If the previously mentioned studies are correct, this indicates that a brow lift in the wrong patient may exacerbate, rather than ameliorate, an aged appearance (as can be seen with an upper blepharoplasty in a hollow orbit as discussed earlier). Careful patient selection then is paramount, as with all procedures.

VOLUME AND CONTOUR OF EYELID

The 3-dimensional appearance of the eyelid is determined by bony support, as well as the soft tissues that fill the upper eyelid space, including eyebrow fat, subcutaneous fat, orbital fat, skin, and orbicularis muscle. Upper eyelid volume

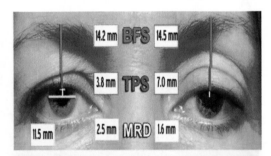

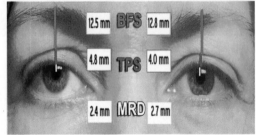

Fig. 18. (*Above*) Demonstration of measurement of brow fat span (BFS), tarsal platform show (TPS), and margin reflex distance (MRD1) on standardized photographs (corneal diameter set at 11.5 mm for scale). (*Below*) In the same patient, following left ptosis surgery and bilateral asymmetric blepharoplasty, TPS symmetry has improved and BFS has shortened. (*From* Goldberg RA, Lew H. Cosmetic outcome of posterior approach ptosis surgery (an American Ophthalmologic Society thesis). Trans Am Ophthalmol Soc 2011;109:157–67; with permission.)

deficiency can be categorized into 4 types as described by Morley and Goldberg[44]: (I) medial A-shaped hollow, (II) generalized hollow, (III) post-blepharoplasty global volume loss, and (IV) upper eyelid hooding with sub-brow volume deflation.[44] Reinflation (and subsequent projection) of the brow and upper lid restores a flat and shadowed surface back into a reflective one. It effaces the

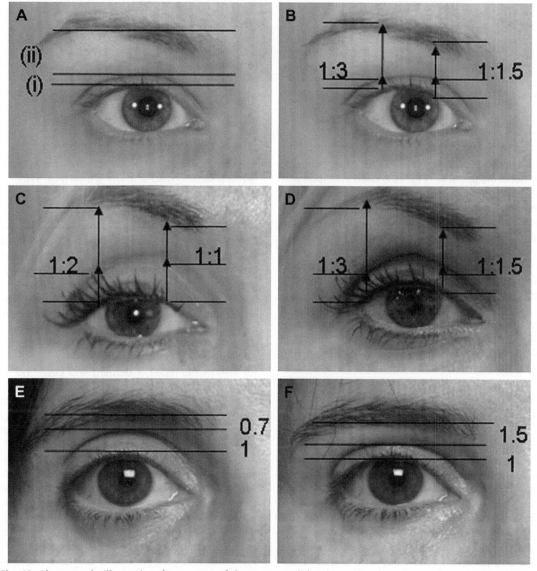

Fig. 19. Photographs illustrating the concept of the upper eyelid ratio and its alteration with age and hyaluronic acid filler treatment (<0.5 mL/eye). (*A*) A youthful upper eyelid (25 years old) showing measurement of the upper eyelid ratio; (i) pretarsal show and (ii) preseptal show. (*B*) The same eyelid as shown in Fig. 19A showing a lateral ratio of 1.0:3.0 and a medial ratio of 1.0:1.5. (*C*) Upper eyelid of a 45-year-old with a lateral ratio of 1:2 and a medial ratio of 1:1. (*D*) The same upper eyelid as in Fig. 19C immediately posttreatment showing a lateral ratio of 1.0:3.0 and a medial ratio of 1.0:1.5. (*E*) Upper eyelid of a 38-year-old with an overall upper eyelid ratio of 1.0:0.7. (*F*) The same eyelid as in Fig. 19E at 4 months posttreatment showing an overall ratio of 1.0:1.5. (*G*) A postblepharoplasty upper eyelid with a lateral ratio of 1.0:1.0 and a medial ratio of 1.0:0.5. (*H*) The same eyelid as in Fig. 19G at 4 months posttreatment showing a lateral ratio of 1.0:1.5 and a medial ratio of 1.0:2.0. (*From* Morley AM, Taban M, Malhotra R, et al. Use of hyaluronic acid gel for upper eyelid filling and contouring. Ophthal Plast Reconstr Surg 2009;25(6):443; with permission.)

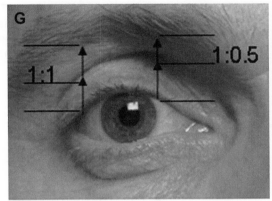
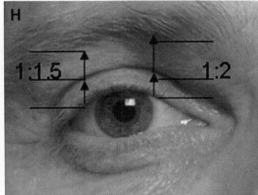

Fig. 19. (*continued*)

shadowed sulcus, whereas the full brow conceals most of the upper lid. **Fig. 16** is used in Matros and Garcia's article[42] to describe 2-dimensional brow measurements, but also illustrates the striking differences in 3-dimensional contour between the youthful and aged periorbital region.

Volume restoration to the region has been recognized and addressed with fat augmentation for several years.[2] Using "off-the-shelf" fillers in this area is a more contemporary concept.[44,45]

Although volumizing the eyebrows is capable of improving skin redundancy caused by deflation of the brow fat, it should not be thought of as a primary tool for brow elevation, as it may lead to an unnatural look if overdone.

The advantages of hyaluronic acid fillers include the following:

- Improved predictability and control
- Reversibility

The use of blunt-tipped cannulas may decrease risk of bruising or vascular compromise. The aforementioned study by Morley and colleagues[44] demonstrated that patients who were Type I to III volume deficient were amenable to nonsurgical rejuvenation. Patients who were Type IV, with pronounced skin redundancy and hooding, were the only patients in the study who stated disappointment with their nonsurgical results. Additional modest lift is possible nonsurgically with chemodenervation, ablative or nonablative laser resurfacing, and energy-based skin-tightening devices (radiofrequency and ultrasound).

Periorbital features, of course, are intimately related. The eyelids cannot be evaluated without addressing the eyebrows and vice versa. For example, lifting a full brow with chemodenervation gives a pleasing result, whereas lifting an empty brow,

whether surgically or nonsurgically, may simply reveal a skeletonized-appearing orbit (**Fig. 17**).

Tarsal Plate Show and Brow Fat Span

The concept of tarsal plate show (TPS) and brow fat span (BFS), as described by Goldberg and Lew,[46] is useful in better understanding the upper eyelid–brow relationship.

TPS is measured as the distance between the eyelid margin and the fold of skin over the eyelid crease. BFS is calculated as the distance from the skin fold to the top of the eyebrow hairs. In a study to better elucidate the posterior approach for lash ptosis repair, Goldberg and Lew[46] noted that margin reflex distance (MRD1; the distance from the light reflex at the center of the pupil to the upper lid margin) failed to adequately take into account several aspects of the surgical results. They therefore added TPS and BFS measurements to better characterize the 3-dimensional relationships in patients with ptosis (**Fig. 18**).

In a follow-up study, the investigators also found that the concept of a TPS-to-BFS (TPS:BFS) ratio was useful for upper eyelid esthetic analysis. They used this ratio to better assess the use of fillers for patients with upper lid volume atrophy (**Fig. 19**).[44] As noted, the youthful eye is long and full, with a parallel lid margin and crease. Youthful eyelids in female patients have a TPS:BFS ratio of 1.0:1.5 in the medial brow and 1.0:3.0 in the lateral brow as it arches upward at the lateral limbus and canthus. In male patients, the ratio is more constant. The aging process changes the relationship depending on the type of volume loss and dermatochalasia. **Fig. 20** illustrates several before and after photographs of patients with mild to moderate upper eyelid volume loss. The TPS:BFS

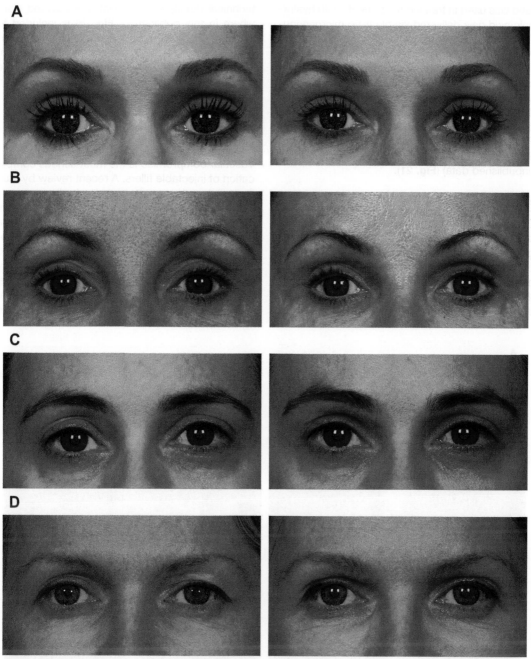

Fig. 20. (*A*) Patient with a prior history of blepharoplasty and browlift with Type III global volume loss. Before (*left*) and 2 months after (*right*) treatment with 1 mL hyaluronic acid gel per side using 27g blunt tipped micro-cannula. (*B*) Patient with Type I A-frame deformity. Before (*left*) and 2 months after (*right*) treatment with 0.5 mL hyaluronic acid gel per side using 27g blunt tipped microcannula. (*C*) Patient with Type I A-frame deformity. Before (*left*) and 2 months after (*right*) treatment with 0.25 mL hyaluronic acid gel per side using 27g blunt tip-ped microcannula. (*D*) Patient with Type I A-frame deformity and hooding of left lid before (*left*) and 3 months after (*right*) glabellar neurotoxin and 0.5 mL hyaluronic acid gel per side using 27g blunt tipped microcannula. Note that the lid margin, lid crease, and the brow are more parallel in all patients after treatment. The ratio of TPS:BFS has improved (<1) in A–C, and the lateral hooding has lifted in D. In A, C, and D, the eyes all appear slightly elongated (less rounded) after treatment. (*Courtesy of* Rebecca Fitzgerald, MD.)

ratio was used in treating the patients with hyaluronic acid gels delivered via blunt-tip microcannulas. Less than 0.5 mL per eye of hyaluronic acid was used in each of these patients.

Goldberg furthermore asserts that the symmetry of TPS may be more important than symmetry of MRD1 in the perception of facial appearance (Robert Goldberg, MD, and colleagues, oral presentation, American Society of Ophthalmic Plastic and Reconstructive Surgery Annual Scientific Meeting, Chicago, IL, October 13, 2010, unpublished data) (**Fig. 21**).

Structures Adjacent to the Eye

Of course, all adjacent structures in the upper third of the face (such as the forehead and temple) greatly affect the esthetics of the eyelids and brows (**Figs. 22–25**). An empty forehead may mimic brow ptosis. Temporal atrophy "clips off" the lateral tail of the brow in frontal view. More detailed descriptions of these areas, as well as

technical details of treatment, are covered elsewhere in this publication. **Fig. 26** is included to illustrate an illusion of "periorbital rejuvenation" done by simply filling in the brow with a ballpoint pen. Note that the fuller brow camouflages the early shadowing at the lid sulcus resulting from deflation.

VASCULAR COMPLICATIONS WITH INJECTABLE FILLERS

Vascular compromise is the most serious complication of injectable fillers. A recent review by Lazzeri and colleagues[47] examined all previously published cases of central retinal artery occlusion. They reported a total of 37 cases; half were secondary to fat augmentation and the rest attributed to filler substances. The investigators noted that both the internal and external carotid artery share anastomoses that lead to the central retinal artery. It was hypothesized that high-pressure injections force product forward that may then

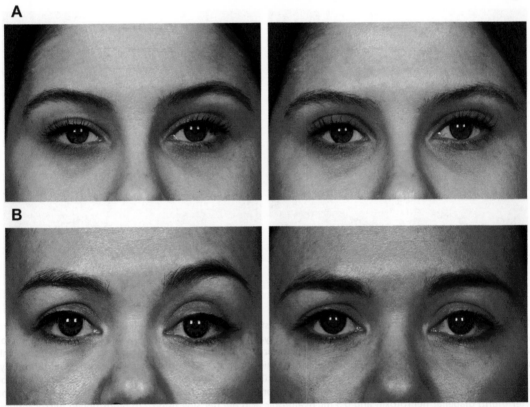

Fig. 21. These before and after pictures demonstrate how asymmetry of TPS can be improved with neuromodulation and fillers. (*A*) Patient with TPS asymmetry (*left*) treated with 0.5 mL hyaluronic acid gel with 27g blunt tipped microcannula to right medial brow fat pad resulting in elevation of right brow and improvement of TPS symmetry (*right*). (*B*) Patient before (*left*) and after (*right*) 2 units onabotulinum toxin type A to left lid margin to correct lid ptosis resulting in lifting of the eyelid. This approach results in relaxation of compensatory brow elevation equalizing TPS. Treatment performed by Robert Goldberg, MD. (*Courtesy of* Rebecca Fitzgerald, MD.)

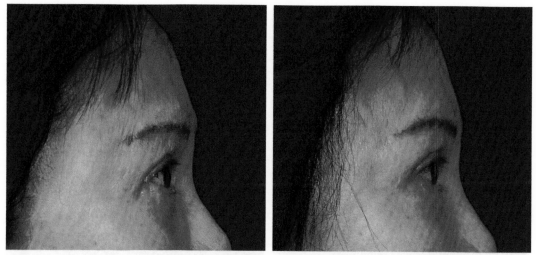

Fig. 22. This Asian woman was treated with glabellar neurotoxin (25 units), poly-L-lactic acid in the temples and supraorbital rim, (3 mL/session/temple; 3 sessions, 9-mL dilution) and hyaluronic acid gel (1 mL/side with a 27g blunt tipped microcannula) in the galeal fat pads of the forehead and brows. Note the projection and the shape of the brow and forehead contour in the posttreatment photograph (*right*). Note also that volume in the temple accentuates the presence of the lateral tail of the brow even in this profile view. (*Courtesy of* Rebecca Fitzgerald, MD.)

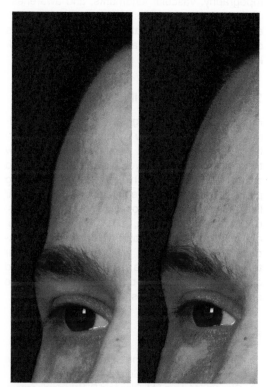

Fig. 23. Treatment of the galeal forehead fat pad with hyaluronic acid (1 mL/side with 27g blunt tipped microcannula) recontours the convexity of the forehead, projects the brow and lifts the upper lid in this young male patient. (*Courtesy of* Rebecca Fitzgerald, MD.)

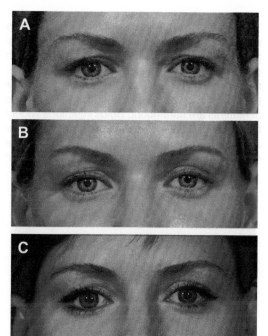

Fig. 24. The underlying contour of the orbital rim must be appreciated in conjunction with the soft tissue coverage to create a natural esthetic outcome in the periorbital region. (*A*) Young woman with periorbital volume deficit, hooding of upper lids, and temple atrophy revealing a prominent lateral orbital rim (pretreatment 2009). (*B*) Three months status post 2 monthly sessions of poly-L-lactic acid (1 vial/session) to lateral zygomatic arch, temples, and supraorbital rim; (*C*) 2.5 years posttreatment (no further treatment). (*Courtesy of* Rebecca Fitzgerald, MD.)

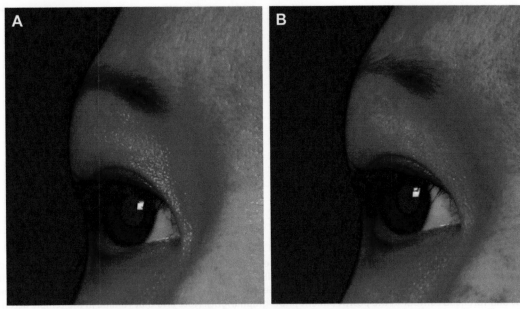

Fig. 25. Woman before (*A*) and after (*B*) injection of 0.5 mL hyaluronic acid (HA) with a 27g cannula to the medial brows and "naso-orbital" line resulting in anterior projection and improved definition of this area.

flow retrograde when pressure from the syringe is released. This subsequent backflow may allow product access to the central retinal artery with devastating consequences. This complication may therefore be avoidable with more thoughtful technique. Slower injections and small volumes of material are paramount. Bolus injections should be avoided. Blunt-tipped microcannulas are now available commercially that may also reduce the risk of penetrating the vessels. Knowledge of facial

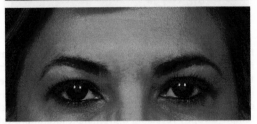

Fig. 26. A ballpoint pen was used here to shape this patient's brows. No other treatment was done. This obviously simulates the "apex lateral" brow of youth. Note also, however, the less obvious effect of camouflage of the deflating lid sulcus shadow.

topography, vascular landmarks, and awareness of "imperfect boundaries" at areas where vessels and nerves traverse anatomic compartments, as discussed earlier, may also help avoid high-risk injections.

SUMMARY/FUTURE DIRECTIONS

Knowledge of facial topography and key facial landmarks serve as a guide to understanding the underlying anatomy of the periorbital region. New technologies have allowed us to recognize and assess 3-dimensional changes during the aging process. Lambros is currently performing a 15-year linear study of 3-dimensional images (Val Lambros, personal communication, 2012). This type of data, along with the ability to make more precise and standardized measurements, will allow the practitioner to better understand the periorbital anatomy and aging process and hence optimize esthetic outcome and reduce complications.

REFERENCES

1. Lambros V. Observations on periorbital and midface aging. Plast Reconstr Surg 2007;120(5):1367–77.
2. Glasgold M, Lam SM, Glasgold R. Volumetric rejuvenation of the periorbital region. Facial Plast Surg 2010;26:252–9.
3. Van den Bosch WA, Leenders I, Mulder P. Topographic anatomy of the eyelids, and the effects of sex and age. Br J Ophthalmol 1999;83:347–52.

4. Lambros V. Volumizing the brow with hyaluronic acid fillers. Aesthet Surg J 2009;29:174.

5. Kirkpatrick SW, Bell FE, Johnson C, et al. Interpretation of facial expressions of emotion: the influence of eyebrows. Genet Soc Gen Psychol Monogr 1996; 122:405.

6. Knoll B, Attkiss KJ, Persing JA. The influence of forehead, brow, and periorbital aesthetics on perceived expression in the youthful face. Plast Reconstr Surg 2008;121:1793.

7. Fisher GJ, Varani V, Voorhees JJ. Looking older: fibroblast collapse and therapeutic implications. Arch Dermatol 2008;144:666–72.

8. Wang F, Garza LA, Kang S, et al. In vivo stimulation of de novo collagen production caused by cross-linked hyaluronic acid dermal filler injections in photodamaged human skin. Arch Dermatol 2007; 143(2):155–63.

9. Pessa JE, Chen Y. Curve analysis of the aging orbital aperture. Plast Reconstr Surg 2002;109:751.

10. Pessa JE. An algorithm of facial aging: verification of Lambros's theory by three-dimensional stereolithography, with reference to the pathogenesis of midfacial aging, scleral show, and the lateral suborbital trough deformity. Plast Reconstr Surg 2000;106:479–88.

11. Shaw RB Jr, Kahn DM. Aging of the midface bony elements: a three-dimensional computed tomographic study. Plast Reconstr Surg 2007;119:675–81.

12. Kahn DM, Shaw RB. Aging of the bony orbit: a three dimensional computed tomographic study. Aesthet Surg J 2008;28:258–64.

13. Shaw RB, Katzel EB, Koltz PF, et al. Aging of the mandible and its aesthetic implications. Plast Reconstr Surg 2010;125:332–42.

14. Sharabi SE, Hatef DA, Koshy JC, et al. Mechanotransduction: the missing link in the facial aging puzzle? Aesthetic Plast Surg 2010;34(5):603–11.

15. Richard MJ, Morris C, Deen B, et al. Analysis of the anatomic changes of the aging facial skeleton using computer-assisted tomography. Ophthal Plast Reconstr Surg 2009;25:382–6.

16. Ellis DA, Masri H. The effect of facial animation on the aging upper half of the face. Arch Otolaryngol Head Neck Surg 1989;115(6):710–3.

17. Pessa J, Zadoo V, Mutimer K, et al. Relative maxillary retrusion as a natural consequence of aging: combining skeletal and soft tissue changes into an integrated model of midfacial aging. Plast Reconstr Surg 1998;101(1):205–12.

18. Le Louarn CL, Buthiau D, Buis J. Structural aging: the facial recurve concept. Aesthetic Plast Surg 2007;31:213–8.

19. Knize D. An anatomically based study of the mechanism of eyebrow ptosis. Plast Reconstr Surg 1996; 97(7):1321–33.

20. Rohrich RJ, Pessa JE. The fat compartments of the face: anatomy and clinical implications for cosmetic surgery. Plast Reconstr Surg 2007;119:2219–27 [discussion: 2228–31].

21. Rohrich RJ, Pessa JE, Ristow B. The youthful cheek and the deep medial fat compartment. Plast Reconstr Surg 2008;121(6):2107–12.

22. Rod J, Rohrich R, Arbique G, et al. The anatomy of suborbicularis fat: implications for periorbital rejuvenation. Plast Reconstr Surg 2009;124:946–51.

23. Pessa JE, Rohrich RJ. Facial topography clinical anatomy of the face. St. Louis, Missouri: Quality Medical Publishing; 2012. p. 36–40.

24. Sadro J, Jaarudi I, Sinhao P. The role of eyebrows in face recognition. Perception 2003;32:285–93.

25. Westmore MG. Facial cosmetics in conjunction with surgery. Course presented at the Aesthetic Plastic Surgery Society meeting. Vancouver, May 7, 1974.

26. Ellenbogen R. Transcoronal eyebrow lift with concomitant upper blepharoplasty. Plast Reconstr Surg 1983;71(4):490–9.

27. Holcomb JD, McCollough EG. Trichophytic incisional approaches to upper facial rejuvenation. Arch Facial Plast Surg 2001;3(1):48–53.

28. Feser D, Grundl M, Eisenmann-Klein M, et al. Attractiveness of eyebrow position and shape in females depends on the age of the beholder. Aesthetic Plast Surg 2007;31:54–160.

29. Price KM, Gupta PK, Woodward JA, et al. Eyebrow and eyelid dimensions: an anthropometric analysis of African Americans and Caucasians. Plast Reconstr Surg 2009;124:615–23.

30. Reid RR, Said HK, Yu M, et al. Revisiting upper eyelid anatomy: introduction of the septal extension. Plast Reconstr Surg 2006;117:65–6 [discussion: 71–2].

31. Odunze M, Rosenberg DS, Few JW. Periorbital aging and ethnic considerations: a focus on the lateral canthal complex. Plast Reconstr Surg 2008; 121:1002–8.

32. Kunjur J, Sabesan T, Hankovan V. Anthropometric analysis of eyebrows and eyelids: an inter-racial study. J Oral Maxillofac Surg 2006;44:89–93.

33. Baker SB, Dayan JH, Crane A, et al. The influence of brow shape on the perception of facial form and brow aesthetics. Plast Reconstr Surg 2007;119(7): 2240–7.

34. Gunter JP, Antrobus SD. Aesthetic analysis of the eyebrows. Plast Reconstr Surg 1997;99:1808–16.

35. Freund RM, Nolan WB. Correlation between brow lift outcomes and aesthetic ideals for eyebrow height and shape in females. Plast Reconstr Surg 1996; 97:1343–8.

36. Schreiber JE, Singh NK, Klatsky SA. Beauty lies in the eyebrow of the beholder: a public survey of eyebrow aesthetics. Aesthet Surg J 2005;25:348–52.

37. Sclafani AP, Jung M. Desired position, shape, and dynamic range of the normal adult eyebrow. Arch Facial Plast Surg 2010;12(2):123–7.

38. Cole EA, Winn BJ, Putterman AM. Measurement of eyebrow position from inferior corneal limbus to brow: a new technique. Ophthal Plast Reconstr Surg 2010;26:443–7.

39. Pham S, Wilhelmi B, Mowlavi A. Eyebrow peak position redefined. Aesthet Surg J 2010;30(3):297–300.

40. Yaremchuk MJ, O'Sullivan N, Benslimane F. Reversing brow lifts. Aesthet Surg J 2007;27:367–75.

41. Lambros V. Discussion changes in eyebrow position and shape with aging. Plast Reconstr Surg 2009;124(4):1302–3.

42. Matros E, Garcia JA, Yaremchuk. Change in eyebrow position and shape with ageing. Plast Reconstr Surg 2009;124:1296–301.

43. Patil SB, Kale SM, Jaiswal S, et al. Effect of aging on the shape and position of the eyebrow in an Indian population. Aesthetic Plast Surg 2011;35:1031–5.

44. Morley AM, Taban M, Malhotra R, et al. Use of hyaluronic acid gel for upper eyelid filling and contouring. Ophthal Plast Reconstr Surg 2009;25:440–4.

45. Choi HS, Whipple KM, Sang-Rog O, et al. Modifying the upper eyelid crease in Asian patients with hyaluronic acid fillers. Plast Reconstr Surg 2011;127:844.

46. Goldberg RA, Lew H. Cosmetic outcome of posterior approach ptosis surgery (an American Ophthalmological Society thesis). Trans Am Ophthalmol Soc 2011;109:157–67.

47. Lazzeri D, Agostini T, Figus M, et al. Blindness following cosmetic injections of the face. Plast Reconstr Surg 2012;129:995.

Preoperative Evaluation of the Brow-Lid Continuum

Craig N. Czyz, DO[a,b], Robert H. Hill, MD[a,c],
Jill A. Foster, MD[a,c,d],*

KEYWORDS

• Brow • Eyelid • Brow-lid continuum • Aging face • Plastic surgery

KEY POINTS

• Neither the eyelid nor the eyebrow can be evaluated in isolation, and should be assessed as a unit: the brow-lid continuum.
• Recognition and documentation of preexisting functional and cosmetic deficits are paramount to creating a surgical plan and setting realistic expectations for surgical outcome.
• Failure to recognize preoperative brow asymmetry in an eyelid procedure may limit the attainment of eyelid symmetry after surgery.
• Preoperative recognition of eyelid ptosis and its impact on the position of the eyelid fold and brow assists the surgeon in surgical planning, and enhances the potential for postoperative symmetry.
• If the superior sulcus is relatively deep preoperatively, excision of orbital fat is contraindicated.

 Videos of complete preoperative evaluation of a male brow and female brow accompany this article.

INTRODUCTION

The periorbital region is often the first facial area to show signs of aging, and patient desires for aesthetic rejuvenation in this area are extremely common in a facial aesthetic surgery practice. Periorbital aging commonly manifests as brow ptosis, dermatochalasis, rhytids, prolapsed orbital fat, and the associated contour irregularities (hollows). To plan appropriate surgical rejuvenation, one must have a thorough understanding of periorbital anatomy and the tissue changes that lead to the perception of aging.

Surgical and nonsurgical rejuvenation is directed toward modification of the anatomic causes of facial aging. The component parts of the upper third of the face, the forehead, brow, and upper eyelid, are all intimately related and have been referred to as a continuum. When evaluating this region, it is important to avoid assessment of structures in isolation. When examining a patient with dermatochalasis, the eyebrow position must also be evaluated to assess its role in the redundancy of upper eyelid tissue. Similarly, any rejuvenative planning must take into account all the anatomic structures (fat, lacrimal gland, and so forth) that may comprise the brow-lid continuum. Failure to do so can result in undesirable outcomes for both surgeon and patient alike. For example, unrecognized upper eyelid ptosis may be the driver for activation of the frontalis muscle, resulting in chronic elevation of the brow. In this set of circumstances, correction of upper lid dermatochalasis or ptosis may unmask latent brow ptosis when the drive to elevate the brow is diminished after upper eyelid surgery.

The majority of perceived facial cosmetic deficiencies are multifactorial in nature; thus, rarely

[a] Division of Ophthalmology, Section Oculofacial Plastic and Reconstructive Surgery, Doctors Hospital/Ohio University, 5100 West Broad Street, Columbus, OH 43228, USA; [b] Department of Ophthalmology, Ohio University College of Osteopathic Medicine, Columbus, OH, USA; [c] Division of Oculofacial Plastic and Reconstructive Surgery, Department of Ophthalmology, The Ohio State University, 915 Olentangy River Road, Columbus, OH 43212, USA; [d] Plastic Surgery Ohio, 262 Neil Avenue, Suite 430, Columbus, OH 43215, USA
* Corresponding author. Plastic Surgery Ohio, 262 Neil Avenue, Suite 430, Columbus, OH 43215, Ohio, USA.
E-mail address: jfoster@jillfoster.com

Clin Plastic Surg 40 (2013) 43–53
http://dx.doi.org/10.1016/j.cps.2012.06.005
0094-1298/13/$ – see front matter © 2013 Elsevier Inc. All rights reserved.

will a single procedure provide maximal improvement. There are multiple purported causes of facial aging, but contemporary thought focuses on 3 primary mechanisms:

1. Changes related to volume loss or deflation, including loss of bone (remodeling) and fat atrophy
2. Tissue descent
3. Skin changes including rhytids, solar damage, thinning and laxity, and loss of dermal collagen

This context is especially true in relation to the brow and upper eyelid, where combined procedures addressing all 3 factors leading to periorbital aging are often needed.

There are multiple options for repositioning and modifying the shape of the brow, including:

- Neuromodulators
- Fillers
- Fat grafting
- Internal or external browpexy
- Direct browplasty
- Forehead plasty
- Endoscopic brow lift

Neuromodulators can be used to selectively treat opposing muscle groups to elevate the brow. Fillers and grafts add volume to the brow, particularly laterally, giving a fuller appearance while causing a mild contour elevation. Surgical brow lift techniques are used to elevate and reshape the forehead and eyebrow while also repositioning the soft tissue of the brow superiorly out of the upper eyelid sulcus. Initial assessment of the brow includes evaluation of height, contour, and the relationship of the brow fat pad to the upper lids. The function of the forehead and brow muscles and their contribution to wrinkling or unevenness of the skin is noted. The underlying structure of the frontal bone, which also contributes to the aesthetic assessment of the brow, is documented.

Blepharoplasty surgery is indicated when the eyelids require recontouring. Blepharoplasty techniques may be used to excise redundant skin and redistribute or remove orbital fat. The assessment of the eyelids includes a layered evaluation of the skin, orbicularis muscle, prolapsed fat, the position of the lacrimal gland, the function of the elevator muscles of the eyelid, and the position of the upper eyelid relative to the globe.

It is necessary to select the appropriate procedure(s) that will provide the optimal results for each individual patient. This process involves not only a clear understanding of the etiology of each patient's cosmetic deficit(s) but also requires the surgeon to have experience in a variety of different surgical and nonsurgical techniques to enhance the outcome. Also, realizing the effect of any procedure(s) on the brow-lid continuum can reduce the need to perform further corrective procedures.

CLINICAL ANATOMY RELEVANT TO EVALUATION OF BROW-LID CONTINUUM
Forehead and Eyebrows

The forehead possesses certain anatomic features that are intimately associated the eyebrow and eyelid **Fig. 1**A. The forehead encompasses the area between the hairline and brows, with the horizontal boundaries being the tail of the brows. The position of the hairline varies between individuals, but is usually higher in men than women. Contraction of the underlying frontalis muscles (the paired eyebrow elevator muscles) causes horizontal rhytids of the forehead. The relative distance ratios between the hairline, temporal tuft, and brow can be manipulated with brow and face-lifting surgery. The surgeon must account for these structures when creating a surgical plan.

Eyebrow contour and height
The eyebrow is made up of a head, body, and tail. It generally has an upward contour at the head and a downward contour at the tail. The brow skin has a full complement of layers and appendages that blend gradually into the single layer skin of the upper eyelid. The male and female eyebrows differ in vertical location and contour. In general, the male brow is lower than the female brow, usually at the level of the superior orbital rim. The female brow is slightly higher and has more of a temporal arch.[1] These subtle distinctions are important to recognize, especially during surgical planning for browplasty. With respect to cosmetic outcome, the resultant contour of the eyebrow is just as important as the height. Preoperative assessment will include whether the brow will be lifted symmetrically, or if an attempt to overcome relative medial or lateral brow ptosis will be attempted.

The vertical height of the eyebrow shows more natural variability than the eyelid. For documentation of the original position of the eyebrow, one can assess the margin-brow distance (MBD) from the nasal canthus to the middle of the brow cilia, from the center of the pupil to the middle of the brow cilia, and from the lateral canthus to the middle of the brow cilia (**Fig. 1**B). Although sometimes helpful for research or to objectively document eyebrow position, these measurements are relatively too time-consuming to be practical in a clinical practice. However, for the novice surgeon they may be of benefit until more experience is attained with surgery.

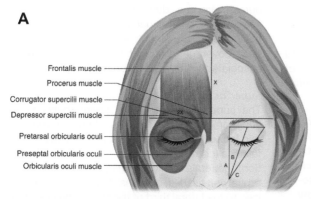
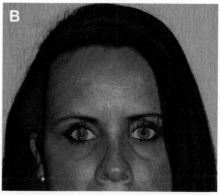

Fig. 1. (*A*) Facial musculature pertinent to the brow-lid continuum. Markings on the forehead indicate what some consider the "ideal" brow contour. The forehead should be 2× in horizontal length as vertical height (×). The lines drawn from the nasal ala through the periocular landmarks to the brow represent the idea position of (A) brow origin (medial canthus); (B) maximal arch (lateral limbus); C. Brow tail termination (lateral canthus). (*B*) Vertical height of eyebrows. Black = VPF; Red = MRD; Purple = MBD.

Frontalis muscle

The frontalis muscle is the elevator of the brow and extends from the brow to the forehead, where it merges with the galea aponeurosis.[2] The frontalis muscle is innervated by the frontal branch of the facial nerve.

> *SURGICAL NOTE: Familiarity with the course of the frontal (temporal) branch of the facial nerve is essential to performing formal brow-lifting surgery, because damage to the nerve can lead to significant morbidity.* See the article on anatomy by Lam and colleagues elsewhere in this issue for full a description and depiction of facial nerves.

Because the width of the frontalis stops short of the tail of the brow, the temporal brow lacks a primary elevator. This factor, in association with gravity, squinting, and involutional volume loss, predisposes to the typical brow ptosis of aging. As a consequence of these changes, there is accentuation of the skin fold in the temporal portion of the upper lid, which is commonly misinterpreted by the patient as redundant eyelid skin. Aggressive attempts to remove this skin can cause worsening temporal brow ptosis.

The depressors of the brow include the orbicularis, procerus, and the corrugator muscles.

- The orbicularis muscle closes the eyelid and pulls the eyebrow inferiorly.
- The procerus muscle has vertical fibers, and contraction causes horizontal rhytids in the glabellar area when depressing the medial head of the eyebrow.
- The corrugator muscle pulls the head of the brow medially and inferiorly, causing vertical rhytids in the glabella.

These rhytids are a common concern for patients and are often amenable to neuromodulation, filler treatment, and/or surgical intervention.

In patients in whom the contraction of the muscles is causing bothersome wrinkling, one may consider weakening these muscles by teasing them away from the skin during forehead/brow surgery.

> *SURGICAL NOTE: Glabellar muscle modification—interrupting the muscle fibers from their skin attachments—helps to diminish rhytid formation. Complete removal of the muscles may be associated with a variety of contour issues, splaying of the brows, and neurosensory deficits. As such, it is best to treat these muscles with a combination of less aggressive surgical muscle modification and neuromodulators.*[3]

Rhytid threading or grafting using superficial musculoaponeurotic system (SMAS) tissue harvested during a facelift can aid in softening deep, static rhytids. For patients in whom SMAS grafting is not an option, fillers can be used. Caution should be used with filler selection for this area, as recent studies have shown the potential for severe complications.[4]

Eyelids

Eyelid skin has no subcutaneous fat and is the thinnest of all body skin. Laxity of the upper eyelid skin is due in part to involutional and extrinsic aging and mechanical factors (the constant movement of the upper eyelids and skin tension). The upper eyelids have potential spaces within their architecture, related to the firm attachment of pretarsal skin to the underlying soft tissue, and the loose attachment of similar preseptal tissue. These potential spaces are susceptible to fluid accumulation from involutional changes, sleep position, and/or other insults. The resulting repetitive and chronic skin stretching eventually leads to loss of elasticity, apparent skin redundancy, and a "puffy" eyelid appearance.

> *SURGICAL NOTE: Whereas the eyelid skin is thin, the eyebrow skin is not. This difference in skin thickness becomes apparent if the upper limb of the blepharoplasty incision is too close to the eyebrow. The subsequent closure will result in thick eyebrow skin annealed to the thin skin of the eyelid, creating a "stepping-off defect" at the incision. This anomaly should be avoided by not placing the upper limb of the incision too close to the brow.*

Eyelid crease

The position and symmetry of the upper eyelid crease and fold are important aesthetic features of the appearance of the upper eyelid. The upper eyelid crease is created by the anterior insertion of the levator aponeurosis to the orbicularis muscle and dermis. These attachments prevent the descent of the orbital fat and project tissue anteriorly as the eyelid fold above the crease. The crease is usually 9 to 12 mm above the central lid margin in adult occidental females, and 8 to 10 mm above the lid margin in adult occidental males.[5] The upper lid crease in Asian individuals is lower, usually in the range of 2 to 5 mm from the eyelid margin. In this population, the orbital septum and the orbital fat extend further inferiorly in the eyelid, creating the appearance of a fuller upper eyelid fold than that of the Occidental eyelid. There are additional anatomic differences between Asian and Occidental eyelids, which are important for the surgeon to evaluate and understand when performing eyelid surgery on Asian patients.[6,7] The review on Asian blepharoplasty by Lee and Ahn elsewhere in this issue details these differences in depth.

Eyelid fold

The lid fold represents the skin, orbicularis muscle, and fat that together drape over and obscure the lid crease when the eye is in primary position. Excessive folding or hooding may result from dermatochalasis, steatoblepharon, brow ptosis, or a combination of all 3 (**Fig. 2**). Affected individuals may perceive a sensation of lid "heaviness," early fatigue with reading or watching television, and even loss of superior and/or peripheral vision. To determine an objective measure of the impact of the upper eyelid position on vision, the visual field

defect may be demonstrated with automated (Humphrey) or manual (Goldmann) visual field testing. This documentation is required if insurance coverage is sought to cover the expenses associated with upper blepharoplasty.

Superior sulcus

The superior sulcus is the region between the superior orbital rim and the globe. In young or thin individuals, the sulcus is typically flat. Sulcus fullness (convex) may be due to orbital fat herniation, generalized lid edema, expansion of the orbital soft tissues, or a mass lesion. Fullness localized to the lateral third of the sulcus may be attributed to lacrimal gland prolapse (**Fig. 3**) or extension of the preaponeurotic fat. Lacrimal gland prolapse is considered an involutional process,[8] yet an estimated 10% to 15% of young individuals undergoing blepharoplasty have symmetrically or asymmetrically displaced lacrimal glands.[9] A physiologic extension of the preaponeurotic fat can protrude anteriorly under the inferior border of the lacrimal gland clinically, resulting in a bulge or fullness in the upper eyelid.[10] Individuals with symmetrically full sulci can undergo fat excision as part of the blepharoplasty procedure. In other patients, an asymmetric contour of the fat may result from involutional changes that include atrophy of the central fat with retention and prolapse of the nasal fat pad (**Fig. 4**A).

> *SURGICAL NOTE: The surgeon should identify this situation of involutional changes preoperatively and, rather than removing the nasal fat, consider transposing it as a pedicle to the central fat location.[11]*

It is important to understand that excessive fat removal can cause a "skeletonized" or gaunt appearance. In individuals who have a deep (concave) sulcus with this skeletonized appearance, various techniques can be used to replace the volume deficiency (see **Fig. 4**A–C).[12] In patients with both concave and convex areas of the sulcus, liposculpting, fat transposition, or fat grafting can be performed to smooth the sulcus contour and avoid exacerbating a deep or full appearance.[13–15]

Eyelid measurements

Eyelid measurements are valuable in the recording and interpretation of eyelid position (see **Fig. 1**). The average distance between the upper and lower eyelids, the vertical palpebral fissure (VPF), is 8 to 10 mm in primary (straight) gaze.[16] Significant variation from the average measurements may be an indication of eyelid retraction or ptosis. These conditions may to be addressed in association with or independently of the aesthetic

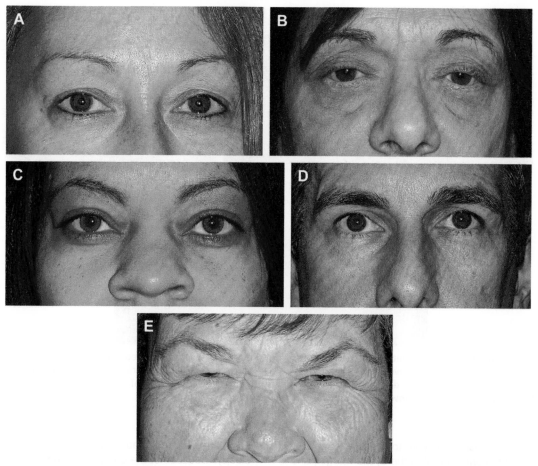

Fig. 2. (*A*) Bilateral upper eyelid dermatochalasis. The amount in skin redundancy is mild in this younger patient. (*B*) Bilateral upper eyelid dermatochalasis with underlying fat atrophy. (*C*) Bilateral upper eyelid steatoblepharon. Note there is also steatoblepharon of the bilateral lower eyelids. (*D*) Bilateral brow ptosis in a middle-aged male. As the male brows are relatively flat and lower set than in the female, ptosis often goes overlooked or misdiagnosed as dermatochalasis of the lid. (*E*) A patient displays bilateral brow ptosis, dermatochalasis, and steatoblepharon. There is also potential for lacrimal gland prolapse, adding to her lateral fullness. Note the patient's eyebrows display an "arch" contour; however, this is from brow-hair grooming and frontalis activation, not anatomic location.

intervention, but require recognition and intervention for the patient to achieve the desired result. The average upper eyelid margin rests approximately 2 mm below the superior corneal limbus. The lower eyelid margin should be at or 1 mm above the inferior corneal limbus so that no sclera is visible between the limbus and the lower eyelid.

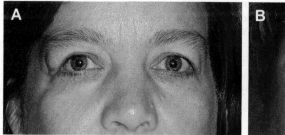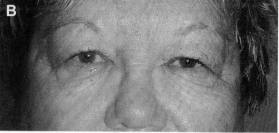

Fig. 3. (*A*) Unilateral lacrimal gland prolapse (*right*) in a patient with bilateral dermatochalasis and mild brow ptosis. (*B*) Bilateral lacrimal gland prolapse in a patient with bilateral dermatochalasis and moderate brow ptosis.

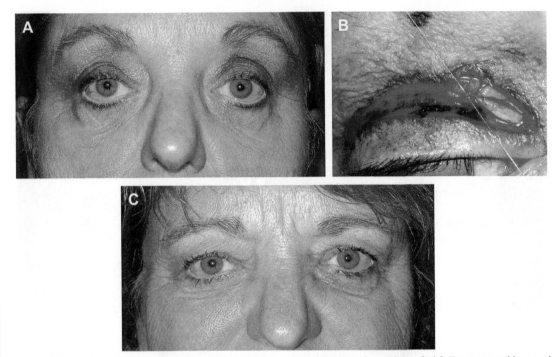

Fig. 4. (A) A patient with bilateral deepened sulcus from central fat atrophy with medial fullness caused by nasal fat prolapse. (B) Intraoperative photograph depicting pedicalization and lateral transfer of the deep medial fat. Note the white color of the deep medial fat in comparison with the yellow color of the central fat. (C) Six-year follow-up of the patient shown in A following fat transposition of the upper lid.

Eyelid position relative to the eye is measured from the central pupil to the eyelid margin, and is referred to as the margin-reflex distance (MRD). "Reflex" refers to the light reflection at the center of the cornea when a light is held parallel to the eye. The MRD_1 denotes that this measurement is to the upper eyelid margin, whereas MRD_2 signifies the distance from the central pupil to the lower eyelid margin (see **Fig. 1**). Thus, MRD_1 plus MRD_2 equals VPF. These measurements add to the interpretation of the VPF. For example, although a patient with both ptosis and lower lid retraction might have a normal value for VPF, the MRD_1 and MRD_2 will be abnormal.

> ***SURGICAL NOTE: Abnormalities in the upper eyelid position should be recognized before surgery because underlying etiology may require further evaluation and correction.***

Normal eyelid levator function is 12 to 16 mm, and is defined as the excursion of the upper eyelid margin from downgaze to upgaze with the frontalis immobilized.[17] Individuals with eyelid retraction have a lid margin that rests higher than normal (increased MRD_1), and may have a "staring" or "surprised" appearance. Those individuals with

ptosis have a decreased MRD_1, and may appear "sleepy" because of the drooping of the lids.

PATIENT EVALUATION BEFORE SURGICAL INTERVENTION
Medical History and Review of Systems

Before surgical intervention, preoperative counseling and setting of realistic expectations are of paramount importance. Identifying systemic and/or morphologic factors that can predispose the patient to adverse outcomes should be done preoperatively. This identification is especially critical in patients with facial asymmetry, whether natural or from previous surgery, trauma, or facial nerve deficits. These individuals should be cautioned that their results may be limited because of their existing conditions.

A general medical history should be taken, with particular attention paid to symptoms of a thyroid disorder, environmental allergies, or episodic eyelid swelling that may suggest blepharochalasis syndrome, a variant of hereditary angioedema.[18,19]

- Chronic eyelid swelling may result in stretching and wrinkling of the eyelid skin, ultimately leading to dermatochalasis.

- Patients should be questioned about hypertrophic scar or keloid formation, especially patients younger than 30 years or with darkly pigmented skin.[20]
- A history of rheumatoid arthritis, other autoimmune disease, or laser vision correction may be associated with coexisting dry-eye syndrome, which can be exacerbated by surgery. A history of dry-eye syndrome, a basal tear secretion test (Schirmer test), and/or evaluation of the ocular surface is of value to assess the increased postoperative risks of dry-eye syndrome.
- Systemic motor deficits (weakness), especially in the presence of ptosis or diplopia, should be investigated for myasthenia gravis (MG). If there is a clinical suspicion of MG, appropriate referral to a neuro-ophthalmologist is warranted.
- To assess the relative risk for excessive intraoperative or postoperative bleeding, patients should be questioned about hematologic disorders, use of aspirin, nonsteroidal anti-inflammatory agents, anticoagulants, chronic oral steroids, vitamin E, St John's wort, garlic, fish oils, and other supplements.[21] The decision to discontinue prescription anticoagulative agents preoperatively and in the early postoperative period should be made in conjunction with the physician in charge of the patient's systemic management.

Previous Treatments

Previous treatments, both surgical and nonsurgical, are documented including time of treatment (last treatment and duration where applicable), patient perceived results, and any adverse reactions or complications. For purposes of brow-lid continuum evaluation, particular focus should be directed toward concurrent or previous neuromodulator treatment as this can affect brow and lid position and contour. It may be in the best interest of the surgeon to re-evaluate any patient seeking surgical rejuvenation who is actively being treated with neuromodulators by another physician once an appropriate time has passed for the effects to be neutralized.

Physical Examination of the Lid and Brow

A detailed physical examination will identify specific anatomic deficits that can be addressed with rejuvenative surgery.

See video of preoperative examination of a male brow and a female brow.

Visual examination

The patient evaluation begins with a measurement of visual acuity using a standard eye chart or near card. Pupil reactivity and eye motility should also be evaluated to document any preoperative abnormalities. Finally, a slit-lamp evaluation is important to rule out ocular surface disease that may predispose an adverse outcome. For those specialists not familiar with these examinations modalities, a preoperative assessment from an ophthalmologist may be beneficial.

Patient photographs

Photographs of the patient in frontal, oblique (three-quarter), and lateral views are taken in a standardized manner. Additional photographs illustrating functional deficits, such as asymmetric lid height, may also be acquired. This important step helps in preoperative planning and can also be used as a reference in the operating room. Photographic documentation further assists in reviewing procedural results with the patient postoperatively, and allows for critical review of surgical outcomes for the physician. Photographic documentation is also a part of the patient's medical record in a plastic surgery practice.

External assessment

The external assessment begins by noting the skin texture, color, and abnormalities such as scars or lesions. The eyebrow position is then evaluated with the patient seated upright, chin level, and the eyes in primary gaze. The patient is asked to activate the frontalis muscle to view the amount and symmetry of brow elevation and dynamic rhytids of the forehead. The surgeon should inspect brow height in relation to the orbital rim, brow shape, and upper eyelid sulcus contour, including fullness from descent of the retro-orbicularis oculi fat (ROOF) pad or lacrimal gland prolapse. Recall that the male brow is less arched and slightly lower than the female brow. One method to gauge brow height is to palpate the superior orbital rim and note the brow position in reference to the rim. A more objective method involves measuring the distance from the inferior corneal limbus to the brow.[22] The height of the eyebrow can also be described with an MBD measurement from the upper eyelid margin to the center of the brow hair, as previously described. This measurement is performed in 3 locations: lateral canthal angle, central pupil, and medial canthal angle (see **Fig. 1**).

Various descriptions of the ideal brow position have been proposed and are reviewed in depth elsewhere in this issue. (See the article on anatomy by Lam and colleagues for a full description and graphic depictions of facial nerves.)

Brow asymmetry

In addition to position, height, and contour, identifying brow asymmetry is important in attaining successful surgical outcomes. Brow asymmetry is quite common and can be easily overlooked in the initial patient assessment. Failure to recognize these differences may negatively affect the outcome of eyelid symmetry, and lead to patient dissatisfaction.

Brow furrows

The depth and location of furrows above the brow are noted, as these can be an indication that the patient is elevating the brow in an attempt to lift a ptotic eyelid, whether true eyelid ptosis or pseudoptosis related to dermatochalasis. In the appropriate patient, these furrows can be a convenient place to mask a surgical scar on elevation of the brow.

Brow horizontal and vertical lines

Asymmetric horizontal lines in the forehead may be an indication of long-standing eyelid asymmetry (ptosis or dermatochalasis in one eyelid relative to the other). Recognizing this will influence the surgical plan and should be explained to the patient before surgery. Identification of vertical glabellar lines should be noted, as the patient may desire surgical effacement of these dynamic rhytids at the time of surgery.

Hairline position

In patients with brow ptosis who desire an elevation, the hairline position and the length of the forehead should be noted. These factors help determine the type of lift to be performed. Brow lifting is described in detail in other articles in this issue by Nahai, Terrella and Wang, and Walrath and McCord. During the evaluation, the physician will discuss incision/technique options with the patient realizing that if the hairline is particularly high, it will be challenging to manipulate the endoscope over the curve of the forehead, and the incisions may need to be in bare scalp. Modification of the high hairline may be accomplished with a pretrichial approach. The disadvantage of the pretrichial technique is an increased likelihood of sensory nerve deficits in the scalp. In the male patient, preexisting forehead lines, the brow cilia, the position of the hairline, and the heaviness of the forehead tissue are all assessed to factor into decisions regarding technique and incision options (**Fig. 5**).

Globe position

The position of the globe is noted relative to the orbital rim. In the setting of a flattened malar eminence, a shallow orbit, or axial myopia (nearsighted patient with increased anterior to posterior

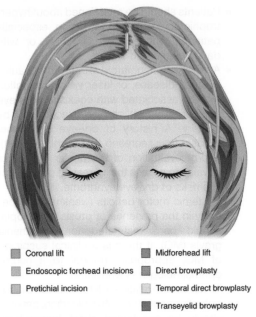

■ Coronal lift	■ Midforehead lift
■ Endoscopic forehead incisions	■ Direct browplasty
■ Pretichial incision	■ Temporal direct browplasty
	■ Transeyelid browplasty

Fig. 5. Browplasty surgical options.

globe length), the globe will appear to protrude forward (proptosis) causing the upper and lower eyelids to appear retracted. In such cases, removal of tissue from the eyelids must be performed with great care as the proptotic appearance of the globe may be accentuated, creating an aesthetically unacceptable startled or staring appearance (**Fig. 6**), and possibly limiting the ability of the eyelids to fully close (lagophthalmos). The presence of actual proptosis is evaluated by exophthalmometry measurements and, if present, requires a medical workup to determine etiology and appropriate management.

Upper eyelid

Attention is then turned to the upper eyelid. The eyelid contour and position is observed. The presence of eyelid retraction or ptosis is noted (**Fig. 7**). To standardize eyelid measurements, the brow should be in a neutral position when evaluating lid position. If the patient is unconsciously elevating the brow with frontalis contraction, the examiner should ask the patient to "relax" the brow. If the patient is unable to comply, the examiner should then place his or her thumbs on the patient's brow to secure it in a neutral position. The skin is inspected for evidence of medial canthal webbing, epicanthal folds, wrinkling, previous surgical scars, pigmentation, and lesions or other defects.

An important consideration in performing removal of upper eyelid dermatochalasis is identification of concurrent true eyelid ptosis. Mechanical ptosis may be improved with removal of

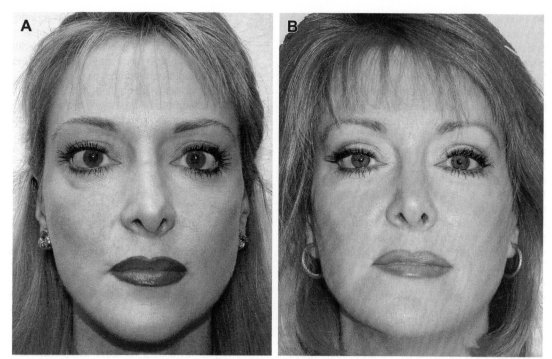

Fig. 6. (*A*) A patient with bilateral prominent globes. (*B*) The patient shown in *A* at 5-year follow-up after bilateral upper and lower blepharoplasty, orbital rim augmentation with implants, and hard palate mucosal grafts to the lower lids.

unnecessary skin and fat, but true myogenic ptosis will persist as a postoperative problem. Patients are unaware of what makes their eyelids look heavy or "baggy," simply wanting an improvement. Failure to recognize preexisting ptosis is probably the most common cause of postoperative ptosis, and is a preventable event with an appropriate preoperative evaluation. As mentioned, compensatory brow elevation may be a hint to the presence of ptosis and should be sought out. Moreover, elevating the eyelid skin to assess the position of the eyelid margin relative to the pupil (MRD$_1$) (see

the section on clinical anatomy) will help to identify whether ptosis is present. Once identified, a discussion with the patient is needed to review that the eyelid malposition exists and to determine whether the patient desires correction.

Upper eyelid crease

The position and definition of the upper eyelid crease and fold are then observed. The crease is the line in the skin that is seen when the patient is asked to look downward, measured as the margin to crease distance, or MCD, measured in

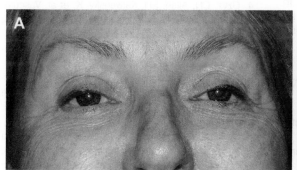

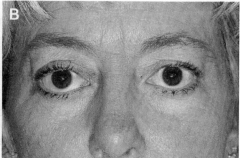

Fig. 7. (*A*) Bilateral myogenic upper eyelid ptosis. The patient is shown compensating for the ptosis with frontalis/brow elevation and head tilt. (*B*) A patient with unilateral upper eyelid retraction (*left*) resulting in eyelid fold asymmetry.

downgaze. The eyelid fold is the redundancy of skin that occurs in the upper eyelid when the lid is in primary position, measured as the margin to fold distance, or MFD. Even small asymmetries in the MFD are noticeable to patients. If the eyelid crease is poorly defined, or if there is asymmetry in crease height between the eyelids, the patient should be made aware of this before surgery. Elevation or blunting of the lid crease may be associated with ptosis and levator aponeurosis dehiscence. Patients are more likely to notice a difference in eyelid symmetry after surgery than beforehand, because of the careful attention typically given to the lids during the postoperative recovery period. As previously described, the normal position of the upper eyelid crease is higher in females, but varies from patient to patient regardless of gender. There are significant anatomic differences between Asian and Occidental eyelids,[7] which are reflected in eyelid crease position, prominence, and contour. There can be great psychosocial significance placed on this feature by many Asian societies, therefore these differences must be recognized and respected. In general, surgical techniques that include the need to modify the eyelid crease or fold make upper eyelid surgery technically more challenging and the results less predictable.

Upper eyelid fat

There are 2 main fat pads of the upper eyelid. Modification of one, both, or neither may be required to achieve the proper lid contour in upper blepharoplasty. Gentle pressure on the globe through a closed eyelid will demonstrate the position of the central and nasal fat pads of the upper lids and accentuate prolapse. Fullness of the lateral third of the upper lid can be caused by lacrimal gland or fat prolapse, and when possible, differentiation should be made to facilitate appropriate surgical planning. If the superior sulcus is relatively concave preoperatively, the excision of orbital fat is contraindicated, as it will produce further skeletonization of the superior fornix. In this setting, fat transposition or grafting may be required to achieve a cosmetically appealing sulcus contour.[11,15]

SUMMARY OF PREOPERATIVE EVALUATION OF THE LID BROW

- The eyes are a focal point of the aesthetic composite of the face. Blepharoplasty is one of the most commonly requested and performed aesthetic procedures.
- The appearance of the eyelids is critically dependent of the on the height, contour, and position of the brows. For this reason,

the brow must be considered in evaluating the patient presenting for blepharoplasty surgery. Hence the practice of considering the brows and eyelids as an aesthetic unit: the brow-lid continuum.

- With the brow-lid continuum in mind, the physician obtains a detailed history, review of systems, and physical examination of the patient before proceeding with surgery, thus allowing for a meticulous and individualized patient analysis and surgical plan.
- Based on findings from physical examination and review of systems, in conjunction with the patient's desires, appropriate preoperative counseling and setting of realistic expectations can ensue.
- Preexisting issues that may lead to surgical limitations are explained to the patient. In a patient with significant preexisting abnormality or unrealistic expectations, the patient should be counseled to seek a second opinion.
- Successful cosmetic blepharoplasty is highly rewarding for both the patient and the surgeon.

VIDEOS

Videos related to this article can be found online at http://dx.doi.org/10.1016/j.cps.2012.06.005.

REFERENCES

1. Gunter JP, Antrobus SD. Aesthetic analysis of the eyebrows. Plast Reconstr Surg 1997;99(7):1808–16.
2. Nerad J. Techniques in ophthalmic plastic surgery. Philadelphia: Elsevier Inc; 2010.
3. Huang W, Rogachefsky AS, Foster JA. Browlift with botulinum toxin. Dermatol Surg 2000;26:55–60.
4. Czyz, CN, Allen, SH, Kalwerisky, K, et al. Vascular compromise following facial dermal filler injection: review of the literature and proposed treatment algorithms. American Academy of Facial Plastic & Reconstructive Surgery Fall Meeting 2011. September 8-11, 2011, San Francisco, CA.
5. Callahan M, Beard C, editors. Beard's ptosis. 4th edition. Birmingham (AL): Aesculapius Publishing; 1990. p. 1–50.
6. Doxanas MT, Anderson RL. Oriental eyelids: an anatomic study. Arch Ophthalmol 1984;102:1232–5.
7. Chen WD. Comparative anatomy of the eyelids. In: Chen WD, editor. Asian blepharoplasty: a surgical atlas. Boston: Butterworth-Heinemann; 1995. p. 1–19.

8. Massry GG. The incidence of lacrimal gland prolapsed in the functional blepharoplasty population. Ophthal Plast Reconstr Surg 2011;27(6):410–3.

9. Smith B, Lisman RD. Dacryoadenopexy as recognized factor in upper lid blepharoplasty. Plast Reconstr Surg 1983;71:629–32.

10. Persichetti P, Di Lella F, Delfino S, et al. Adipose compartments of the upper eyelid: anatomy applied to blepharoplasty. Plast Reconstr Surg 2004;113(1): 373–8.

11. Massry GG. Nasal fat preservation in upper eyelid blepharoplasty. Ophthal Plast Reconstr Surg 2011; 27:352–5.

12. Maniglia JJ, Maniglia RF, Jorge dos Santos ME, et al. Surgical treatment of the sunken upper eyelid. Arch Facial Plast Surg 2006;8:269–72.

13. Proffer PL, Czyz CN, Cahill KV, et al. Addition of dermis-fat graft to diminish cable visibility in frontalis suspension for patients with pre-existing deep superior sulci. Ophthal Plast Reconstr Surg 2009;25(2): 94–8.

14. Seiff SR. The fat pearl graft in ophthalmic plastic surgery: everyone wants to be a donor! Orbit 2002;21(2):105–9.

15. Czyz, CN, Foster, JA, Cahill, KV, et al. Orbital superior sulcus volumetric rejuvenation utilizing dermis fat graft. American Academy of Cosmetic Surgery 25th Anniversary Scientific Meeting. January 18, 2009. Phoenix, AZ.

16. Read SA, Collins MJ, Carney LG, et al. The morphology of the palpebral fissure in different directions of vertical gaze. Optom Vis Sci 2006; 83(10):715–22.

17. American Academy of Ophthalmology. Orbit, eyelids, and lacrimal system. Basic and clinical science course 2007-2008. San Francisco, CA: American Academy of Ophthalmology: 223.

18. Collin JR. Blepharochalasis. A review of 30 cases. Ophthal Plast Reconstr Surg 1991;7:153–7.

19. Koursh DM, Modjtahedi SP, Selva D, et al. The blepharochalasis syndrome. Surv Ophthalmol 2009; 54(2):235–44.

20. Juckett G, Hartman-Adams H. Management of keloids and hypertrophic scars. Am Fam Physician 2009;80(3):253–60.

21. Czyz CN, Lam VB, Foster JA. Management of complications of upper eyelid blepharoplasty. In: Massry GG, Murphy M, Azizzadeh B, editors. Master techniques in blepharoplasty and periorbital rejuvenation. New York: Springer; 2011. p. 109–23.

22. Cole EA, Winn BJ, Putterman AM. Measurement of eyebrow position from inferior corneal limbus to brow: a new technique. Ophthal Plast Reconstr Surg 2010;26(6):443–7.

Nonsurgical Rejuvenation of the Upper Eyelid and Brow

Hema Sundaram, MD[a],*, Monika Kiripolsky, MD[b]

KEYWORDS

- Noninvasive facial rejuvenation • Dermatology • Fillers • Neuromodulators • Laser devices

KEY POINTS

- Nonsurgical rejuvenation of the upper eyelid and brow regions can produce profound improvement in overall facial appearance.
- A comprehensive understanding of structural and functional facial anatomy and ideal facial proportions is essential to evaluate each patient effectively, select the appropriate treatments, and devise an optimal treatment plan.
- Nonsurgical treatments can be classified into 1 of 3 major categories based on mechanism of action: soft tissue fillers, neuromodulators, and laser and light energy–based devices. Adjunctive treatments include chemical peels and topical therapies.
- Facial aging is characterized by volume loss from multiple tissue planes (bone, muscle, subcutaneous fat, and skin). Identification and correction of volume loss from the upper eyelid and brow is a prerequisite for effective rejuvenation of these regions.
- Combination of soft tissue fillers with neuromodulators may be appropriate for many patients and yield enhanced results. Hyaluronic acid fillers may be considered the best option for volume restoration to the upper eyelid and brow.
- Since volume loss is a cardinal feature of facial aging, adoption of a predominantly volumetric rather than ablative approach to the upper eyelid and brow may yield the best results.

BACKGROUND ON NONSURGICAL TREATMENT OF THE AGING FACE

Facial aging is also characterized by decreased tissue quality, which has manifestations including loss of elasticity, dyschromia, and textural anomalies. An integrative approach to nonsurgical rejuvenation incorporates improvement in skin quality and reflectance as a valuable adjunct to volume replacement and neuromodulation.

Age-related changes in the eyebrows can be corrected via brow repositioning and shaping with various nonsurgical rejuvenation treatments, including neuromodulators, soft tissue fillers, and radiofrequency. This can produce a beneficial, secondary improvement in upper eyelid hooding.

The ideal approach to nonsurgical rejuvenation of the upper eyelid and brow involves familiarity with the multiple treatment modalities that are currently available. An appropriate *combination* of treatments, tailored specifically for each patient to address individual aging patterns, may be synergistic and more efficacious than any one treatment alone.

When evaluating and treating the upper lid and brow, it is useful to visualize a "periorbital frame" that is bordered by the eyebrows, glabella, temporal fossa, and superior mid face. Nonsurgical treatments can be directed *within* the periorbital frame with the aim of replacing volume, regenerating tissue quality, rebalancing facial vectors and proportions, and improving skin reflectance. Treatments directed *outside* the periorbital frame can produce a secondary vectoring effect on the upper eyelid and brow, and include light energy-based modalities, such as fractionated radiofrequency

[a] 11119 Rockville Pike, Suite 205, Rockville, MD 20852, USA; [b] Scripps Health, 351 Santa Fe Drive, Suite 101, Encinitas, CA 92024, USA
* Corresponding author.
E-mail address: hemasundaram@gmail.com

Clin Plastic Surg 40 (2013) 55–76
http://dx.doi.org/10.1016/j.cps.2012.08.009
0094-1298/13/$ – see front matter © 2013 Elsevier Inc. All rights reserved.

(RF), microfocused ultrasound (MFU), and lasers, as well as soft tissue fillers and neuromodulators.

INTRODUCTION AND RATIONALE FOR COMBINED TREATMENTS

If, as the poets say, the eyes are the window to the soul, then the eyebrows and the eyelids may be considered the all-important frame to that window. Studies of how we view others' faces show that an observer's gaze consistently falls first on the eyes and the area surrounding them, before tracking to other parts of the face with repeated returns to the eyes and periorbital region. Given this focus, it is hardly surprising that rejuvenation of the brow and upper eyelid region, with consequent improvement in appearance of the eyes, can have a dramatic impact on how the whole face is perceived.

Although there is significant individual variation in patterns of facial aging, the early manifestations may often be seen in the eyebrows and eyelids (**Fig. 1**).

Eyebrow and Lid Ptosis

Conventionally, eyebrow ptosis and/or upper eyelid ptosis (blepharoptosis) have been described. Both may be considered to be due to volume loss from multiple tissue planes, including the underlying fat compartments and bony structures, as well as an increase in skin laxity and some degree of muscular imbalance. Over time, the eyebrow tends to lose its lateral arch, and it appears somewhat flattened in older patients. It is essential to differentiate true, primary eyelid ptosis affecting the (tarso) levator muscle from eyelid ptosis that is unveiled as a secondary consequence of eyebrow ptosis. Each can present as excess folding of upper eyelid skin, but the appropriate treatment strategy for one differs from that of the other. In some patients, preexisting congenital eyelid ptosis, mechanical factors, such as repeated insertion and removal of contact lenses, or neurogenic factors may also be contributory. Based on this model, rejuvenation strategies have focused on mechanical elevation of either the eyebrows or the upper eyelids, or both.

With the understanding that these are the age-related changes that are conventionally described, careful inspection of older faces and comparison with photographs taken in youth reveal that some actually display an elevation in the eyebrows with age. The most obvious example is when

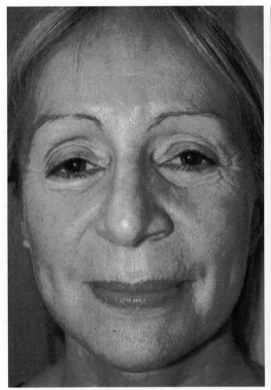
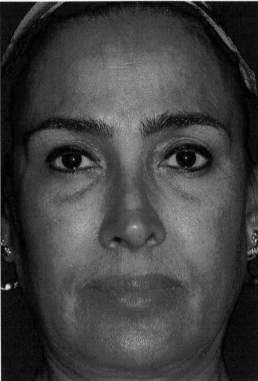

Fig. 1. Variation in individual aging patterns. Both women are 57 years old. The woman on the left, with Fitzpatrick skin phototype I, has a distinctly different pattern of facial aging to the woman on the right, with Fitzpatrick skin phototype IV. Both have bilateral upper eyelid ptosis and some degree of eyebrow asymmetry. (Patient on right has permanent makeup to the eyebrows and upper eyelids.) (*Courtesy of* Hema Sundaram, MD.)

upper eyelid ptosis that is more apparent on one side is secondarily offset to some extent by contraction of the frontalis muscle, resulting in one eyebrow that lies higher than the other. It is our observation that most patients exhibit some degree of partially compensated eyelid ptosis when examined closely enough both in repose and in animation. This can be obscured when the compensatory contraction by frontalis is relatively symmetric on both sides of the forehead, and also to some extent in women by differential tweezing of each eyebrow (**Fig. 2**).

Variance in Ideal Eyebrow Position

Ideal, youthful eyebrow position and shape vary from individual to individual, and even on the basis of hereditary and ethnic factors. However, it is instructive to study the faces of children and young adults. Their eyebrows are frequently less arched and less elevated than those of older individuals who have undergone cosmetic procedures with the aim of rejuvenation. As with many aspects of our field, we still have much to learn. In the quest to correct age-related changes to the upper face, it is important not to lose sight of what looks most natural and to hoist the eyebrows high in an esthetically unappealing attempt to offset redundant upper eyelid folds. As we continue to advance our knowledge of how facial architecture changes with age, we must also strive for a better understanding of the functional changes, and incorporate both structural and functional considerations into treatment planning.

The 4 Pillars of Rejuvenation: 4 R's Method-Based Classification

An integrative approach to facial rejuvenation has been described as being composed of 4 main pillars[1] or 4 R's:

1. Relaxation of muscles with neuromodulators
2. Refilling with injectable fillers
3. Resurfacing of skin, e.g. with lasers or light energy-based devices, chemical peels
4. Redraping of tissue with surgery, lasers or light energy-based devices

This classification is method-based, in that it is founded on the procedures that may be used to achieve improvement.

For many patients, a combination of procedures represents the best, multimodal approach to nonsurgical rejuvenation of the eyebrow and upper eyelid. For example, an injectable botulinum toxin neuromodulator can be administered to the superolateral aspect of the orbicularis oculi muscle to raise the lateral aspect of the brow (Relaxation). The same patient may also benefit from strategic placement of a hyaluronic acid filler above and under the eyebrow and to the upper eyelid (Refilling), and also from fractional bipolar RF to the upper face, including the region just above the eyebrows (Redraping and Resurfacing).

The 4 Pillars of Rejuvenation: 4 R's Outcome-Based Classification

Although a method-based classification is certainly helpful, an outcome-based classification that relates to desired objectives is also of value because it facilitates the formulation of effective, patient-centric treatment plans. Using the 4 R's formula, we might consider the pillars of an outcome-based classification to be the following:

1. Replacement of tissue volume
2. Regeneration of tissue quality
3. Rebalancing of facial vectors and proportions
4. Improvement of skin Reflectance

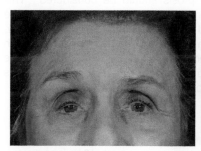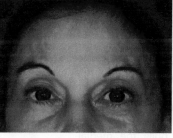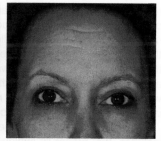

Fig. 2. Asymmetrical eyebrow elevation in compensation for upper eyelid ptosis. (*Left*) Obvious manifestation, with significant elevation of the right eyebrow and accentuation of horizontal rhytides on the right side of the forehead. Despite this partial compensation, the patient's bilateral upper eyelid ptosis is still slightly more pronounced on the right side in repose. (*Middle*) Less obvious manifestation, with elevation of the right eyebrow and slight residual right upper eyelid ptosis in repose. (*Right*) More subtle manifestation with slight elevation of the right eyebrow, accentuation of the horizontal rhytides on the right side of the forehead, and no greater ptosis of the right upper eyelid than the left in repose. (*Courtesy of* Hema Sundaram, MD.)

The synergistic potential of combining multi-tasking nonsurgical procedures is apparent if we now examine the treatment plan listed previously through the prism of this classification. The injected neuromodulator effects a rebalancing of facial vectors and proportions. The filler also rebalances facial vectors and proportions by lifting and contouring. In addition, fillers replace tissue volume, regenerate tissue quality via stimulation of collagenesis, and can improve skin reflectance, especially if a multiplane "sandwich" implantation technique is used. RF can rebalance facial vectors and proportions, improve skin reflectance, and also contribute to regeneration of tissue quality and replacement of tissue volume.

BRIEF ANATOMIC OVERVIEW

Anatomic considerations for the upper eyelid and brow are addressed in detail elsewhere in this issue; therefore, a brief overview is provided here.

Like the rest of the face, the upper periorbital region (upper eyelid, orbital sulcus, and eyebrow) is best viewed as a 3-dimensional structure. The upper eyelid should have a well-defined supratarsal crease. Age-related loss of bone contributes significantly to an inward caving of the supraorbital fossa, and supraorbital hollowing, which is a principal feature of facial aging. Supraorbital hollowing has been described as occurring in 4 main zones, as a result of varying degrees and patterns of volume loss. From medial to lateral, these zones are the medial fat pad, the hollow overlying the supraorbital foramen, the middle fat pad, and the lateral fat pad.[1] (See the articles by Lam and colleagues, and Terella and Wang, elsewhere in this issue, for detailed anatomic description and graphics.)

The tissue planes underlying the brow from most superficial to most deep are the epidermis, dermis, subcutaneous fat, superficial fascia and musculature, subgaleal loose areolar tissue, periosteum (deep fascia), and bone. Eyelids also have several layers. The middle layer, known as the orbital septum, is a connective tissue sheet that thickens as it extends toward the bony orbit and is ultimately referred to as the arcus marginalis where it inserts into the orbital rim. Fat at the roof of the orbit lies beneath the arcus marginalis.

Key musculature of the upper eyelid and brow includes the procerus (which pulls the medial aspect of the brow downward); the corrugator supercilii and depressor supercilii bilaterally (which pull the medial brow downward and medially); and the orbicularis oculi, the sphincteric ring around the bony orbit that approximates the upper and lower eyelids when contracted and whose medial portion serves as a medial brow depressor. The eyebrows are elevated by contraction of the frontalis muscle, which is in the form of bifid muscle bellies or a continuous sheet that extends over the forehead to join with the occipitalis muscle on the scalp (**Fig. 3**).

PRETREATMENT EVALUATION

The ideal eyebrow shape for a woman is quite different from the ideal for a man. In both, the medial brow should transition smoothly into the skin at the root of the nose, creating a continuous, gently curved line from the nose to the orbit. Youthful female eyebrows arch gracefully, with the arch positioned such that it directly overlies the superciliary groove of the orbital foramen. The peak of the arch should be positioned above the lateral limbus of the iris, and the eyebrow should then slope downward as it passes toward the lateral canthus. Ideally, the most lateral portion of the female eyebrow (the "tail") lies on a horizontal plane that is 1 to 2 mm above the lowest portion of the medial eyebrow. The ideal female eyebrow has been described as resembling the wing of a gull.[2] In contrast, the male eyebrow should have less of an arch, and be positioned at approximately the level of the superior bony orbital margin, ie, lower on the superciliary arch than in females (**Fig. 4**).

Symmetry and Height Measurements

Before treatment, the patient's eyebrows should be evaluated for symmetry of height as well as for degree and position of the arch. Eyebrow ptosis can be determined by measuring the distance from the central inferior edge of the brow to the central upper lid margin. If this distance is much less than 10 mm, the diagnosis of eyebrow ptosis should be considered.[3] This measurement can also be performed for the medial and lateral aspects of the eyebrow. Comparison of these 3 measurements for each eyebrow and comparison between the eyebrows can help to determine whether or not there is eyebrow ptosis or asymmetry of the eyebrows.

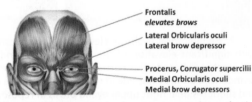

Fig. 3. Elevator and depressor muscles of the eyebrows. (*Courtesy of* Hema Sundaram, MD.)

Female brow	Male brow
Gentle curve with arch ¾ length above orbital rim	Straight line at or slightly below orbital rim

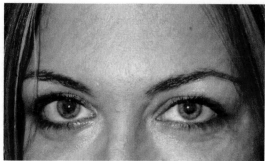 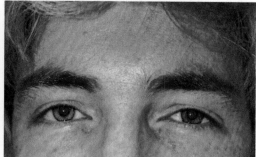

Fig. 4. The ideal brow. (*Courtesy of* Hema Sundaram, MD.)

Ptosis Evaluation

Upper eyelid ptosis (blepharoptosis) can be detected by measuring either the palpebral fissure width (also known as the palpebral fissure height) or the margin reflex distance-1 (MRD_1). The palpebral fissure width is the distance between the margins of the central upper eyelid and the central lower eyelid; ideally, this should be approximately 10 mm on each side.[3] The MRD_1 is evaluated with the patient in a primary gaze position, by shining a light placed between the examiner's eyes directly toward and parallel to the patient's eyes at the same level. MRD_1 is the distance from the central upper eyelid margin to the center of the pupillary light reflex. Measurement of the MRD_1 allows more accurate assessment of upper eyelid ptosis than measurement of the palpebral fissure width, as the MRD_1 is independent of lower eyelid position. A normal MRD_1 is approximately 4.0 to 4.5 mm. Measurements smaller than the lowest limit of normal can signify upper eyelid ptosis. A difference between the MRD_1 measurements of each eye signifies upper eyelid asymmetry.

Upper Eyelid Crease Measurement

The upper eyelid crease is quantified by the marginal crease distance (MCD), which is the distance from the central portion of the upper lid margin to the central aspect of the crease in downward gaze. To measure the MCD, the patient is asked to look downward, then slightly upward, then downward again. A normal central MCD has been defined for women as 8 to 10 mm, and for men as 5 to 7 mm; however, a central MCD as high as 9 to 11 mm may be considered within normal limits.[3] A disinsertion or dehiscence of the levator aponeurosis causing acquired upper eyelid

ptosis results in an MCD that is much greater than normal. In contrast, patients with congenital ptosis often have an indistinct upper eyelid crease.

Recognition of eyebrow elevation may be more difficult unless there is asymmetrical compensated eyelid ptosis, as it requires knowledge of the patient's own baseline: her eyebrow position in youth. Comparison of the patient's current appearance with photographs taken before the age of 30 may be helpful in this regard.

PATIENT ASSESSMENT AND ESTABLISHMENT OF REALISTIC EXPECTATIONS

The patient can be provided with a mirror and asked to point out what she specifically dislikes about the area around her eyes, and what she expects rejuvenation procedures to accomplish. Comparison with photographs from the patient's youth may give a clearer picture of individual patterns of aging and what is realistically achievable.

Patients invariably desire treatments that are safe, effective, long-lasting, as painless as possible, and have the least possible postprocedural recovery time. Establishment of realistic expectations during pretreatment consultation is key to achieving patient satisfaction. It is important to discuss the nature of facial aging, and what can truly be defined as rejuvenation, ie, the achievement of a more youthful appearance. In our opinion, this does not include the obliteration of lines of expression or facial mobility, both of which are present even in children, the most shining examples of youthful beauty. Nor does it include the raising of the eyebrows to a level that is higher than is typically seen in children and young adults, in an attempt to offset loss of tissue volume, skin elasticity, and/or muscle tone. Patients may be best advised that well-performed procedures can help them to look their best for their age, rather than fueling an ill-advised and ultimately futile attempt to look a different age.

The practitioner can provide an approximate prediction of how much improvement in quality of upper eyelid skin might be accomplished through each laser and light energy-based device that is being considered for this purpose. Similarly, it is informative to define the extent to which eyebrows can repositioned or reshaped through the use of neuromodulators, fillers, and laser or light energy-based devices in the upper face. Finally, patients can be counseled if they probably will not achieve the outcome they desire with nonsurgical procedures alone, and if more invasive measures, such as blepharoplasty or endoscopic brow lifting, are appropriate.

NONSURGICAL REJUVENATION PROCEDURES

As noted previously, it is important to understand both structural anatomy and the functional interplay of eyebrows and eyelids when considering treatment strategies. Volume loss in all tissue planes ascending from the bone to the epidermis is now recognized as a cardinal feature of the aging process.[4] In addition, skin elasticity decreases and there are changes in muscle tone, both in repose and in animation. These manifestations of aging can be addressed via nonsurgical procedures, with the caveat that the goal should always be to achieve natural-looking results, even if this entails compromising on the extent of improvement that is sought.

Treatment of the upper face with a combination of nonsurgical rejuvenation techniques can improve brow position, and correct upper eyelid hooding to some extent. These techniques can be divided into 1 of 4 categories:

1. Neuromodulators
2. Soft tissue fillers
3. Laser and light energy-based devices
4. Adjunctive treatments, including chemical peels and topical therapies

A further subdivision can be made according to the area to which the treatments are applied: within or outside the periorbital frame.

The Periorbital Frame

It may be helpful to assess the eyes within a "periorbital frame," which we define as encompassing the eyebrow, the upper eyelid, the lower eyelid, and also the glabella and superior mid face. An individualized strategy for injection of neuromodulators

within the periorbital frame can be formulated by coupling evaluation of each patient's muscle mass and activity, and the extent and pattern of hyperdynamic and static rhytides, with a thorough understanding of facial anatomy and the patient's treatment objectives.

Strategies for soft tissue fillers and lasers or light energy-based devices are determined by evaluation of periorbital volume loss, loss of skin elasticity, and dyspigmentation (most commonly, hyperpigmentation). Other treatment modalities that may be considered for integrative rejuvenation of the periorbital frame include chemical peels with glycolic acid, salicylic acid, or trichloroacetic acid; cosmetic tattooing (permanent makeup); semipermanent eyelash extensions; and eyebrow and eyelash tinting. Although some of these procedures may seem minor, and even trivial, they can produce gratifying results at a reasonable cost and with little or no recovery time (**Fig. 5**).

Neuromodulators

The injectable neuromodulators that are currently approved by the United States Food and Drug Administration (FDA) for esthetic use are abobotulinumtoxin A (Dysport; Medicis, Scottsdale, AZ), incobotulinumtoxin A (Xeomin; Merz Aesthetics, San Mateo, CA), and onabotulinumtoxin A (Botox Cosmetic; Allergan, Irvine, CA).

Dysport and Botox are classified as complexed toxins because they are manufactured with the 150-kDa botulinum toxin A (BoNT-A) molecule bound covalently in a complex to accessory proteins, which are believed to dissociate from the toxin molecule within minutes of being exposed to physiologic pH during the reconstitution and/or injection process.[5]

Xeomin consists of the BoNT-A molecule alone and is classified as a naked toxin.

Controlled studies of evidence level II have shown the safety and efficacy of Dysport, Xeomin,

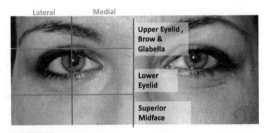

ASSESS FOR:
Volume loss: degree and pattern
Muscle imbalance
Loss of skin elasticity

Fig. 5. The periorbital frame. (*Courtesy of* Hema Sundaram, MD.)

and Botox all to be excellent. Dosage units of Botox and Xeomin are clinically equivalent, whereas the dosage units for Dysport are distinct. Although there may be some variation in the equivalence of Dysport units with Botox or Xeomin units at different dosages, for practical purposes 2.5 Dysport (Speywood) units may be considered equivalent to 1 Botox or Xeomin unit.

Brow Shaping

When performed appropriately, eyebrow shaping has a profound effect on the face, both for women and men. In women, restoration of graceful arches to the eyebrows can partially relieve upper eyelid hooding and increase the emphasis of the eyes. This, in turn, increases the prominence of the upper one-third of the face relative to the lower two-thirds, which shifts facial proportions back toward the youthful ideal of the heart shape or inverted egg. Brow shaping with neuromodulators is often combined with neuromodulator treatment of the glabella, forehead, and crow's feet to optimize patient satisfaction. In appropriately selected patients who have retained good skin elasticity and do not have a bulging pretarsal orbicularis oculi, it may also be valuable to add a small dose of neuromodulator to this zone of the orbicularis sphincter in the midpupillary line, with the aim of lowering the inferior ciliary margin by a fraction of a millimeter to produce an appealing, wide-eyed look.

Successful brow shaping with neuromodulators requires an understanding of the fascinating interplay among the following:

- Frontalis muscle, which serves as the brow elevator
- Superolateral portion of orbicularis oculi, which is the lateral brow depressor
- Procerus, corrugator supercilii, depressor supercilii, and medial portion of orbicularis oculi, which are the medial brow depressors

Technique

- To elevate the lateral portion of the eyebrows, a small dose of neuromodulator is injected subdermally at a single point into the superolateral portion of the orbicularis oculi on each side. Weakening of this lateral brow depressor allows the relatively unopposed frontalis muscle to better elevate the lateral eyebrow.
- The appropriate injection site can be identified by palpating the belly of orbicularis oculi under the lateral arch of the eyebrow in maximal contraction (frowning). The injection can then be performed with the patient in repose.

Surgical note: The eyebrows themselves cannot serve as an accurate guide to placement of this injection, as there is great individual variation in eyebrow shape and position, often amplified by tweezing in women.

- Injection of neuromodulator into the procerus and the corrugator and depressor supercilii muscles similarly weakens the medial brow depressors and allows the frontalis to elevate the medial portion of the eyebrows.
- If the frontalis is injected concurrently, its pattern of injection also influences eyebrow position and shape.
- To enhance the arch of the eyebrows, the lateral injection point on each side of the frontalis can be placed slightly higher than the medial injection point at mid-forehead level, to weaken the lateral portion of the frontalis less than the medial portion. A higher dose of neuromodulator over the medial and lateral portions of the eyebrows and a lower dose over the middle portion will magnify this effect (**Figs. 6** and **7**)

Cryoneuromodulation (Myoscience, Redwood City, CA) is a nonchemical neuromodulator option that is currently under study in the United States and approved in Europe for temporary improvement of dynamic rhytides of the forehead. The handheld percutaneous device targets the temporal branch of the facial nerve to prevent signal transduction. The results are reported to be comparable in longevity to those of botulinum toxin neuromodulators, and can include improvement in the position and shape of the eyebrows.

Soft tissue fillers

Placement of soft tissue fillers just below or just above the eyebrow can improve its shape and position, and yield secondary improvement in upper eyelid hooding. Very small volumes of filler (typically no more than 0.1 mL each side) can also be implanted directly into the upper eyelid with serial microthreading technique for restoration of volume.

The periorbital frame is both anatomically and esthetically unforgiving. Fillers must be implanted with great care and with appropriate injection technique and depth to avoid contour irregularities. Injection of a fraction of a milliliter too much filler or even the slightest misplacement can transform an attractive result into a disaster, and may even

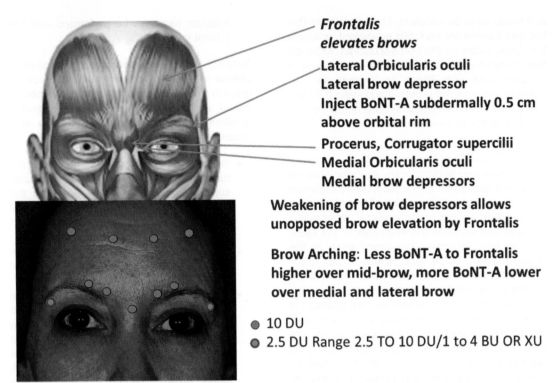

Frontalis
elevates brows

Lateral Orbicularis oculi
Lateral brow depressor
Inject BoNT-A subdermally 0.5 cm
above orbital rim

Procerus, Corrugator supercilii
Medial Orbicularis oculi
Medial brow depressors

Weakening of brow depressors allows
unopposed brow elevation by Frontalis

Brow Arching: Less BoNT-A to Frontalis
higher over mid-brow, more BoNT-A lower
over medial and lateral brow

● 10 DU
● 2.5 DU Range 2.5 TO 10 DU/1 to 4 BU OR XU

Fig. 6. Brow shaping with botulinum toxin neuromodulator. It is recommended that small doses of neuromodulator are injected into the superolateral aspect of orbicularis oculi to avoid an unnatural appearance owing to overelevation of the lateral portion of the eyebrow. If further brow lifting is felt to be esthetically appropriate at follow-up at least 2 to 3 weeks after treatment, additional neuromodulator can be injected. BU, Botox units; DU, Dysport (Speywood) units; XU, Xeomin units. (*Courtesy of* Hema Sundaram, MD.)

cause complications, such as prolonged periorbital swelling, which is often presumed to be a manifestation of obstruction of lymphatic outflow.[6]

For these reasons, we strongly recommend hyaluronic acid (HA) products as the fillers of choice for structures within the periorbital frame, including the brow and upper eyelid. The excellent safety profile and efficacy of HA fillers and the ability to inject them precisely through small-gauge needles through microcannulas permit the achievement of optimal results. Their complete reversibility via injection of hyaluronidase or simple extrusion enables corrections to be made, if needed.

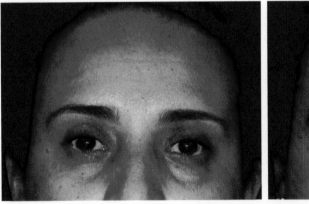
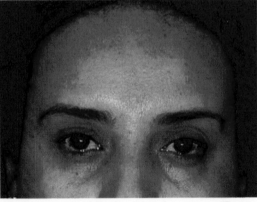

Fig. 7. A 45-year-old woman in repose before and 33 days after brow shaping and eye opening with botulinum toxin neuromodulator. Patient received injection of neuromodulator (abobotulinumtoxin A) to the frontalis, superolateral, lateral canthal, and pretarsal orbicularis oculi, procerus, corrugator supercilii ,and depressor supercilii muscles. (*Courtesy of* Hema Sundaram, MD.)

HA filler products that are currently approved by the FDA for esthetic use may be divided into 4 families based on their manufacturing processes and physicochemical characteristics:

1. The NASHA (nonanimal stabilized HA) products are Restylane and Perlane (Medicis)
2. Hylacross products are Juvéderm Ultra and Ultra Plus (Allergan)
3. Cohesive Polydensified Matrix HA is Belotero Balance (Merz)

These 3 product families all have a high total HA concentration, between 20 and 24 mg/mL, and therefore a high water-binding capacity[7] and the property of binding further water after injection. Controlled, Evidence Level II show them to have comparable safety, efficacy, and longevity.

4. Prevelle Silk (Mentor, Santa Barbara, CA)

The fourth type of HA product has a lower total HA concentration of 5.5 mg/mL and therefore a lower water-binding capacity. It may be classified as hydrated HA because it will not tend to absorb further water after injection. Hydrated HA has about half the longevity of the other HA products because of its lower HA concentration.

The rheologic (flow-related) properties of these HA fillers are of utility in determining their appropriate applications.[8] NASHA fillers have a high elastic modulus (G prime), and thus high lifting capacity and the ability to resist the forces of gravity and facial movement. They are firm products best suited to subdermal implantation, and provide maximal lift when implanted in the preperiosteal or subcutaneous tissue planes. NASHA products also have high viscosity, which confers resistance to spread and results in contour stability after implantation. Hylacross HA fillers, which have lower elastic modulus and viscosity, are softer products with more propensity to spread within tissue after implantation. They contain particles that vary more in shape and size than the particles in NASHA products[9] and, like NASHA products, are best implanted subdermally. Cohesive polydensified matrix HA has the lowest elastic modulus and viscosity, and is the softest product with the least lift and the most tissue spread after implantation. It has little or no tendency to cause the Tyndall effect when implanted superficially, because it lacks the prominent particulate phase that is required to scatter short-wavelength blue light and create bluish skin discoloration. This, together with its softness, makes cohesive polydensified matrix HA appropriate for intradermal implantation. Hydrated HA, which has low elasticity and viscosity, is also a soft, spreading product and carries little or no risk of the Tyndall effect after superficial implantation because of its low concentration of particles (**Figs. 8** and **9**).[6,10]

The clinical relevance of these rheologic data is underscored by histopathologic and ultrasound studies that confirm the direct correlation between HA product viscosity and its tissue distribution after intradermal implantation.[11] NASHA remains as a well-defined bolus, Hylacross HA distributes somewhat more diffusely within the dermis, and cohesive polydensified matrix HA has homogeneous intradermal distribution.

Facial Volume Loss in all Tissue Planes

Age-related loss of facial volume is understood to occur in all tissue planes, ascending from the bone to the subdermal soft tissues to the dermis and epidermis.[12] Volume loss from the subdermal soft tissues is characterized by depletion of the superficial and deep fat compartments of the face,[13] a process that is discussed in detail elsewhere in this issue. Because volume loss occurs in multiple tissue planes, it is logical to replace volume in a multiplane or "sandwich" pattern.[10,14]

Subdermal Filler

Deep (subdermal) filler implantation into the forehead will offset loss of volume from the central and lateral-temporal fat compartments of the forehead and produce outward and upward vectoring that lifts and contours the eyebrows. We categorize this as "deep lifting volumetry."

For deep volume restoration around the eyebrow, NASHA or Hylacross HA fillers (Restylane or Juvéderm Ultra) can be implanted supraperiosteally or subcutaneously into the supraorbital sulcus. This may be accomplished via serial or linear threading with a blunt microcannula or small-gauge sharp needle. Serial microaliquots of filler may also be deposited deeply with a sharp needle.

NASHA or Hylacross HA can also be implanted with the same techniques just above the lateral two-thirds of the eyebrow, where a sulcus often develops with age, due to loss of volume and tissue quality. Implantation of filler to re-inflate this sulcus enhances the shape of the eyebrows and produces a consummately natural-looking eyebrow lift. Here, the anatomically safe and esthetically preferred tissue plane for deep implantation, as for the whole forehead, is the subgaleal glide plane.[15] The use of a blunt microcannula for subdermal (subcutaneous or supraperiosteal) filler implantation may decrease the risks of inadvertent intravascular injection and ecchymosis.[16,17]

A number of HA fillers that are available outside the United States are suitable for deep implantation

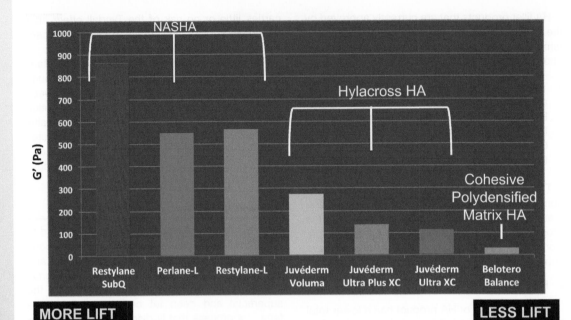

Fig. 8. Elastic modulus (G') of HA fillers. Measured at 0.7 Hz. HA products are grouped by generic family name. (*Data from* Sundaram H, Voigts B, Beer K, et al. Comparison of the rheological properties of viscosity and elasticity in two categories of soft tissue fillers: calcium hydroxylapatite and hyaluronic acid. Dermatol Surg 2010;36(Suppl 3):1859S–65S; and Sundaram H, Flynn T, Cassuto D, et al. New and emerging concepts in soft tissue fillers. J Drugs Dermatol 2012;11(8):s12–25.)

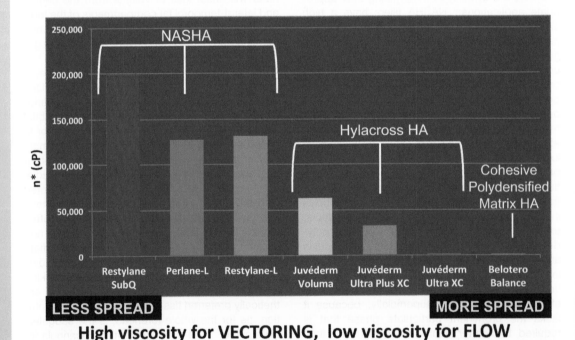

Fig. 9. Complex viscosity of HA fillers. Measured at 0.7 Hz. HA products are grouped by generic family name. (*Data from* Sundaram H, Voigts B, Beer K, et al. Comparison of the rheological properties of viscosity and elasticity in two categories of soft tissue fillers: calcium hydroxylapatite and hyaluronic acid. Dermatol Surg 2010;36(Suppl 3):1859S–65S; and Sundaram H, Flynn T, Cassuto D, et al. New and emerging concepts in soft tissue fillers. J Drugs Dermatol 2012;11(8):s12–25.)

into the brow and other areas of the forehead, by virtue of their properties of flow and cohesivity, which make them firm but moldable. These include Emervel Deep and Emervel Volume (QMed/Galderma, Uppsala, Sweden), Juvéderm Voluma (Allergan), Belotero Intense (Merz) and Modélis Shape (Anteis, Geneva, Switzerland). Some of these fillers are currently under study in the United States, and thus are on the horizon for American injectors.

Superficial Fillers

Superficial volume restoration to the upper eyelid and under or above the eyebrow will produce some outward and upward vectoring. There is also significant horizontal vectoring parallel to the skin surface, as the fillers selected for intradermal or superficial subdermal implantation are softer and tend to have a predominance of flow over elasticity.[10] We characterize this as "superficial flow volumetry"; clinically, it results in improvement of both crepey skin and skin reflectance.

Based on their softness and flow characteristics, cohesive polydensified matrix HA (Belotero Balance) and hydrated HA (Prevelle Silk) are products that are currently approved in the United States and appropriate for superficial implantation with serial puncture or threading technique. They also carry little or no risk of the Tyndall effect even when implanted superficially into the thin-skinned periocular region. Transient skin blanching after implantation is both a manifestation and a confirmation of superficial filler placement. Because the skin of the upper eyelid is extremely thin, very small volumes of filler (typically no more than 0.1–0.2 mL) should be implanted with micro-threading technique.

As with the deep approach, a blunt microcannula optimizes safety and potentially decreases the incidence of ecchymosis in the entire periocular region.[16–18] However, filler may be placed more precisely with a sharp needle within the superficial dermis, which is of higher resistance than the deeper dermis. Best practice techniques for multi-plane volume restoration with blunt microcannulas alone and in combination with sharp needles have been reviewed recently.[19]

Patients with fair to good retention of skin elasticity and with volume loss from the medial aspect of the upper eyelid will tend to achieve the best results from filler injection. HA fillers that are currently approved for use outside the United States and may subsequently become available to American injectors for superficial implantation include Belotero Soft (Merz), Emervel Touch and Restylane Fine Lines (both QMed/Galderma), Teosyal First Lines (Teoxane, Geneva, Switzerland) and Surgiderm 18 (Allergan). In addition, HA products that are injected superficially to improve dermal hydration and elasticity (ie, tissue quality) rather than to restore volume are available in Europe and elsewhere; examples include Restylane Vital (QMed/Galderma) and Juvéderm Hydrate (Allergan) (**Figs. 10–12**).

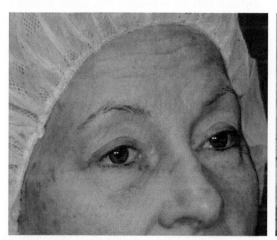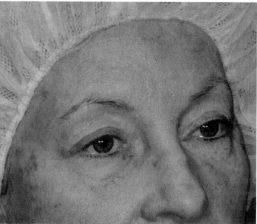

Fig. 10. Before and 30 minutes after injection of cohesive polydensified matrix HA (Belotero Balance) to glabella and forehead with superficial blanch injection technique. Non-Tyndall cohesive polydensified matrix HA was injected with retrograde technique via a sharp needle into the intradermal and superficial subdermal tissue planes. Transient skin blanching at the point of these superficial injections has resolved 30 minutes after injection. Note natural-looking improvement in eyebrow shape and position after superficial volume replacement to the forehead and glabella. This patient has bilateral eyebrow elevation, as partial compensation for her upper eyelid ptosis. Botulinum toxin neuromodulator injection would not have addressed her fundamental problem of volume loss. It would also have carried the risk of exacerbating her pre-existing upper eyelid ptosis by weakening the compensatory mechanism of frontalis contraction. (*Courtesy of* Hema Sundaram, MD.)

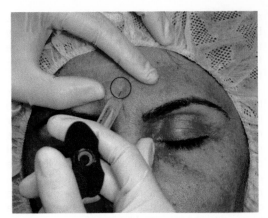

Fig. 11. Superficial blanch injection technique for glabellar and forehead rhytides. Retrograde intradermal injection of non-Tyndall HA with light crosslinking and small gel calibration (Emervel Touch). Transient skin blanching at the point of injection (*circled*) is a result of intradermal placement of the filler. Stretching of the skin with the fingers of the nondominant hand in a perpendicular direction to the rhytides facilitates this intradermal placement. (*Courtesy of* Hema Sundaram, MD.)

The benefits of combining HA fillers with a botulinum toxin type A (BoNT-A) neuromodulator are well documented.[20,21] In the eyebrow and eyelid regions, as elsewhere on the face, the 2 treatment modalities can produce a synergistic improvement. In addition, the neuromodulator may potentially prolong the longevity of the filler by decreasing the shearing forces on it owing to hyperdynamic facial musculature (**Figs. 13** and **14**).

Lasers and light energy-based devices

Considerable interest has focused on the notion of tightening skin of the upper eyelid and brow to improve their position and shape, and a number of laser and light energy-emitting devices are commonly used with this stated aim. They include nonablative erbium-doped mid-infrared (IR), IR, and near-IR lasers; sublative fractionated radiofrequency (RF) devices; ablative fractionated carbon dioxide and fractionated erbium:YAG lasers; and devices that emit microfocused ultrasound (MFU).

When considering which of these devices truly improves the shape and position of the eyebrows and upper eyelid, it is important to distinguish between postprocedural edema, which may last for several months, and true regeneration of tissue quality. Both can produce upward vectoring and consequently a lifting effect, but edema is transient and not related to meaningful structural changes in the treated tissue. Similarly, when assessing collagenesis and/or elastogenesis with any devices, it is ideal to examine the tissue 12

months or more after treatment, as upregulation of collagen and elastin production can occur in the first few weeks to months after treatment simply as a manifestation of the immediate wounding response, rather than as a predictor of long-term clinical improvement.

From an anatomic perspective, it is logical that long-term lifting requires structural changes in the deeper tissues: the mid to deep dermis and hypodermis. Devices that predominantly ablate tissue may be considered to cause inward vectoring owing to contracture, whereas devices that predominantly regenerate tissue will cause outward vectoring. These considerations may be of more utility than the notion of skin tightening, which is actually scientifically inaccurate even though it may be helpful when discussing procedures with patients.

The relatively long wavelength of radiofrequency (RF) allows it to penetrate into the dermis and hypodermis. RF devices that cause 3-dimensional volumetric heating of the deeper tissues and stimulate collagenesis and/or elastogenesis may be viewed as providing upward and outward vectoring. Infrared (IR) devices can also provide some degree of volumetric heating but their vectoring force is principally inward owing to tissue contracture.

MFU deposits discrete points of microthermocoagulation at specific depths in the deeper tissues, to provide upward and inward vectoring due to discrete points of tissue contracture. Fine rhytides can be improved and some degree of vectoring obtained with lasers and light energy devices that deliver thermal energy more superficially, including fractionated laser resurfacing devices that target a specific fraction of the skin surface area, while leaving intervening islands of normal skin untouched.

Because numerous devices are available within these various genres, an overview is provided here of some representative technologies.

RF DEVICES

Fractional bipolar RF is a chromophore-independent method of volumetrically heating the dermis to cause collagen coagulation and potentiate collagenesis.[22,23] It has been described as a "sublative" procedure for skin resurfacing and wrinkle reduction because most of the RF energy passes through the epidermis and is delivered to the dermis. The resultant limited epidermal ablation with sublative resurfacing optimizes therapeutic effects and comfort, and reduces or even eliminates the risk of postinflammatory hyperpigmentation for diverse skin types, even up to

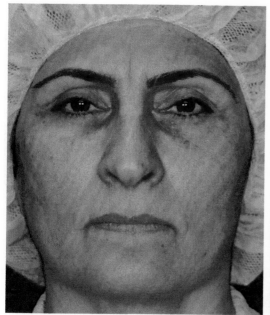 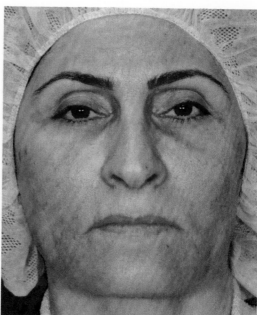

Fig. 12. Deep and superficial vectoring with HA fillers. Same patient as in **Fig. 11**: A 53-year-old woman before and 30 minutes after pan-facial deep and superficial volumetry using a range of HA products (Emervel, generic name HA$_E$) that are customized for specific clinical applications by variation of gel calibration (particle size) and crosslinking. Deep lifting volumetry for upward and outward vectoring of the eyebrows was achieved by pre-periosteal implantation of the product with heavy crosslinking and large gel calibration (HA$_E$ Volume) to the temporal fossae. Superficial flow volumetry for horizontal and outward vectoring was achieved by intradermal implantation of the product with light crosslinking and small gel calibration (HA$_E$ Touch) into the glabella. The Emervel products are currently approved for esthetic use in Europe and elsewhere, and are under study in the United States. (*Courtesy of* Hema Sundaram, MD.)

Fitzpatrick skin phototype 6.[24,25] A device that emits fractional bipolar RF (eMatrix, Syneron Medical Ltd, Yokneam, Israel) has disposable tips composed of rows of electrode pins in a bipolar array. These pins function as positively and negatively charged electrodes to deliver RF energy through the epidermis and deeper into the dermis between each pair of positive and negative electrodes to form a closed circuit loop of RF current.

The superficial, dry stratum corneum exerts high impedance, which allows the RF energy to follow each pin by itself (as in monopolar RF), resulting in limited surface ablation. The dermis has lower impedance because it contains more water and electrolytes, which allows the RF energy to flow as a current between the positive and negative electrode pins; the resultant bipolar RF creates a diffuse zone of thermocoagulation and necrosis with relatively low tissue ablation. The overall effect is to deliver fractionated RF energy to the skin in the shape of an inverted cone, such that the dermal effect is high relative to the epidermal effect. The temperature of the targeted tissue is raised to between 45° and 65°C for thermally induced remodeling of existing dermal collagen fibers, and stimulation of collagenesis.

Fractional Bipolar RF Device Settings

Device settings can be varied with respect to the depth of ablative zones, the extent of surrounding coagulated tissue, and the proportions of coagulation, necrosis, and ablation. RF energy of up to 62 mJ per electrode pin can be delivered, with ablation/coagulation/necrosis and subnecrosis up to a maximum depth of approximately 450 μm and epidermal ablation of 5% to 7%. The number of electrode pins on the tip can be varied. For a given RF fluence, the smaller the number of pins, the greater the depth of penetration of the closed loops of RF current. A tip with 8 × 8 array of 64 electrode pins is commonly used, and a smaller 44-pin tip is also available for focused treatment and for smaller areas. If a greater effect on the epidermis is required, multiple passes over the targeted tissue can be performed with the 64-pin tip (**Fig. 15**).

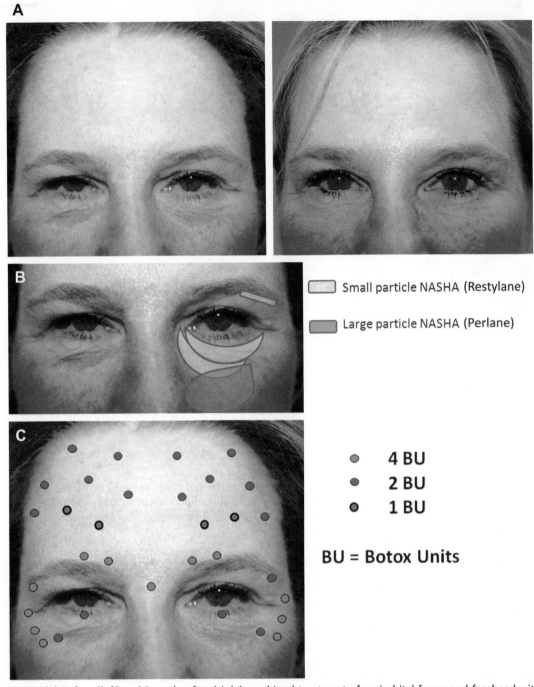

Fig. 13. (*A*) Before (*left*) and 3 weeks after (*right*) combined treatment of periorbital frame and forehead with NASHA fillers (Restylane and Perlane) and onabotulinumtoxin A (Botox Cosmetic). (*B*) Filler injection strategy for periorbital frame. Small particle NASHA (Restylane) was injected with anterograde technique, pre-periosteally to the lower eyelids and under the eyebrows and also into the superficial subdermis of the lower eyelid. Large-particle NASHA (Perlane) was injected with anterograde technique to the midface. (*C*) Neuromodulator injection strategy for periorbital frame and forehead. Onabotulinumtoxin A (Botox Cosmetic) was injected to the procerus, corrugator supercilii, depressor supercilii, frontalis, and orbicularis oculi muscles. Injection of frontalis was with microdroplet technique.

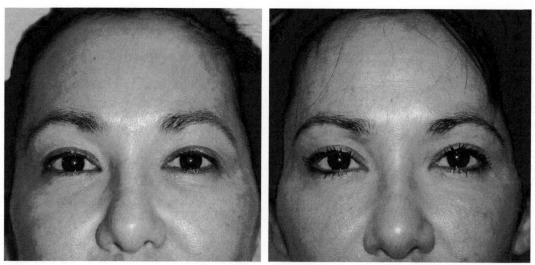

Fig. 14. Before and 5 weeks after combined treatment of periorbital frame and forehead with NASHA fillers (Restylane and Perlane) and abobotulinumtoxin A (Dysport). (*Courtesy of* Hema Sundaram, MD.)

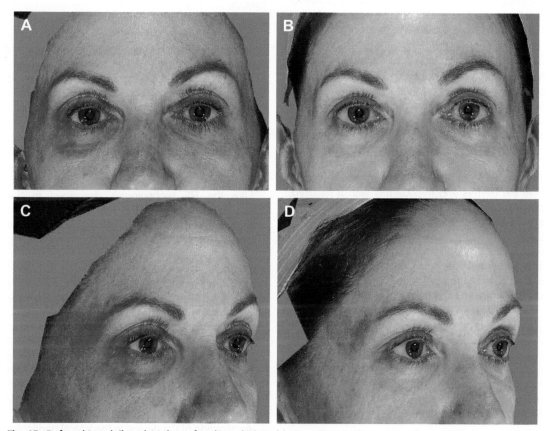

Fig. 15. Before (*A* and *C*) and 14 days after (*B* and *D*) "sublative rejuvenation" with a fractional bipolar RF device (eMATRIX) using a varied intensity treatment protocol. In this early stage after treatment, improvement is noted in eyebrow shape and position and also in lower eyelid contour, rhytids and hyperpigmentation. Additional images several months after treatment would be needed to clarify the extent of long term improvement. (*Courtesy of* Hema Sundaram, MD.)

Fractional Bipolar RF Device Results

Treatment of the upper eyelid and brow region with this fractional bipolar RF device may be viewed as producing a volumetric improvement in that there is tissue regeneration rather than tissue ablation. This manifests as decreased skin laxity, fine rhytides, hyperpigmentation, and improved skin reflectance.[26] Sublative resurfacing can be combined during the same treatment session with another device that integrates bipolar RF and IR energies for controlled, deep dermal heating of targeted facial zones (Sublime or Refirme, Syneron Medical Ltd.) to address deep skin folds and provide a contouring effect. Greater precision of RF delivery with the newer of these devices (Sublime), which is operated from the same platform as the sublative treatment, allows the maximum RF energy to be reduced to 100 J/cm^3, with clinical results as good as or better than with the other device (Refirme), which has a maximum energy of 120 J/cm^3. Multiple single passes can be performed for heat stacking, to provide upward and outward vectoring effect at the temples and superolateral mid face before treatment of the full face, including the forehead, with sublative resurfacing.

Other RF Devices

Multisource phase-controlled RF uses multiple electrodes and RF generators that operate in specific algorithms to deliver RF energy into the deep dermis and hypodermis with relative sparing of the epidermis.

A device that features this technology (EndyMed 3 DEEP, Caesarea, Israel) uses a matrix array of up to 112 electrodes and 6 RF generators to volumetrically heat the dermis and hypodermis with a focused, controlled flow of RF energy. Multiple electrical fields are created that repel each other, which drives the energy vertically into the targeted tissue and reduces the flow of energy through the skin surface. This epidermal sparing optimizes safety, comfort, and efficacy of the treatment in diverse skin types, without the need for adjunctive cooling.[27]

Combined monopolar and bipolar RF can be delivered simultaneously for deep and superficial volumetric heating of tissue. A device with this technology (Accent, Alma Lasers, Ltd, Caesarea, Israel) uses a dual-purpose platform supplying monopolar RF for deep tissue heating and bipolar RF for superficial heating.[28]

Continuous monopolar RF may also be used for eyebrow and eyelid rejuvenation via subdermal heating (eg, Pelleve, Ellman International, Oceanside, NY).[29]

Fractional bipolar RF with microneedling entails the delivery of RF energy directly to the reticular dermis via an array of microneedles. One device (ePrime, Syneron) has an array of ten 32-gauge needles arranged in 5 paired sets. When treatment is performed to stimulate volumetric rejuvenation of the mid face, this may have a beneficial secondary outward and upward vectoring effect on the periorbital frame.

MICROFOCUSED ULTRASOUND

A MFU device (Ulthera, Inc, Mesa, AZ) is cleared by the FDA as a Class II medical device for nonsurgical brow lifting. Transducers generate ultrasound energy at a frequency of 4 to 7 MHz, which is focused to yield discrete zones of thermal microcoagulation spaced 1.0 to 1.5 mm apart, along defined tissue planes within the dermis and hypodermis.[30] This device has an energy of up to 1.2 J. Lower frequency transducers deliver energy to a tissue depth of 4.5 mm, which is at the level of the subcutaneous muscular aponeurotic system (SMAS) and platysma, and higher frequency transducers deliver energy to a depth of 3 mm, which is within the deep dermis, while sparing the epidermis. There is simultaneous ultrasound imaging of the tissue planes that are being targeted. The thermal energy delivered to specific tissue planes within the dermis and hypodermis causes collagen contracture, resulting in upward and inward vectoring for a lifting effect, and can potentiate collagenesis. The tissue between, above, and below thermal coagulation points is spared, resulting in less recovery time after the procedure.[31]

Like the RF technologies described in the preceding section, MFU is suitable for patients with diverse Fitzpatrick skin phototypes because it spares the epidermis, thus reducing or eliminating the risk of postinflammatory hyperpigmentation.[32]

For lifting of the eyebrows, the device is applied to the lateral part of the forehead, including the region just above the lateral two-thirds of the eyebrows and MFU energy is delivered at a depth of 3 mm. This lifting effect has been quantified in the Evidence Level II studies,[33] in which 89% of study subjects had clinically significant brow lifting 90 days after a single treatment session with a mean brow elevation of 1.7 mm. Subsequent research has been performed with higher-energy protocols.

Application of the device to the lateral periocular region also contributes to the vectoring effect. Because MFU induces tissue ablation, it may be best used in conjunction with volumetric methods of improving tissue quality such as soft tissue fillers and radiofrequency, in order to avoid exacerbating pre-existing age-related volume loss.[34,35]

OTHER LASER AND LIGHT ENERGY DEVICES

Devices that target the epidermis and superficial subdermal tissue may be combined with RF and/or MFU in appropriately selected patients.

Fractionated ablative laser treatment uses selective photothermolysis to target water as the chromophore. The overall efficacy of rhytid reduction and improvement in skin laxity is greater with ablative than with nonablative resurfacing lasers; however, a balance must be found for many patients between this greater efficacy and the significantly greater postprocedural recovery time. The reader is directed to a review article further detailing the individual parameters of various nonablative laser and IR devices, such as specific depths of dermal penetration, energy column width, and vertical thermal injury (microthermal zones or MTZs).[36]

Ablative fractional resurfacing lasers include the 10,600-nm carbon dioxide (CO_2) (eg, Pixel Perfect, Alma Lasers, Ltd., Buffalo Grove, IL; Fraxel Re:pair, Solta Medical, Hayward, CA; DEKA Smartxide DOT, DEKA, Calenzano, Italy; and UltraPulse, Lumenis, Santa Clara, CA), which can be applied to the forehead including the area just above the eyebrows.

The 2940-nm Erbium:Yttrium Aluminum Garnet (Er:YAG) (eg, Pixel2940, Alma Lasers, Ltd.) can also be used for the forehead and, in addition, for the eyelids.

Subtypes of these lasers vary according to their optimal pulse duration, depth of penetration, beam diameter, residual thermal damage (RTD), and the necessary fluence that each must emit to achieve optimal pulsed laser ablation. Many current thought leaders consider CO_2 laser ablation to provide more tissue contraction and improvement in rhytides than Er:YAG ablation.[37,38] For the eyelids and eyebrows, as for other facial regions, selection of the appropriate device is determined by the areas to be treated, the clinical needs for each patient, and the postprocedural recovery time that can be tolerated.

Devices that target varying levels within the dermis and emit fractional (1540 and 1550 nm) erbium-doped midinfrared energy can be used with the aim of addressing skin laxity of the upper lid and brow (eg, Fraxel SR and SR1500, Solta Medical, Hayward, CA, and Lux 1540 Fractional, Palomar Medical Technologies, Burlington, MA).

Devices emitting noncoherent (825–1350 nm) IR light penetrate into the reticular dermis. Bipolar RF may be added to the IR for synergistic effect (eg, Matrix IR, Syneron Medical Ltd.) or the IR may be applied alone (eg, StarLux, Palomar). Q-switched (1064 nm) near-IR Nd:YAG lasers have also been shown to elicit some dermal remodeling (eg, GenesisPlus, Cutera Inc, Brisbane, CA).[39,40]

Another fractional nonablative resurfacing device uses 2 separate, sequentially emitted wavelengths (1320 and 1440 nm) to focus energy into both the superficial and deep dermis (Affirm Multiplex, Cynosure Inc, Westford, MA).

See **Figs. 15–18** for pretreatment and posttreatment images. These are images of all the laser and light technologies not just for the last device discussed.

AFTER CARE

Most nonsurgical treatments to the upper lid and brow have little or no recovery time and do not require complex after care. Patients can be encouraged to return to normal daily activities almost immediately. To minimize the potential for

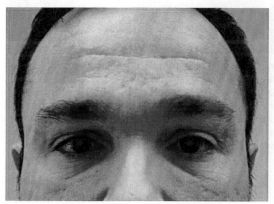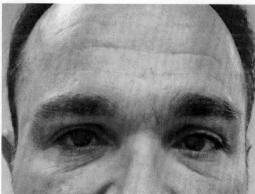

Fig. 16. Before and 4 months after "sublative rejuvenation" with a fractional bipolar radiofrequency device (eMATRIX): 5 weeks after third treatment and 4 months after first treatment. (*Courtesy of* Hema Sundaram, MD.)

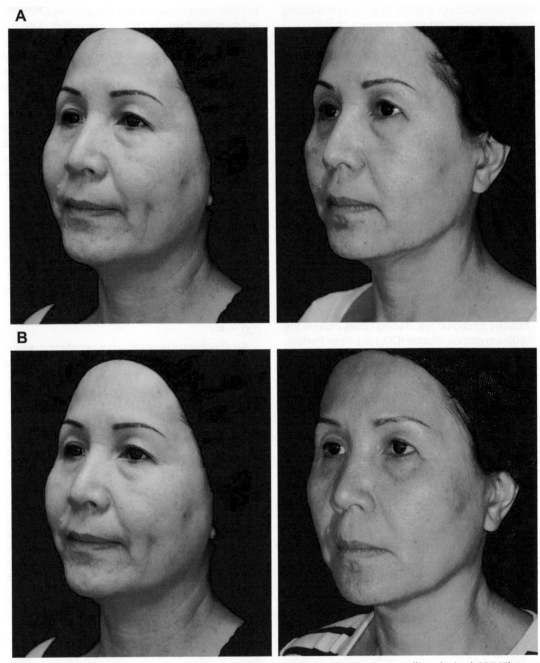

Fig. 17. (*A*) Before and 3 weeks after treatment with a fractional bipolar RF microneedling device (ePRIME): treatment has been applied to the mid and lower face including the temporal region and has a secondary upward and outward vectoring effect on the periorbital frame. (*B*) Same patient before and 14 weeks after fractional bipolar RF microneedling (ePRIME), 11 weeks after incobotulinumtoxin A (Xeomin) and calcium hydroxylapatite filler (Radiesse). Incobotulinumtoxin A was injected to orbicularis oculi (including the superolateral portion for lateral brow elevation), procerus, corrugators, frontalis and nasalis muscles, and also to the depressor anguli oris, mentalis and masseters. Filler was injected to the pre-jowl sulcus. (*Courtesy of* Hema Sundaram, MD.)

posttreatment edema, cool compresses can be applied while the patient is in the office and then for up to several days as needed after the patient returns home.

When injecting botulinum toxin neuromodulators or soft tissue fillers, ecchymosis can be diminished by the application of ice packs during and after treatment, and by the topical application of

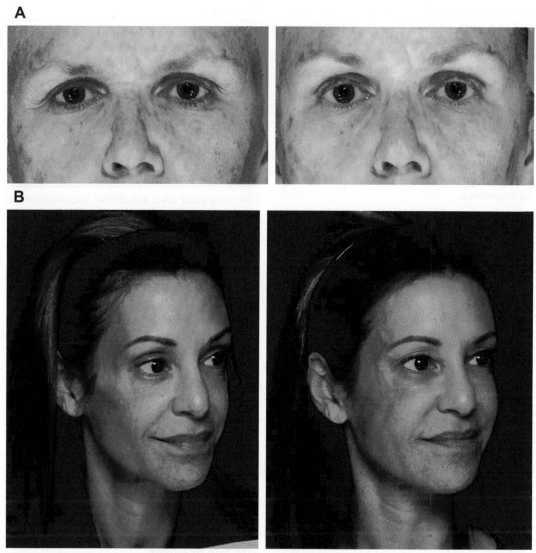

Fig. 18. (*A*) Before and 180 days after MFU (Ulthera). Multiplane delivery of ultrasound energy at tissue depths of 4.5 mm, 3 mm and 1.5 mm. (*B*) Before and 3 weeks after MFU (Ulthera), abobotulinumtoxin A (Dysport) and calcium hydroxylapatite (Radiesse) and hydrated hyaluronic acid (Prevelle Silk) filler. MFU was applied to the upper face, botulinum neurotoxin was injected to the orbicularis oculi in the crow's feet region, and fillers were injected with multiplane "sandwich" technique to the mid and lower face using blunt cannulas and sharp needles. Note volume loss throughout the periorbital frame of the first patient (*A*) and temporal hollowing in the second patient (*B*). To achieve optimal results, both patients would benefit from soft tissue filler implantation to the regions treated with MFU. (*Courtesy of* Hema Sundaram, MD.)

vitamin K oxide or arnica creams for several days following the procedure. Some patients may also benefit from sublingual arnica tablets. Thorough, sterile preparation of the skin before commencement of soft tissue filler injection and maintenance of scrupulous sterile technique during the procedure will minimize or eliminate the risk of infection or biofilm development.

Patients undergoing fractionated ablative laser treatments are instructed to perform vinegar and water soaks followed by topical application of

a petrolatum-based ointment every 4 to 6 hours for several days after the procedure, until the skin reepithelializes completely.

The recommended schedule for follow-up appointments varies according to the procedures that were performed. Patients who received fractionated ablative laser treatments can return for reevaluation 1 to 2 days afterward, to ensure the treatment sites are healing without evidence of secondary infection or other complications. A telephonic follow-up 2 to 5 days after the procedure is reassuring for patients who have received treatment with fillers, neuromodulators, nonablative or sublative lasers, RF, or MFU, and allows any immediate concerns to be addressed. These patients can then return for in-person follow-up 2 to 4 weeks after the procedure.

COMPLICATIONS

Complications arising from nonsurgical rejuvenation treatments of the upper eyelid and brow are minimized when the procedures are appropriately performed by clinicians with the requisite training and experience.

Ecchymosis

Ecchymosis and temporary tissue tenderness or swelling can arise following injection of a filler or neuromodulator.[41,42] The incidence and extent of ecchymoses can be minimized by the measures described previously, including cold compresses or ice packs before and after injection. Significant ecchymoses can be treated during the acute stage with the pulsed dye laser or yellow-green intense pulsed light, to hasten their resolution.[43]

Ptosis

Upper eyelid ptosis caused by neuromodulator injection is considered attributable to diffusion or spread of the neuromodulator through the orbital septum after injection of the glabella, such as when targeting the medial brow depressors. The incidence of ptosis is low and comparable with abobotulinumtoxin A, incobotulinumtoxin A, and onabotulinumtoxin A. The risk of ptosis may be minimized by avoidance of inappropriately high doses of neuromodulator to the glabella, and possibly by avoidance of forceful pressure on the treated areas immediately after injection.

Intravascular or Nerve Damage

The risk of intravascular filler injection or accidental nerve damage can be minimized by a thorough knowledge of facial anatomy and by application of injection techniques that are appropriate for the selected filler products and the regions to be injected, e.g. insertion of the needle at the appropriate tissue level to avoid vital structures in each facial region. Pulling back on the syringe plunger after needle insertion and before filler injection has been advocated as a method of detecting inadvertent entry of the needle into a large blood vessel. However, reflux of blood may not be apparent even if the needle is within a vessel, owing to collapse of the vessel walls under the negative pressure generated when the plunger is pulled back.

Compression

Compression of blood vessels or other vital structures is perhaps a more common concern than intravascular injection. The risk of vascular compromise due to compression can be decreased by slow, careful injection of small microaliquots of filler rather than large boluses. Selection of high-G prime fillers for facial regions where a lifting effect is required allows volume-efficient filling and removes the need for large boluses of filler.

Filler Migration

Filler migration after subdermal implantation can also be minimized by avoidance of large bolus injections and instead the use of microaliquot or serial threading technique.

Contour Irregularities

Contour irregularities, most commonly, convexities, are best prevented by avoidance of overcorrection during the procedure. Minor contour irregularities may be improved by point pressure and tissue molding. Convexities during the first 1 to 3 days after injection, especially when associated with focal tenderness and fluctuance, may be because of an underlying hematoma. Resolution of a hematoma can be hastened by following the previous recommendations for management of ecchymoses. Convexities after visible ecchymosis has resolved can be addressed by injection of hyaluronidase to dissolve the unwanted HA. The Lambros method, in which the hyaluronidase is diluted with lidocaine, has been reported to cause fewer reactions than the Vartanian method, which uses undiluted hyaluronidase.[44,45]

Infection or Biofilm

Acute or subacute infection may present as erythema, swelling, or tenderness of an area previously injected with a soft tissue filler. Biofilms, collections of bacteria that secrete a protective and adhesive matrix that is relatively impervious to antibiotics and other therapies, may present in a similar manner but with a longer incubation period. Biofilms are currently considered a rare complication of filler injections and are difficult to diagnose via standard bacterial cultures. If infection or biofilm are suspected, initiation of systemic antibiotics is the first line of treatment; macrolide antibiotics, such as clarithromycin or azithromycin, may be of particular efficacy by virtue of their effects on leukocyte chemotaxis and phagocytosis.[46] It may also be helpful to remove the injected substance, eg, through injection of hyaluronidase or even through incision and drainage or excision.

Diagnosis may be facilitated by aspiration or lesional biopsy, where appropriate.

Risk Factors for Lasers and Light Energy-Based Devices

Fractionated lasers may be preferred over nonfractionated lasers because they yield more predictable, controlled results, faster skin-healing time, and reduced risk of adverse events, such as scarring, dyschromia, and postprocedural infections.[36] For each patient, the selected device represents a balance between safety and efficacy.

Patients treated with fractionated ablative lasers (ie, CO_2 and Er:YAG) can develop secondary infections with bacteria (including atypical mycobacteria) or herpes simplex viral outbreaks following treatment. Bacterial and viral cultures (vs direct immunofluorescence) should be performed in any patient suspected of having a secondary infection following laser treatment. Appropriate empiric treatment with systemic antibiotics or antiviral medications can be initiated while awaiting culture results. *Candida* can also colonize skin after treatment with ablative lasers, and should be considered in any patient with persistent, facial erythema or an eruption of small pustules despite negative bacterial cultures and/or a course of systemic antibiotics.

SUMMARY

Nonsurgical rejuvenation of the upper eyelid and brow can yield dramatic improvement in overall facial appearance via comfortable techniques with minimal postprocedural recovery time. An appropriate *combination* of treatments, tailored specifically for each patient, is often more efficacious than any one particular treatment alone. Treatments that improve skin quality are a valuable adjunct to volume restoration to optimize eyebrow position and shape and decrease upper eyelid hooding. These results can be achieved by targeting tissue within or outside the periorbital frame. The key to formulating an effective, individualized treatment plan is to perform a thorough structural and functional analysis of each patient's face during the pre-treatment consultation. Our current understanding is that multi-level volume loss is a cardinal feature of facial aging. It therefore follows that careful assessment for volume loss and adoption of a predominantly volumetric rather than ablative approach to rejuvenation of the face, including the upper eyelid and brow, may represent a restorative strategy that yields the best results.

REFERENCES

1. Wu WT. Periorbital rejuvenation with injectable fillers. In: Cohen SR, Born TM, editors. Facial rejuvenation with fillers. Elsevier Limited; 2009. p. 93–105.
2. Benedetto AV. Cosmetic uses of botulinum toxin A in the upper face. In: Botulinum Toxins in Clinical Aesthetic Practice (Series in Cosmetic and Laser Therapy). 2nd edition. Taylor & Francis Group; 2011.
3. Putterman A. Evaluation of the cosmetic oculoplastic surgery patient. In: Cosmetic oculoplastic surgery. New York: Grune & Stratton, Inc; 1982. p. 11–26.
4. Lambros V. Observations on periorbital and midface aging. Plast Reconstr Surg 2007;120(5):1367–76.
5. Eisele KH, Fink K, Vey M, et al. Studies on the dissociation of botulinum neurotoxin type A complexes. Toxicon 2011;57(4):555–65.
6. Sundaram H, Monheit G, Goldman M, et al. Clinical experiences with hyaluronic acid fillers. J Drugs Dermatol 2012;11(3):s15–27.
7. Kablik J, Monheit G, Yu L, et al. Comparative physical properties of hyaluronic acid dermal fillers. Dermatol Surg 2009;35(Suppl 1):302S–12S.
8. Sundaram H, Voigts B, Beer K, et al. Comparison of the rheological properties of viscosity and elasticity in two categories of soft tissue fillers: calcium hydroxylapatite and hyaluronic acid. Dermatol Surg 2010;36(Suppl 3):1859S–65S.
9. Stocks D, Sundaram H, Michaels J, et al. Rheological evaluation of the physical properties of hyaluronic acid dermal fillers. J Drugs Dermatol 2011; 10(9):974–80.
10. Sundaram H, Flynn T, Cassuto D, et al. New and emerging concepts in soft tissue fillers. J Drugs Dermatol 2012;11(8):s12–25.
11. Flynn T, Sarazin D, Bezzola A, et al. Comparative histology of intradermal implantation of mono and biphasic hyaluronic acid fillers. Dermatol Surg 2011;37:637–43.
12. Shaw RB Jr, Kahn DM. Aging of the midface bony elements: a three-dimensional computed tomographic study. Plast Reconstr Surg 2007;119(2):675–81.
13. Rohrich RJ, Pessa JE. The fact compartments of the face: anatomy and clinical implications for cosmetic surgery. Plast Reconstr Surg 2007;119(7):2219–27.
14. Fagien S. New and emerging concepts in soft tissue fillers: personal perspective. J Drugs Dermatol 2012;11(8):s25.
15. Sundaram H, Carruthers J. 2013. Glabella and central brow in soft tissue augmentation ed. Carruthers J. and Carruthers A, Proc Cosmetic Derm ed. Dover J. [Elsevier].
16. Zeichner JA, Cohen JL. Use of blunt tipped cannulas for soft tissue fillers. J Drugs Dermatol 2012;11(1):70–2.
17. Cassuto D. Blunt-tipped microcannulas for filler injection: an ethical duty? J Drugs Dermatol 2012; 11(8):s42.

18. Berros P. Periorbital contour abnormalities: hollow eye ring management with hyalurostructure. Orbit 2010;29(2):119–25.

19. Sundaram H, Weinkle S, Pozner J, et al. Blunt-tipped microcannulas for the injection of soft tissue fillers: a consensus panel assessment and recommendations. J Drugs Dermatol 2012;11(8):s33–9.

20. Carruthers J, Carruthers A. A prospective, randomized, parallel group study analyzing the effect of BTX-A (Botox) and nonanimal sourced hyaluronic acid (NASHA, Restylane) in combination compared with NASHA (Restylane) alone in severe glabellar rhytides in adult female subjects: treatment of severe glabellar rhytides with a hyaluronic acid derivative compared with the derivative and BTX-A. Dermatol Surg 2003;29(8):802–9.

21. Klein AW, Fagien S. Hyaluronic acid fillers and botulinum toxin type A: rationale for their individual and combined use for injectable facial rejuvenation. Plast Reconstr Surg 2007;120(Suppl):81S.

22. Dierickx C. The role of deep heating for noninvasive skin rejuvenation. Lasers Surg Med 2006;38:700–807.

23. Hruza G, Taub A, Collier S, et al. Skin rejuvenation and wrinkle reduction using a fractional radiofrequency system. J Drugs Dermatol 2009;8(3):259–65.

24. Man J, Goldberg DJ. Safety and efficacy of fractional bipolar radiofrequency treatment in Fitzpatrick skin types V-VI. J Cosmet Laser Ther 2012;14(4):179–83.

25. Lee HS, Lee DH, Won CH, et al. Fractional rejuvenation using a novel bipolar radiofrequency system in Asian skin. Dermatol Surg 2011;37(11):1611–9.

26. Sundaram H, Truslow S. Clinical and histopathological evaluation of a fractional bipolar radiofrequency device for facial skin ablation and resurfacing. Chicago (IL): American Society for Dermatologic Surgery (ASDS) 2010 Annual Meeting.

27. Sadick N, Sato M, Palmisano D, et al. In vivo animal histology and clinical evaluation of multisource fractional radiofrequency skin resurfacing (FSR) applicator. J Cosmet Laser Ther 2011;13:204–9.

28. Friedman DJ, Gilead LT. The use of hybrid radiofrequency device for the treatment of rhytids and lax skin. Dermatol Surg 2007;33:1–9.

29. Javate RM, Cruz RT Jr, Khan J, et al. Nonablative 4-MHz dual radiofrequency wand rejuvenation treatment for periorbital rhytides and midface laxity. Ophthal Plast Reconstr Surg 2011;27(3):180–5.

30. White M, Makin I, Barthe P, et al. Selective creation of thermal injury zones in the superficial musculoaponeurotic system using intense ultrasound therapy: a new target for noninvasive facial rejuvenation. Arch Facial Plast Surg 2007;9(1):22–9.

31. White M, Makin I, Slayton M, et al. Selective transcutaneous delivery of energy to porcine soft tissues using intense ultrasound (IUS). Lasers Surg Med 2008;40(2):67–75.

32. Harris M, Sundaram H. Skin of color. American Academy of Facial and Plastic Reconstructive Surgery (AFPRS) 2012 Annual Meeting, Washington, DC.

33. Alam M, White LE, Martin N, et al. Ultrasound tightening of facial and neck skin: a rater blinded prospective cohort study. J Am Acad Dermatol 2010;62:262–9.

34. Sundaram H. Micro-focused ultrasound: a new technology for rejuvenative procedures. www.DermQuest.com. 2012. Available at: http://www.dermquest.com/Expert_Opinions/Surgery__Cosmetics/Microfocused_ultrasound_a_new_technology_for_rejuvenative_procedures.html. Accessed November 20, 2012.

35. Sundaram H. Blinded evaluation of nonsurgical lifting of the face and submental region in diverse skin types utilizing micro-focused ultrasound with novel multi-plane tissue targeting and enhanced energy delivery. Kissimmee (FL): American Society of Laser Medicine and Surgery (ASLMS) 2012 Annual Meeting.

36. Alexiades-Armenakas M, Dover J, Arndt K. The spectrum of laser skin resurfacing: nonablative, fractional, and ablative laser resurfacing. J Am Acad Dermatol 2008;58(5):719–37.

37. Rostan E, Fitzpatrick R, Goldman M. Laser resurfacing with a long pulse erbium:YAG laser compared to the 950 ms CO2 laser. Lasers Surg Med 2001;29:136–41.

38. Ross E, Miller C, Meehan K, et al. One-pass CO2 versus multiple-pass Er:YAG laser resurfacing in the treatment of rhytides: a comparison side-by-side study of pulsed CO2 and Er:YAG lasers. Dermatol Surg 2001;27:709–15.

39. Goldberg D, Whitworth J. Laser skin resurfacing with the Q-switched Nd:YAG laser. Dermatol Surg 1997;23:903–7.

40. Sumian C, Pitre F, Gauthier B, et al. Laser skin resurfacing using a frequency doubled Nd:YAG laser after topical application of an exogenous chromophore. Lasers Surg Med 1999;25:43–50.

41. Lemperle G, Rullan PR, Gauthier-Hazan N. Avoiding and treating dermal filler complications. Plast Reconstr Surg 2006;118:92S–107S.

42. Gladstone HB, Cohen JL. Adverse effects when injecting facial fillers. Semin Cutan Med Surg 2007;26:34–9.

43. DeFatta RJ, Krishna S, Williams EF. Pulsed-dye laser for treating ecchymoses after facial cosmetic procedures. Arch Facial Plast Surg 2009;11(2):99–103.

44. Lambros V. The use of hyaluronidase to reverse the effects of hyaluronic acid filler. Plast Reconstr Surg 2004;114:277.

45. Andre P, Levy PM. Hyaluronidase offers an efficacious treatment for inaesthetic hyaluronic acid overcorrection. J Cosmet Dermatol 2007;6(3):159–62.

46. Gao X, Ray R, Xiao Y, et al. Macrolide antibiotics improve chemotactic and phagocytic capacity as well as reduce inflammation in sulfur mustard-exposed monocytes. Pulm Pharmacol Ther 2010;23(2):97–106.

Esthetic Rejuvenation of the Temple

Amy E. Rose, MD[a], Doris Day, MD, MA[a,b],*

KEYWORDS

- Temple hollowing • Soft tissue fillers • Temple augmentation

KEY POINTS

- Loss of volume in the temples is an early sign of aging that is often overlooked by both the physician and the patient.
- Augmentation of the temple using soft tissue fillers improves the contours of the upper face with the secondary effect of lengthening and lifting the lateral brow.
- After replacement of volume, treatment of the overlying skin with skin tightening devices or laser resurfacing help to complete a comprehensive rejuvenation of the temple and upper one-third of the face.

INTRODUCTION

The approval by the Food and Drug Administration (FDA) of the first injectable hyaluronic acid in 2003 (Restylane; Medicis, Scottsdale, AZ) marked the beginning of the modern era of global or pan-facial soft tissue augmentation. Since 2003, the armamentarium of available fillers has expanded exponentially and the emphasis has shifted from a relatively myopic view of filling lines, such as the nasolabial folds, to a more global one that values the face as a complete, cohesive esthetic unit. Esthetic physicians began to appreciate that completely effaced nasolabial folds appear unnatural. Furthermore, a perfectly corrected lower face appears mismatched in the setting of a neglected middle and upper face. This type of esthetic has been termed the "Picasso Face," in that one area of the face is overexaggerated and stylized compared with a neighboring area of the face that has not been addressed at all.[1] Included in a more global view of facial rejuvenation is increased attention to volume restoration of the upper and lateral face in areas such as the

temples. The temples are often neglected by both physicians and patients when planning a strategy for global volume restoration. Temporal rejuvenation, however, has the potential to make a major impact in terms of imparting a more youthful shape to the face.

The youthful temple is convex and continuous with the zygomatic arch, such that the outline of the lateral orbital rim is not appreciable and the entire length of the eyebrow is visible from the frontal view. With age, the temporal fossa becomes concave, which emphasizes the bony outline of the lateral orbital rim and pulls the tail of the lateral eyebrow posteriorly, contributing to an overall skeletonized and peanut-shaped appearance of the face (Fig. 1). Hollowing of the temples is a change that often occurs at a relatively young age in thin patients but rarely represents a specific chief concern of a patient seeking cosmetic consultation. Patients more often notice and seek treatment for the fine lines and wrinkles without an appreciation that these are merely a symptom of a larger issue of global volume depletion. Additionally, there are no soft tissue

a The Ronald O. Perelman Department of Dermatology, New York University Langone Medical Center, 550 1st Avenue, New York, NY 10016, USA; b Day Dermatology and Aesthetics, 10 East 70th Street, 1C, New York, NY 10021, USA
* Corresponding author.
E-mail address: doris.daymd@gmail.com

Clin Plastic Surg 40 (2013) 77–89
http://dx.doi.org/10.1016/j.cps.2012.09.001

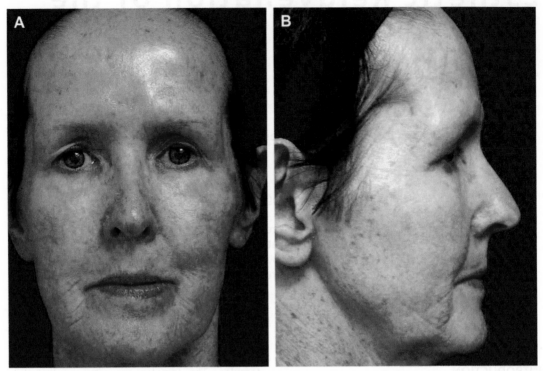

Fig. 1. Volume loss in the temples (*A*) and jawline (*B*) cause the face to appear less wide than it truly is. (*From* Obagi S. Specific techniques for fat transfer. Facial Plast Surg Clin N Am 2008;16:403; with permission.)

fillers that have FDA approval for use in the temples, which may explain, at least in part, some of the reluctance to treat this area.

The ideal esthetic appearance of a youthful face is not a static image but rather one that changes to reflect the societal values and popular culture of the time. In the mid-1990s, the "heroin chic" esthetic popularized by designer Calvin Klein and super model Kate Moss emphasized features of wasting and cachexia reminiscent of drug addiction. Pale skin, dark under-eye circles, and temporal hollowing were key elements of this esthetic. By the end of the 1990s, the heroin chic era had largely ended after the overdose of fashion photographer Davide Sorrenti and the rise in popularity of Gisele Bundchen and other models with more "healthy" proportions of the face and body. Additionally, with the development of protease inhibitors for the treatment of HIV, facial wasting became socially stigmatizing, leading to FDA approval of both poly-L-lactic acid (PLLA) and calcium hydroxylapatite (CaHA) for the treatment of HIV-associated lipodystrophy. It is still important to obtain an adequate sense of the patient's esthetic ideals before augmenting any area of the face, as there are patients who prefer a more hollowed out look with prominent facial bones.

Age-related changes in the face affect the overlying epidermis, dermis, subcutaneous fat, muscle, and bone. A comprehensive approach to rejuvenation of the temples must take into account all of these changes. Augmentation with soft tissue filler primarily addresses the age-related changes of the bone, muscle, and fat, whereas laser-resurfacing and skin-tightening devices can address the overlying changes in the dermis and epidermis.

CLINICAL ANATOMY OF THE TEMPORAL FOSSA
Bony Landmarks

One of the reasons why dermal fillers are underused in the temporal fossa may be an unfamiliarity or uncertainty with the underlying anatomy. The term "temples" typically refers to the temporal fossa, which is a shallow depression on the lateral sides of the skull between the forehead and the cheek. The bony landmarks of the temple include the superior temporal line, the frontal process of the zygomatic bone anteriorly, and the zygomatic bone inferiorly.[2] Clinically, the hairline marks the posterior-most aspect of the temple.

Fascial Layers

The layers of the temple from superficial to deep include the skin, subcutaneous fat, temporoparietal fascia, deep temporal fascia, temporalis muscle, and temporal bone. The superficial temporal artery and vein course through and are the vascular supply to the temporoparietal fascia, which is immediately deep to subcutaneous fat and is the equivalent of the superficial musculoaponeurotic system (SMAS) below the zygomatic arch. Superiorly, the temporoparietal fascia integrates with the epicranial aponeurosis of the forehead and scalp.[2] The temporal branch of the facial nerve, which innervates the frontalis, corrugator supercilii, procerus, and obicularis oculi, also traverses the temporal fossa, where it lies within the temporoparietal fascia. This is in contrast to areas below the zygomatic arch, where the branches of the facial nerve are deep to the SMAS.

Below the temporoparietal fascia is the deep temporal fascia, which contains the middle temporal artery, a branch of the superficial temporal artery. The deep temporal fascia divides into a superficial and deep layer that envelopes the temporal fat pad approximately 2 to 3 cm above the zygomatic arch.[2] Arising from the deep temporal fascia is the temporalis muscle, which fans out over the surface of the temple (**Fig. 2**). The temporalis muscle lifts and retracts the mandible.

EVALUATION

Age-related changes occur at all levels of the temple from the bone up to the epidermis. Loss of bony substance in the temple, in conjunction with atrophy of the temporalis muscle and wasting of the temporal fat pad, contribute to a gaunt,

skeletonized appearance in which the bony outline of the zygomatic arch and the temporal line become more pronounced. These changes become even more prominent in patients who have been previously augmented over the zygoma. Important factors to assess before initiating a strategy for facial rejuvenation include skin elasticity, loss of subcutaneous volume, adherence of the skin to the SMAS, and loss of skeletal support.[3] A complete medical and medication history should be obtained with particular attention to history of autoimmune disease, keloids, current pregnancy, breast feeding, and herpetic infection. Medications known to increase the risk of postprocedure bleeding and bruising include nonsteroidal anti-inflammatories, aspirin, vitamin E, garlic, gingko, ginger, St John's wort, gingseng, fish oil, and other herbal supplements.[4] If medically reasonable, these medications should be stopped 2 weeks before treatment and the intake of alcohol should be minimized before and after treatment.[5]

History of prior brow lift or facelift can affect the strategy for injection, as the development of scar tissue in the temple can alter the integrity of the fascial planes. It is also important to evaluate the temporal skin, as the presence of overlying rhytides and photodamage can negate or significantly detract from the rejuvenation obtained from soft tissue augmentation. It is important to listen carefully to patients' preferences; gain an appreciation of their esthetic ideals; and educate them on the risks, benefits, and alternatives of temple rejuvenation.

It is generally advised that the patient be evaluated and marked in an upright sitting position that captures the effects of gravitational forces on the anatomy, contour, and shadowing of the face. Preexisting asymmetry should be

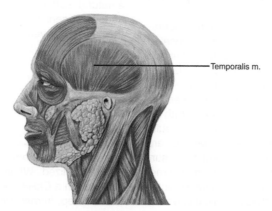

Temporalis m.

Fig. 2. Muscles of facial expression. (*From* Azzizadeh B, et al. Master techniques in facial rejuvenation. Philadelphia, PA, USA: Elsevier; 2007; with permission.)

documented and discussed thoroughly with the patient. Written informed consent should be obtained, and off-label use of the products disclosed. Preprocedure and postprocedure photography is a key component to managing patient expectations. In the case of temporal augmentation, it is particularly important to take pictures from several angles other than the frontal view to fully demonstrate the improvement in the contour. It has been suggested that oblique views with standardized lighting are best, while recognizing that the subtle 3-dimensional changes can often only be fully appreciated in person.[6]

PATIENT PERSPECTIVE

Although most patients do not specifically recognize or request temporal augmentation, it likely contributes to their overall sense of appearing older. Common chief complaints of patients with temporal wasting include "looking tired" or an impression that the "face is falling."[7] Although the ideal facial shape differs among cultures, a heart-shaped contour that is widest at the temples and narrowest at the chin is often a cosmetically desirable result and can be obtained via augmentation of the temples. Before injection of the temples with filler, local anesthetic or saline can be injected to give the patient a preview of the expected result.[8] Loss of volume in the temples also contributes to the appearance of brow ptosis, as the lateral tail of the eyebrow descends into the hollowness of the temple. Augmenting the temples has the additional effect of bringing the tail of the brow anteriorly, which makes it appear longer and higher when the patient is viewed from the front. Augmentation of the temples should be one part of a global strategy for improving the volume loss of the upper and middle face.

When selecting a filler for temporal augmentation, patients should be thoroughly counseled regarding the differences between hyaluronic acid (HA) fillers and biostimulatory injectables, such as CaHA and PLLA. Particularly with PLLA, patients should understand that the effect is gradual and requires a series of injections. With regard to skin-tightening procedures, the results using nonablative laser or energy devices are subtle compared with those obtained from surgical lifting, but have considerably less downtime. It is crucial that patients have appropriate expectations and understand that these medical interventions are an alternative, not a substitute, for plastic surgery.

PROCEDURE
Temporal Augmentation with Soft Tissue Fillers

Augmentation of the temples can be achieved using autologous fat or fillers, such as HA, CaHA, PLLA, or silicone. Currently, none of the fillers have an FDA indication for augmentation of the temples, and thus patients must be informed that this is an off-label use. The temple, however, serves as an ideal area of the face for an FDA indication, because it is a discrete anatomic location with well-defined borders. The bony landmarks of the temple form a discrete indentation similar to a pool or lake and thus the degree of filling or hollowing can easily be appreciated based on how close the "water" is to being level with the surrounding ground. We propose a scale of temporal hollowing, graded from 0 through 4, with 0 representing a completely contiguous and smooth transition between the zygoma and the lateral temporal line and 4 representing severe atrophy with prominence of the zygoma and bones of the lateral orbit.

Factors to consider when selecting a filler for the temporal region include the onset of the effect, the texture of the product, the longevity of the result, and the safety profile. HA fillers result in an immediate augmentation, have a soft and natural appearance under the skin, and last for approximately 12 months.[6] They are generally considered to be safe, with few serious adverse reactions reported in the literature and no immunogenicity. Additionally, one key advantage of HA fillers is that they are easily reversible with hyaluronidase in the event of vascular occlusion or patient dissatisfaction. PLLA (Sculptra Aesthetic; Sanofi-Aventis, Bridgewater, NJ) is also commonly used for temporal augmentation and provides a gradual volumizing effect over several months. Advantages of PLLA include a natural, soft look that incorporates the endogenous collagen. Disadvantages include cost and the need for several treatments. CaHA (Radiesse, Merz Aesthetics, San Mateo, CA), like Sculptra, is considered a biostimulatory filler with effects that develop gradually over time, but also has an immediately appreciable effect on volume at the time of injection.

Planes of Injection for Augmentation

The appropriate plane of injection depends on the product utilized. When using the semipermanent fillers, such a CaHA and PLLA, the plane of injection is deep, immediately over the periosteum. A deep plane of injection minimizes the chance of inadvertent intravascular injection or injury to the nerves and vasculature as they run significantly more superficial through the temporal fossa. HA fillers may be injected deep or more superficially in the subcutaneous plane with blunt-tip micro-cannulas. Deeper injections of HA fillers typically require more product than superficial.

Hyaluronic Acid

There are currently no controlled clinical studies that evaluate the safety or efficacy of any of the dermal fillers for temporal augmentation. In a retro-spective review of 20 female patients, Moradi and colleagues[7] described their technique for temporal augmentation using Restylane. Patients were prep-ped and treated with topical anesthetic ointment for 15 minutes. A 30-gauge needle was inserted perpendicular to the skin through the dermis, at which point the angle was adjusted to 45° such that the plane of injection of the filler was immedi-ately above the superficial temporal fascia. Approx-imately 0.05 to 0.10 mL of filler was injected at each site using an anterograde, retrograde, or depot injection technique with an average total volume of 0.95 mL needed to fill each temporal fossa. All patients self-reported satisfaction with the augmen-tation, which was sustained for at least 6 months in all cases. There were no adverse events reported other than mild tenderness and bruising.

Ross and Malhotra[6] also reported their experi-ence with temporal augmentation in a series of 20 patients using Perlane (Medicis). After the patient was prepped and anesthetized, a 27-gauge needle was inserted, bevel down, in the plane of the super-ficial temporal fascia. At each of the 3 injection sites, 0.5 mL of product was placed along the ante-rior temple and then massaged to prevent contour irregularities. Patients received a mean of 0.9 mL of filler per temple, with a reported duration of effect of approximately 1 year. Complications included postprocedure prominence of the superficial vein, bruising, and discomfort with chewing.[6]

Poly-L-lactic Acid

PLLA (Sculptra Aesthetic; Sanofi-Aventis) is a biodegradable alpha-hydroxy acid material con-sisting of PLLA microparticles, sodium carboxy-methylcellulose, and mannitol that has been used for other medical applications, such as absorbable sutures, for many years.[3] FDA approved in 2004 for the treatment of HIV-associated lipodystrophy, it was also granted FDA approval in July 2009 for cosmetic indications, including correction of na-solabial fold defects and other facial wrinkles. As with the other soft tissue fillers, use in the temporal region is off-label. PLLA is considered a biostimulatory product that promotes the

deposition of collagen over time by stimulating an inflammatory tissue response. In contrast to HA fillers, the effects of PLLA are more gradual in onset and require 2 to 8 injections every 4 to 6 weeks over the course of several months de-pending on the degree of volume deficit. PLLA lasts longer than HA fillers with a duration of action of up to 2 years.[9]

The biostimulatory effect of PLLA is dependent on the host response; thus, only patients with intact immune systems are good candidates for PLLA injections. The main advantages of PLLA include its biostimulatory method of action and the increased duration of up to 2 years. One of the disadvantages of PLLA is that the correction is gradual and dependent on the robustness of the host response, thus making it difficult for the injector to gauge the appropriate end point for correction at the time of injection. Because of a certain degree of unpredictability with PLLA, great caution must be taken to avoid overcorrec-tion. Another potential deterrent to the use of PLLA is the cost and the need for repeat treat-ments over the course of several months. Although the price of injections varies based on geography and the practitioner, the cost to the patient per vial of PLLA is approximately $900.[3]

Although the package insert recommends reconstitution with only 5 mL of sterile water 2 hours before treatment, most practitioners use a dilution of at least 8 mL with varying combina-tions of sterile or bacteriostatic saline and 1% or 2% lidocaine. The use of epinephrine depends on the preferences of the injector. Some believe that it improves hemostasis while others believe that the vasoconstrictive effect can mask evidence of impending vascular compromise. After reconstitution, the vial is gently swirled with care to avoid rigorous shaking that can lead to formation of foam that can obstruct the needle. Patient preparation includes cleansing the face with soap and water and application of topical anesthetic. It is worth noting that some practitioners do not use topical anesthesia, believing that the proper plane of injection for PLLA is far deeper than can be penetrated by topical medications.[9] A 3-mL syringe with a 25-G or 26-G needle can be used. PLLA is in-jected in the supraperiosteal plane, deep to the temporalis fascia, using a depot technique with boluses of 0.3 to 3.0 mL, followed by firm massage.[1]

Calcium Hydroxylapatite

CaHA (Radiesse, Merz Aesthetics) is considered a "combined filler," with both gradual biostimulatory properties and immediate space-filling effects. The composition of CaHA is 30% CaHA small-particle (25–45 μm) microspheres suspended in 70% aqueous gel composed of 6.4% glycerin and 1.3% sodium carboxymethylcellulose.[10] Because the calcium microspheres are the same as the components of human bone and teeth, CaHA is biocompatible and does not require sensitivity testing before use. The immediate filling effect is a result of the aqueous carrier, which is eventually absorbed over time, leaving behind the calcium microspheres to serve as a scaffold for the growth of new tissue stimulated by the local fibrohistiocytic response. Eventually, at approximately 9 months, the microspheres are also absorbed and eliminated from the body as calcium and phosphate ions through the kidneys. The duration of volume correction after CaHA is reported to be 10 to 14 months, with shorter duration in areas with high mobility and frequent muscle movement, such as the nasolabial fold.[10,11] A "booster" injection 3 months after the initial treatment may prolong the effect for as long as 15 to 18 months.[4] Radiesse gained FDA approval in 2006 for the correction of moderate to severe facial wrinkles and folds and for correction of HIV-associated lipoatrophy. The use of CaHA for temporal augmentation is considered an off-label use.

Like PLLA, the plane of injection for CaHA in the temples is immediately superior the periosteum. Because the plane of injection is deep, pain control is an important consideration, as this affects both the patient's perception of the outcome and his or her desire to return for additional treatment. Compared with HA fillers, injection of CaHA is associated with more discomfort regardless of the plane of injection. In 2009, the FDA officially approved the injection technique of adding lidocaine to the CaHA syringe immediately before injection, which dramatically improved pain control and reduced the need for regional nerve blocks. In this technique, 0.15 to 0.20 mL of 2% plain lidocaine is drawn up in a 3-mL syringe and attached to the 1.3-mL or 1.5-mL syringe of Radiesse using the female-to-female luer lock connector provided separately in the Merz Aesthetics Accessory Kit. The 2 syringes are pushed back and forth, pushing the Radiesse into the lidocaine first, until a smooth mixture is obtained.[11] It should be noted, however, that the addition of lidocaine at a concentration of 0.3% will decrease the viscosity and elasticity of Radiesse to the level of medium-viscosity and elasticity HA fillers such as Restylane and Perlane. This in turn reduces the degree of lifting that can be obtained with a given volume.[12]

CaHA is injected with a 27-gauge, 1.25-inch or 28-gauge, 0.75-inch needle using a variety of injection techniques, including retrograde, linear, fanning, or cross-hatching. For temporal augmentation, many injectors prefer a bolus depot technique followed by firm massage to prevent nodules.[4] CaHA can safely be combined with laser or light therapies such as intense pulsed light (IPL) or nonablative fractional resurfacing to address overlying photodamage. Studies have also shown that CaHA is not altered after radiofrequency heating; thus, combination with skin-tightening procedures is also safe.[10] Similarly, other products, such as HA fillers, can be layered with CaHA to address the more superficial lines that remain after the volume deficit has been addressed.[13] One advantage of CaHA in the temples is that, because of its high viscosity and elasticity relative to HA fillers, a smaller volume is generally required to produce the same degree of correction.[12] Because the temple can sometimes require larger volumes for adequate correction, the semipermanent fillers have the potential to be more cost effective for the patient. A large-particle CaHA has FDA approval for the treatment of urinary incontinence, and there are preliminary data in 3 case reports suggesting that it is safe when injected in the middle face and may have longer-lasting clinical effects relative to the small-particle Radiesse.[14] The larger-size particles, however, necessitated the use of a larger-bore needle (21 gauge) and regional nerve blocks for adequate anesthesia.

Authors' Technique for Temporal Augmentation

For temporal augmentation, the authors have found the semipermanent biostimulatory fillers PLLA (Sculptra) and CaHA (Radiesse) to produce the best results and to be the most time and cost effective for the patient. PLLA is reconstituted at least 24 hours before the procedure with 8 mL of bacteriostatic water. Immediately before injection, 1 mL of 2% lidocaine with epinephrine is added to the vial. Once reconstituted, PLLA should be refrigerated and can be stored for up to 3 to 4 weeks. Using a 3-mL syringe with a 25-gauge, 1.0-inch or 1.5-inch needle, the plane of injection is deep, just above the periosteum with aspiration before injection (**Fig. 3**). A depot bolus technique is used, starting at the front of the hairline and proceeding anteriorly to the medial aspect of the eyebrow, which provides a secondary effect of lifting the tail of the brow. Typically, 2 to 4 injection points are needed for adequate augmentation. Keeping the injecting thumb off the plunger until

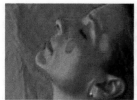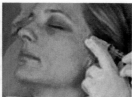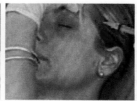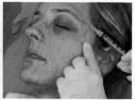

Fig. 3. Series of supraperiosteal injections with PLLA. (*From* Fitzgerald R, Vleggaar D. Using poly-L-lactic acid to mimic volume in multiple tissue layers. J Drugs Dermatol 2009;8(Suppl 10):S10; with permission.)

the needle is in the plane of injection helps to prevent inadvertent deposition of product in the muscle, and brisk injections in succession will avoid clogging of the needle. At the initial visit, 1 to 2 vials are used with no more than 2 vials used in a single visit. Subsequent visits are timed 1 month apart for 1 to 2 visits and then every 6 to 8 weeks for additional visits. Ice packs are applied immediately postprocedure and patients are instructed to massage the area 3 to 5 times per day for 5 minutes for 5 days. Postprocedure complications are minimal with some patients complaining of a mild soreness in the jawline. When using Radiesse, the injection technique is the same, using approximately 0.3 to 0.5 mL of product per side with molding and massage to avoid overcorrection and nodule formation.

Resurfacing and Skin Tightening

Once the underlying contour and volume defects have been corrected, it is important to also address the texture, color, and draping of the overlying temporal skin. Periorbital rhytides may become more prominent after volume correction of the temple and should be treated with botulinum toxin. Additionally, the temples are a common place for acne scars, which may also become more prominent after temporal augmentation and should also be addressed as part of global rejuvenation strategy. The use of laser, light, and other energy sources to address aging skin in a nonablative or fractionally ablative way that spares the epidermis is becoming increasingly popular and serves to complement soft tissue augmentation. There are also many nonsurgical skin-tightening devices that are well suited to address skin laxity in the periorbital and temporal region.

Nonablative and Ablative Fractional Resurfacing

The concept of fractional photothermolysis was a major breakthrough in the field of nonsurgical rejuvenation. Fully ablative CO2 resurfacing, which had been the gold standard for the treatment of photoaging for more than 10 years, was made

virtually obsolete with the introduction of fractional lasers. In contrast to fully ablative CO2, which removes a contiguous layer of the epidermis, fractional lasers create small cores of injury termed microthermal zones with intact skin left between the cores. The 1550-nm erbium-doped laser served as the prototype of fractional resurfacing lasers and is still commonly used, often in combination with other wavelengths that target superficial epidermal pigmentation. Like the CO2 laser (10,600 nm), the target chromophore is also water, but the 1550-nm wavelength is only moderately absorbed relative to the CO2 laser, resulting in what is termed "nonablative" thermal injury.[15] The 1550-nm wavelength creates zones of thermal injury in the dermis topped with epidermal necrotic debris and an intact stratum corneum. Subsequent improvement in skin texture and tightness likely results from the stimulation of normal collagen production as a response to dermal injury. There is virtually no down time associated with the nonablative fractional lasers, and thus it serves as a useful adjunct to temple augmentation in patients with early, mild signs of photoaging in the skin overlying the temples.

The fully ablative CO2 offers the most dramatic results with the most down time, and the nonablative fractional lasers have no down time but have fairly modest results. In 2007, the concept of fractionally ablative CO2 resurfacing emerged as a response to the unmet need for a resurfacing laser with more dramatic results than nonablative lasers but with less downtime than the fully ablative CO2. Fractional ablative lasers have FDA clearance for the treatment of rhytides, textural abnormalities, pigmented lesions, and vascular dyschromia.[15] Like the 1550-nm erbium-doped fractional laser, the CO2 fractional ablative laser also creates microthermal zones of injury, but the core is ablative (rather than thermal) and extends full thickness from the stratum corneum to the dermis with depths of 1300 μm depending on the wavelength and energy.[16] These full-thickness zones of injury yield better skin-tightening results than the nonablative lasers and equivalent or possibly better results than traditional resurfacing because of the greater depth of penetration into the dermis.[17] In addition to the fractional CO2 (10,600 nm), there is also a fractional erbium (Er): YAG (2940 nm) and a yttrium aluminum garnet (YSGG) (2790 nm) that deliver the same type of ablative microscopic columns. All of these wavelengths have water as their target chromophore, thus causing controlled damage to collagen, blood vessels, and epidermal keratinocytes.[15] The CO2 laser has a lower absorption coefficient for water than the Er:YAG laser, resulting in more collateral thermal injury but better hemostasis and, in general, a better clinical result.[18] Some of the fractional CO2 devices have adjustable spot sizes and shapes that allow for more precise coverage of geometric areas of the face, such as periorbital region. The recovery time after fractional CO2 resurfacing is approximately 1 week, with full reepithelialization at 3 to 6 days.[16] A comprehensive approach to rejuvenation of the temples requires attention to the quality and texture of the periorbital skin. Fractional ablative lasers, including the CO2 and Er:YAG lasers have been shown to reduce periorbital rhytides by 10% to 20% in a single treatment, with both types of laser equally effective.[19] Multiple sessions are likely required to maximize results.

Nonablative Radiofrequency Skin Tightening

Radiofrequency (RF) generates an electric current that produces heat via resistance in the dermis and subcutaneous tissue without damage to the overlying epidermis. The depth of penetration into the skin depends on the shape of the handpiece used and the impedance of the tissue. The skin-tightening effect of RF is believed to result from immediate contraction of collagen fibrils that denature on heating with subsequent neocollagenesis as part of a longer-term wound-healing process that occurs over several months.[20] Two commonly used RF devices include Thermage (Thermage, Hayward, CA) and Pellevé (Ellman International, Oceanside, NY). Thermage is a 6-MHz monopolar RF device that is FDA approved for treatment of rhytides and wrinkles, including eyelid treatment and for temporary improvement of cellulite. Pretreatment application of topical lidocaine for 1 hour with or without adjunctive oral analgesia is usually adequate anesthesia for the procedure. The treatment areas are marked in a grid pattern of 1 × 1-cm squares using a template that is supplied by the manufacturer of the device. Coupling gel is applied to the treatment areas, and the tissue is then heated to 65 to 75°C, which is believed to be the critical temperature for denaturization of collagen.[21] A cooling tip

protects the overlying epidermis, and the patient is monitored closely during treatment for any signs of epidermal injury, such as vesiculation. The initial Thermage protocols called for the maximum tolerable energy in a single pass, which was subsequently revised to multiple passes at lower energies after reported cases of tissue depression over the temple and the middle cheek.[22] Treatment end point is based on the patient's feedback regarding the degree of heat sensation and the clinical end point of appreciable skin tightening. The use of Thermage is contraindicated in patients with pacemakers and should not be used over areas that contain metal implants or hardware.

Pellevé can deliver monopolar or bipolar RF depending on the handpiece used and is FDA approved for treatment of mild to moderate facial wrinkles in skin types I to IV. A treatment gel ensures proper coupling of the device, and the Pellevé electrodes are moved in a circular pattern over the skin with 3 to 4 passes that raise the skin temperature to 42°C.[23] The total treatment time for the entire face is approximately 35 minutes. The primary difference between the 2 devices is that the Pellevé delivers the RF continuously in contrast to the Thermage, which delivers pulsed RF. Some argue that the continuous RF allows for a safer, more controlled delivery of RF, although there are no randomized controlled studies that compare the 2 devices. In contrast to Thermage, treatment with Pellevé does not require anesthesia or external cooling of the skin. Patient feedback regarding the sensation of heat is important to prevent overheating, and the temperature of the skin is closely monitored throughout the procedure. Additionally, the Pellevé system has many different sizes and shapes of handpieces, including rounded tips that can be used depending on the anatomic area being treated, and thus is well suited for treatment on the face. Similarly, the Thermage device has 2 levels of shallow-depth tips used to treat the eyelids, periorbital region, hand, and lips; medium-depth tips for the face and neck; and deeper tips for body contouring. Patients typically require 2 to 3 treatments with Pellevé, spaced 1 month apart, with the effect lasting for up to 2 years.[23,24] One advantage of Thermage is that clinical results are usually seen after only a single treatment session. The cost of Thermage is generally more than Pellevé because of increased cost of disposable treatment heads that must be changed with every treatment. Patients must be counseled that the effects of nonablative skin tightening are sometimes subtle and often are combined with fractional resurfacing or other modalities to obtain the best clinical result. Like other nonablative interventions, patients should be counseled that the results are not comparable to those obtained with surgery. Both of the skin-tightening devices serve to complement soft tissue augmentation in the temporal region.

Intense Focused Ultrasound Skin Tightening

Intense focused ultrasound (IFUS) works via acoustic energy that creates friction between molecules and leads to the generation of heat and focal tissue damage.[25] Ultrasound energy has been used for several years in the treatment of benign and malignant tumors of the prostate. More recently, the technology has been refined and adapted for more focal applications at much lower energies. Energy levels of up to 100 J are used to debulk macroscopic tumors compared with the nominal amounts of 0.5 to 8.0 J used in skin-tightening procedures.

Focused ultrasound creates inverted conical-shaped zones of thermal coagulation of approximately 1 mm^3 with a depth of penetration up to 4.5 mm beneath the skin, depending on the settings used.[26] The energy is localized to the dermis and subcutis, sparing of the overlying epidermis and eliminating the need for active cooling. Ulthera (Ulthera Inc, Mesa, AZ) was FDA approved in 2006 for nonsurgical brow lifting and integrates ultrasound visualization, which allows the operator to control the depth of penetration of the energy. In contrast to lasers, ultrasound devices are capable of selectively delivering energy to the subcutis, sparing the overlying dermis and epidermis. Additionally, the absorption of ultrasound energy is based on the inherent properties of the tissue, not a specific chromophore, thus the melanin content of the skin does not play a role in the treatment settings.[26,27] In turn, the use of ultrasound devices are an attractive alternative to laser-based therapies in patients with skin of color.

In 2010, Alam and colleagues[25] specifically evaluated the efficacy of focused ultrasound skin tightening in treating the upper face in the context of full face and neck treatment. The study was a rater-blinded, prospective cohort study of 35 patients treated with IFUS to the forehead, temples, cheeks, submental, and sides of the neck with varying depths (range 3.0–4.5 mm) and energies (range 0.4–1.2 J) depending on the anatomic site. The thickness of the skin in the temples is 6 mm, which is thicker than the forehead, which ranges from 3.5 to 5.0 mm, but is slighter thinner than the cheeks, which are 5 to 8 mm thick. For the forehead and temples, the 7-MHz probe was used, which obtains a depth of 4.5 mm.

Preparation included the application of topical lidocaine/tetracaine for 45 minutes, followed by cleansing of the face with soap and water. The proper coupling of the device to the skin and the depth is confirmed using the ultrasound imaging function. The pulses are delivered in a series of lines, with 17 coagulative zones per line, 2 seconds per line, and spaced 3 to 5 mm apart. Treatment of the entire face was completed in 15 to 25 minutes. Three blinded reviewers were asked to identify the pretreatment and posttreatment (90 days) photographs, with the procedure considered successful if the photographs were identified correctly, a failure if they were identified incorrectly, or no change if there was no appreciable difference. Improvement in brow position was evaluated similarly, with any improvement noted between pretreatment and posttreatment photographs considered to be significant. Of the 35 subjects, 86% had improvement in eyebrow lift with a mean change in brow height of 1.9 mm.[25] Thus, the combination of temporal augmentation, which brings the tail of the brow anteriorly with skin-tightening procedures that lift the brow superiorly, has the potential to provide multidimensional improvement to the upper face.

Combining Procedures

As mentioned previously, a comprehensive approach to rejuvenation of the temples requires attention to all aspects of the upper one-third of the face, particularly the periorbital region. The restoration of the normal contours and volume of the temples must be complemented by other approaches to address periorbital rhytides, photodamage, and laxity. The combination of soft tissue filler, neurotoxin, laser resurfacing, and skin tightening addresses all aspects of the aging temple. Opinions differ, however, regarding the appropriate order and temporal spacing of these procedures. The combination of filler and neurotoxin is commonly used in all areas of the face and can safely be performed at the same office visit. Particularly in the case of temporal augmentation, in which the plane of injection is deep to the subcutaneous tissue, it is unlikely that there would be any complication arising from procedures such as injection of botulinum toxin superficially into the orbicularis occuli or resurfacing procedures. It is worth considering, however, that after injection of PLLA or Radiesse into the temple, there is a significant amount of posttreatment massage, which may increase the possibility, although slim, of diffusion of botulinum toxin across the bony orbit and into the ocular muscles, leading to ptosis. Similarly, it may be prudent to separate temple augmentation from skin-tightening procedures with devices such as Ulthera, which have the capability of penetrating deep to fascia. Patient comfort must of course also be taken into consideration, limiting the number of procedures that can be performed at a single visit.

AFTER CARE

There should be minimal to no downtime associated with temporal augmentation, with only mild swelling postinjection. For patients treated with HA filler, some advocate the application of gentle pressure to the temple intermittently throughout the first evening after injection to reduce the chance of bruising and contour irregularities.[8] Other injectors advise patients to avoid exercise and direct pressure on the temples for at least 72 hours.[6] It is believed that the use of supplements, such as Arnica Montana, bromelain (a derivative of pineapple), and vitamin K may reduce postinjection ecchymosis.[10] Ice packs and analgesics are advised to minimize postprocedure swelling and pain. There are differing opinions with regard to the frequency and duration of massage needed after PLLA to prevent the formation of nodules. Many advocate the "5-5-5" posttreatment schedule: massaging 5 times per day, for 5 minutes, for 5 days. Others believe that immediate posttreatment massage in the office and the same evening is enough to prevent nodules if the injection technique is correct. In a case series of 106 consecutive patients treated with PLLA, Schierle and Casas[3] suggested that pretreatment and posttreatment with nightly 0.025% topical tretinoin dramatically improved outcomes in terms of the skin quality and the degree of neocollagenesis. They hypothesized that there may be a synergistic effect between retinoids and the biostimulatory effects of PLLA, which is perhaps worthy of further study.

Aftercare for nonablative laser therapy is minimal. Patients typically experience erythema and edema 1 to 3 days posttreatment, with subsequent bronzing and light peeling of the skin. Posttreatment care after fractional CO_2 resurfacing involves the application of bland emollients and cold compresses for the duration of the reepithelialization period. Postoperative acneiform eruptions are not uncommon, in which case switching to a nonocclusive emollient and starting a gentle acne regimen can be helpful.[18] Patients should be instructed to avoid rubbing or picking at the treated area, as this will increase the likelihood of scarring. Green-tinted makeup can mask the posttreatment erythema, which can persist for several weeks, and sun protection is critical to reduce the change of postinflammatory hyperpigmentation. After intense focused ultrasound, patients may experience redness or swelling for several days posttreatment but no other specific after care is required.

COMPLICATIONS

Complications of temporal augmentation are typically mild and transient and include bruising of the lower eyelid, headache, local tenderness, and prominence of the superficial vessels the first few days after injection.[8] It is important to assess the superficial vasculature before augmentation, as veins that are lying in the temporal fossa may become more prominent as the overlying skin of the temple is displaced anteriorly after injection. This should be discussed with the patient before the procedure to avoid the impression that the filler caused the vasculature prominence, when in fact, it was present but merely obscured preprocedure. In patients with a history of brow or facelift, the placement of the filler can be more difficult to control because of scarring in the temporal plane. Bruising is a common complication after injection of any of the soft tissue fillers, and can be minimized by keeping the number of injection sites low and taking care to avoid visible vessels. When any bleeding is noted during injection, firm pressure should be applied immediately. The use of blunt cannulas rather than sharp cannulas may also decrease rates of bruising, although this remains controversial. In the event that bruising occurs, it can be masked with green-tinged makeup or treated with pulsed dye laser.

Most of the complications related to soft tissue augmentation with fillers are related to preparation of the product and injector technique. Important consideration should be given to the plane of injection based on the filler that is used, as many complications of soft tissue fillers are related to improper depth of injection. When using PLLA, the plane of injection is deep, below the temporalis muscle. Injection of PLLA into the temporalis muscle can result in the formation of palpable nodules. Other causes of nodule formation after PLLA include uneven injection volumes, inadequate reconstitution volumes, or inflammatory host response.[9] In Schierle and Casas' report[3] of 106 consecutive patients treated with PLLA for full-face volume restoration, the rate of nodule formation was only 4.7%. The investigators speculated that a higher reconstitution volume of up to 9 mL with a longer hydration time of 48 hours reduces the risk of nodule formation after PLLA. In Goldman's report[9] of his experience injecting PLLA over the course of 8 years in more than 1000 patients, he noted that the temple was one of the areas at highest risk of nodule formation.

He recommends conservative volumes, injected deep using a depot technique to minimize the incidence of nodule formation. CaHA (Radiesse) also has a low risk of nodule formation (except when used in the lips, which is discouraged by the manufacturer), and there is no evidence to suggest that, although the microspheres are the same composition as human bone and teeth, that they have any osteoinductive properties.[10] It has also been well demonstrated that Radiesse does not obscure radiographic images.[5] There have been no reported cases of granuloma formation or hypersensitivity reactions after CaHA,[11] and studies of Radiesse in Fitzpatrick Skin Types IV to VI reported no incidents of keloid formation, hypertrophic scarring, or pigmentary alterations.[28]

Another complication of temporal augmentation with fillers is contour defects resulting from uneven injection of the substance or overcorrection. A recent report described the "dilution solution" in which HA is diluted with normal saline in attempt to obtain a smoother augmentation.[8] The technique relies on the concept that filler is more evenly distributed in a larger volume of saline and, as the saline absorbs, the filler concentrates more evenly, resulting in a smoother contour than when straight filler is used. The investigators reported that the most effective dilution per temple was 2 mL of HA, 1 mL of 1% lidocaine with epinephrine, and 3 mL of normal saline. The plane of injection was subcutaneous, adjacent to the superficial temporal fascia and below the visible vessels, with 3 injections proceeding anterior to posterior using a 1.5-inch, 22-guage needle.[8]

Management of nodule formation depends on the type of filler used. Many of the nodules can be flattened with simple massage, although this may be more difficult after Radiesse or PLLA. HA nodules that cannot be massaged flat can be injected with hyaluronidase or excised using a needle. Visible nodules after PLLA usually must be excised, as injection with steroid may lead to atrophy of the fat surrounding the nodule, leading to a donut effect that makes the nodule more noticeable.[9]

The most dreaded complication of soft tissue augmentation is vascular compromise. This can occur either by direct intravascular injection into a vessel or via compression of the vasculature when high volumes are injected into tight anatomic spaces. The superficial temporal artery is generally easily palpable and thus can be avoided. There are currently no reports of intravascular incidents during temporal augmentation in the literature. For all injection techniques, the needle is inserted deep to the major vessels and movement of the needle while injecting may help to prevent intravascular injection. Several injectors advocate aspiration before injection, although this may prove difficult when using HA fillers with high viscosity. For areas such as the temple that may require high volumes, it is better to have multiple sessions with lower volumes at each session than high volumes in fewer sessions. Signs of intravascular injection include blanching of the skin followed by blue-gray discoloration and exquisite pain. If there is a concern of vascular occlusion, treatment measures include the application of warm compresses to promote vasodilation, nitroglycerine paste covering 3 cm of the surrounding area, 75 U of hyaluronidase, and daily subcutaneous injections with low molecular weight heparin to prevent thrombosis.[29] Skin prick testing is generally recommended before use of hyaluronidase because of rare cases of anaphylaxis, but many practitioners do not perform skin testing, especially in an acute situation. In the event of occlusion after CaHA or Sculptra, the area should be treated with nitroglycerin paste and the material excised from the area of impending occlusion if possible. The use of hyperbaric oxygen has also been reported as effective in halting impending necrosis and is performed daily for a minimum of 30 sessions.[29]

Reports of complications after fractional CO2 resurfacing are often related to overly aggressive settings in anatomic sites with thin skin, such as the eyelid and the neck. Long pulse durations and high densities of treatment coverage in these sites have resulted in both hypertrophic scarring on the neck and erosions with subsequent ectropion periorbitally.[17] Delayed-onset hypopigmentation 6 to 12 months posttreatment has also been reported.[16] Bacterial infection and reactivation of herpes simplex following fractional CO2 resurfacing have also been reported. Prophylaxis with antivirals, especially for patients with a known history of herpes simplex, is generally recommended, with the consensus on postprocedure prophylactic antibiotics less clear.

Side effects after RF skin tightening include transient erythema for a few hours and mild edema lasting for 1 to 2 days.[23] Reported complications after Thermage include transient crusting, skin depression resolving in 3 weeks, uneven brow position, tenderness around the jawline, and transient dysesthesias, including anesthesia of the earlobe and trigeminal neuralgia.[21,30] There have been subjective reports of temporal wasting by investigators who reviewed the posttreatment photographs provided by the manufacturer of Thermage, although this has not been officially documented by the physicians who performed the treatment.[30] These same investigators suggested that lower treatment settings be used in the temporal region to avoid injury to the underlying temporal fat pad. Geronemus and colleagues[21] recommend avoiding Thermage over areas that have been augmented with silicone because of a case of a postprocedure biopsy-proven silicone granuloma in a patient with a history of silicone in the nasolabial folds. Other studies suggest, however, that Thermage can be used safely in combination with other soft tissue fillers.[21,22]

Complications of focused ultrasound are also minimal and include posttreatment erythema and edema lasting for no longer than 1 week. Alam and colleagues[25] reported the development of white striations on the necks of 2 patients treated with the 3.0-mm probe that resolved with the use of topical steroids and left no residual pigmentary or textural abnormalities. They hypothesized that the complication was a result of inadequate coupling to the skin during the procedure, resulting in dermal injury. They subsequently used only the 4.5-mm probe in the neck, which deposits energy deeper in the subcutis, sparing the overlying papillary dermis.

SUMMARY

Loss of volume in the temples is an early sign of aging that is often overlooked by both the physician and the patient. Augmentation of the temple using soft tissue fillers improves the contours of the upper face with the secondary effect of lengthening and lifting the lateral brow. After replacement of volume, treatment of the overlying skin with skin-tightening devices or laser resurfacing help to complete a comprehensive rejuvenation of the temple and upper one-third of the face.

REFERENCES

1. Fitzgerald R, Vleggaar D. Using poly-L-lactic acid (PLLA) to mimic volume in multiple tissue layers. J Drugs Dermatol 2009;8(Suppl 10):s5–14.
2. Sykes JM. Applied anatomy of the temporal region and forehead for injectable fillers. J Drugs Dermatol 2009;8(Suppl 10):s24–7.
3. Schierle CF, Casas LA. Nonsurgical rejuvenation of the aging face with injectable poly-L-lactic acid for restoration of soft tissue volume. Aesthet Surg J 2011;31(1):95–109.
4. Redbord K, Busso M, Hanke CW. Soft-tissue augmentation with hyaluronic acid and calcium hydroxyl apatite fillers. Dermatol Ther 2011;24:71–81.
5. Ridenour B, Kontis TC. Injectable calcium hydroxylapatite microspheres (Radiesse). Facial Plast Surg 2009;25(2):100–5.
6. Ross J, Malhotra R. Orbitofacial rejuvenation of temple hollowing with perlane injectable filler. Aesthet Surg J 2010;30(3):428–33.
7. Moradi A, Shirazi A, Perez V. A guide to temporal fossa augmentation with small gel particle hyaluronic acid dermal filler. J Drugs Dermatol 2011; 10(6):673–6.
8. Lambros V. A technique for filling the temples with highly diluted hyaluronic acid: the "dilution solution". Aesthet Surg J 2011;31(1):89–94.
9. Goldman M. Cosmetic use of poly-L-lactic acid: my technique for success and minimizing complications. Dermatol Surg 2011;37(5):688–93.
10. Lizzul P, Narurkar VA. The role of calcium hydroxylapatite (Radiesse) in nonsurgical aesthetic rejuvenation. J Drugs Dermatol 2010;9(5):446–50.
11. Busso M. Calcium hydroxylapatite (Radiesse): safety, techniques, and pain reduction. J Drugs Dermatol 2009;8(10):s21–3.
12. Sundaram H, Voigts B, Beer K, et al. Comparison of the rheological properties of viscosity and elasticity in two categories of soft tissue fillers: calcium hydroxylapatite and hyaluronic acid. Dermatol Surg 2010;36:S3.
13. Beer K. Dermal fillers and combinations of fillers for facial rejuvenation. Dermatol Clin 2009;27: 427–32.
14. Alam M, Havey J, Pace N, et al. Large-particle calcium hydroxylapatite injection for correction of facial wrinkles and depression. J Am Acad Dermatol 2011;65(1):92–6.
15. Allemann I, Kaufman J. Fractional photothermolysis—an update. Lasers Med Sci 2010;25:137–44.
16. Tajirian A, Goldberg DJ. Fractional ablative laser skin resurfacing: a review. J Cosmet Laser Ther 2011;13:262–4.
17. Tierney E, Eisen RF, Hanke CW. Fractionated CO2 laser skin rejuvenation. Dermatol Ther 2011; 24:41–53.
18. Alexiades-Armenakas M, Sarnoff D, Gotkin R, et al. Multi-center clinical study and review of the fractional ablative CO2 laser resurfacing for the treatment of rhytides, photoaging, scars and striae. J Drugs Dermatol 2011;10(4):352–62.
19. Karsai S, Czarnecka A, Jünger M, et al. Ablative fractional lasers (CO2 and Er:YAG): a randomized controlled double-blind split-face trial of the treatment of peri-orbital rhytides. Lasers Surg Med 2010;42(2):160–7.
20. Rusciani A, Curinga G, Menichini G, et al. Nonsurgical tightening of skin laxity: a new radiofrequency approach. J Drugs Dermatol 2007;6(4): 381–6.
21. Sukal S. Thermage: the nonablative radiofrequency for rejuvenation. Clin Dermatol 2008;26:602–7.
22. Burns J. Thermage: monopolar radiofrequency. Aesthet Surg J 2005;25(6):638–42.

23. Javate R. Non-ablative treatment for periorbital rhytides and midface laxity. Oceanside, New York: Ellman International; 2011.

24. Petrou I. RF device's steady vs pulsed waves heat the way to less painful facial rejuvenation. Cosmet Surg Times 2009;12:28–9.

25. Alam M, White LE, Martin N, et al. Ultrasound tightening of facial and neck skin: a rater-blinded prospective cohort study. J Am Acad Dermatol 2010;62(2):262–9.

26. Laubach H, Makin IR, Barthe PG, et al. Intense focused ultrasound: evaluation of a new treatment modality for precise microcoagulation within the skin. Dermatol Surg 2008;34(5):727–34.

27. White M, Makin IR, Barthe PG, et al. Selective creation of thermal injury zones in the superficial musculoaponeurotic system using intense ultrasound therapy. Arch Facial Plast Surg 2007;9(1):22–9.

28. Marmur E, Taylor SC, Grimes PE, et al. Six month safety results of calcium hydroxylapatite for treatment of nasolabial folds in Fitzpatrick skin types IV-VI. Dermatol Surg 2009;35:1641–5.

29. Kassir R, Kolluru A, Kassir M. Extensive necrosis after injection of hyaluronic acid filler: case report and review of the literature. J Cosmet Dermatol 2011; 10(3):224–31. http://dx.doi.org/10.1111/j.1473-2165. 2011.00562.x.

30. Bassichis B, Dayan S, Thomas JR. Use of a nonablative radiofrequency device to rejuvenate the upper one-third of the face. Otolaryngol Head Neck Surg 2004;130:397–406.

Laser Skin Resurfacing, Chemical Peels, and Other Cutaneous Treatments of the Brow and Upper Lid

Jeremy A. Brauer, MD[a],*, Utpal Patel, MD, PhD[b], Elizabeth K. Hale, MD[a,b]

KEYWORDS

- Laser resurfacing • Chemical peels • Aging face • Facial rejuvenation
- Noninvasive cosmetic surgery

KEY POINTS

- Evaluation and treatment of the eyebrow and upper eyelid must include thorough appreciation of their relationship to the forehead and periorbital complex.
- The upper third of the face consists of the forehead, temples, glabella, eyebrows, and upper eyelids, with varying skin textures, and many important skeletal landmarks and interconnecting muscle groups.
- A thorough past medical and surgical history as well as review of all topical and oral medications and allergies is imperative when evaluating a patient for potential rejuvenative treatment.
- Dermabrasion, chemical peels, laser, light, and energy devices, as well as neuromodulation and fillers, are used to varying degrees as first-line resurfacing and rejuvenation techniques for the eyebrow and upper eyelid.

INTRODUCTION

The focus of this article is treatments of the brow and upper lid; yet, one cannot evaluate and treat these target areas without appreciating their relationship to the forehead and periorbital complex.

With age, there is a loss of the supporting framework of collagen, elastin, and hyaluronic acid, as well as losses of bone and fat. Increased skin laxity results, with redundancy, accentuated skin folds, and uneven texture. Nature's course can be further expedited by exogenous factors, such as chronic sun exposure, cigarette smoking, and other insults to the skin and underlying structures, resulting in further wrinkling and dyspigmentation.

Resurfacing of the skin of the brow and upper lid may be achieved by mechanical dermabrasion, application of chemical peels, laser surgery, and treatment with energy devices, including radiofrequency and focused ultrasound. We focus on treatments designed to stimulate collagen synthesis, as well as improve fine lines, wrinkles, and overall appearance of the skin.

ANATOMY OF THE UPPER EYELID, EYEBROW, AND FOREHEAD

The upper third of the face consists of the forehead, temples, glabella, eyebrows, and upper eyelids.[1] We focus on the skeletal landmarks,

a Laser & Skin Surgery Center of New York, 317 East 34th Street, New York, NY 10016, USA; b The Ronald O. Perelman Department of Dermatology, New York University Langone Medical Center, 550 1st Avenue, New York, NY 10016, USA
* Corresponding author.
E-mail address: jbrauer@laserskinsurgery.com

Clin Plastic Surg 40 (2013) 91–99
http://dx.doi.org/10.1016/j.cps.2012.08.006
0094-1298/13/$ – see front matter © 2013 Elsevier Inc. All rights reserved.

muscles, and skin and subcutaneous tissue of the upper lid, brow, glabella and forehead for our purposes here.

Skeletal Landmarks

Bony landmarks of this anatomic location include the following[1]:

- lateral, supra, and infraorbital margins
- supra and infraorbital and zygomaticofacial foramina
- superciliary and zygomatic arches
- superior and inferior temporal lines
- frontal and malar eminences

The supraorbital margin is composed of the frontal bone with the often palpable supraorbital notch, or foramen, located approximately 2.5 cm (ranging from 1.5 to 3.8 cm) from the facial midline.[1] This is where the supraorbital nerve exits the orbit to join the supraorbital artery and vein and innervate the forehead, scalp, and upper eyelid.

The superciliary arch lies above and parallel to the supraorbital margin, underneath the eyebrow and above the frontal sinus. This arch may be absent in women. Above this arch, the frontal eminence of the anterior scalp and forehead may be palpable.

The infraorbital margin is composed medially of the maxillary bone and laterally by the zygomatic bone.

Approximately 2.5 cm from the facial midline and 1.0 cm inferior to the infraorbital rim is the infraorbital foramen, where additional vessels and nerve are located.

Laterally, the frontal process of the zygomatic bone forms the orbital margin.

Along the supralateral rim, across the temple and parietal scalp, it is possible to palpate the superior attachment of the temporalis muscle. It is at this point of attachment that the inferior and superior temporal lines on the frontal and parietal bones may be noted.

Although the supraorbital and infraorbital and lateral orbital margins are distinctly defined by bony structures, the medial orbital margin is less so, being formed by the frontal bone superiorly and maxilla inferiorly.

The cheekbone, or malar eminence, is formed by the zygomatic bone, with its fullness attributed to the overlying buccal fat pad.

The widest part of the cheek, and face, is the zygomatic arch, formed by the temporal process of the zygomatic bone and the zygomatic process of the temporal bone. It is located between the malar eminence and superior border of the external auditory meatus.

Muscles

The muscles of the eye, including the upper eyelid, consist of the following[1]:

- orbicularis oculi
- procerus
- corrugators supercilii
- levator palpebrae superioris

The orbicularis oculi muscle complex is one of the superficial muscles of facial expression, lying beneath and acting on the eyelid and periorbital skin. The voluntary and involuntary palpebral portion of the muscle overlies the tarsal plate and orbital septum, and may act independently of or together with the purely voluntary orbital portion. This latter portion originates superiorly on the anterior part of the supraorbital rim, medial to the supraorbital foramen, and connects with other superficial muscles of facial expression. These include the frontalis, procerus, and corrugators supercilii superiorly; the superficial temporalis fascia laterally; and the muscles of the quadratus labii superioris and the zygomaticus complex inferiorly. The upper pretarsal and preseptal muscles depress the upper lid, whereas the levator palpebrae superioris muscle contributes to the raising of the upper eyelid. It is the fibrous elements of this muscle aponeurosis that create the smooth, taut appearance of the eyelid margin skin.[1]

The glabellar complex consists of the corrugator supercilii and procerus muscles. The corrugator supercilii is small and deep, originating from and located directly on the frontal bone of the medial superior orbit. The repeated activity of this muscle is responsible for the vertical furrows, or "11 lines," located at the root of the nose. This muscle inserts into eyebrow skin and interdigitates with the frontalis and orbicularis oculi. In fact, a part of this muscle is derived from fibers of the orbital portion of the orbicularis. As a brow depressor, contraction draws the eyebrow downward and medially, resulting in a "scowl." The procerus muscle originates at the lower nasal bone and nasal cartilage, attaching to the skin at the nasal root. Its fibers similarly are interwoven with the frontalis, orbicularis oculi, and corrugator supercilii. Contraction of this muscle results in inferior movement of the forehead and eyebrows. This muscle is responsible for the transverse wrinkles at the root of the nose and the "bunny lines."

Eyebrows are elevated and held in position by the main forehead muscle, the frontalis. This muscle originates in the galea aponeurotica just at the anterior hairline, with insertions into the skin of the forehead and eyebrows, as well as with the orbicularis oculi and glabellar complex. Contraction raises the eyebrows, responsible for the horizontal creases of the forehead, as well as aids in widened opening of the eye. Loss of function or paralysis results in a flat forehead and drooping eyebrow.

Skin and Subcutaneous Tissue

Eyelid skin is the thinnest on the body, with minimal subcutaneous tissue underlying the preseptal and pretarsal skin, the upper lid with greater redundancy than the lower.[1] In undamaged, youthful skin, there should be a seamless transition from this thin eyelid skin to the thicker skin of the eyebrow. The subcutaneous tissue consists of loose connective tissue with a notable absence of fat in the skin overlying the tarsal plate. Eyelashes serve a protective and sensory function, and the upper eyelid has more than 100 follicles arranged in multiple rows. Unlike other terminal hair follicles, they are not associated with arrector pili muscle. Additionally, eyelashes have a shorter anagen and greater telogen phase, and are not sensitive to androgens.

The dense fibrous tissue of the tarsal plate provides eyelid support, with the posterior margins adjoining conjunctivae. The orbital fat overlying the intraocular muscles is held in place by the multilayered orbital septum, a connective tissue structure that extends from the aponeurosis to the tarsal plate. The upper eyelid fat pad is located between this septum and aponeurosis, divided into the central and medial compartments. The retro-orbicularis fat is directly above, under the orbital portion of orbicularis oculi.

The forehead encompasses the thicker skin from the hairline to eyebrows and laterally at the temporal ridges, just medially to the lateral eyebrow.

EVALUATION
Functional and Esthetic

Aging of the upper third of the face results in functional changes in addition to the cosmetic concerns. As individuals age, the location of the eyebrow lowers from its original position at or above the supraorbital rim.[1] This can result in ptosis, and becomes even more of a concern when an individual also develops redundancy of upper eyelid skin. Functionally, this may affect upward gaze and superior field of vision. In compensating for this, often the frontalis muscle is overused, and more prominent transverse forehead creases result. In youth, the forehead is free of deep horizontal wrinkles that come with age and prolonged use. Ptosis of the glabella deepens the vertical and horizontal frown lines associated with the corrugator supercilii and procerus muscles. Additionally, as we age, fat is redistributed, and along with gradual weakness of the underlying connective tissue, results in increased prominence of transitions between the cosmetic units of periorbital and surrounding skin.

To effectively evaluate the upper eyelid and brow, it is imperative to note the positioning of the two relative to one another as well as the forehead. Esthetically, the upper eyelid should be full, with greater density laterally. The lengthwise upper eyelid skin crease, located between the medial canthus and the lateral orbital rim, should be well demarcated, dividing the eyelid with a more prominent superior component that seamlessly flows laterally into the temporal region. The visible distance between the upper eyelid margin and the superior palpebral sulcus should be 3 to 6 mm. Regarding the aperture, the upper eyelid margin should cover 1 to 2 mm of the iris.

In addition to shape, location, and symmetry of the eyebrows, differences in gender and in the shape and size of one's face and eyes dictate what is considered to be a culturally acceptable and esthetically pleasing brow. In men, the brow appears heavier and should be located at the supraorbital rim with less of an arch when compared with women. In women, the eyebrow should be located above the supraorbital rim. There are considered to be 5 basic shapes of eyebrow: curved, sharp angled, soft angled, rounded, and flat.[2] The ideal eyebrow is defined by the following landmarks (**Fig. 1**):

1. A vertical plane containing the edge of medial eyebrow, medial canthus, and the alar base
2. A horizontal plane containing the medial and lateral eyebrow edges
3. An oblique plane containing the lateral edge of eyebrow and the lateral canthus
4. A vertical plane containing the peak of the eyebrow and lateral limbus

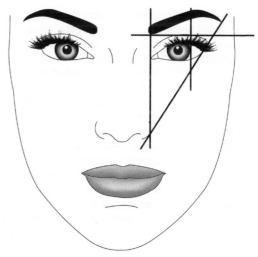

Fig. 1. Ideal brow position.

Additionally, elevation of eyebrows gives the perception of having smaller eyes. This is especially true in individuals with deep-set eyes, because elevation of eyebrow will make the supraorbital rim more prominent and exacerbate a hollow appearance. On the other hand, eyebrows that are set too low will obstruct superior visual field.

Past Medical and Surgical History

In addition to the physical evaluation of the patient from a functional and esthetic perspective, it is equally, if not more, important to adequately screen all patients by obtaining a thorough past medical and surgical history as well as review of all topical and oral medications and allergies. In particular, history of infectious disease, including oral herpes simplex virus, connective tissue disease or other diseases of impaired wound healing, active skin condition in area of treatment, history of Bell palsy, and prior surgical and nonsurgical procedures are necessary in your initial consultation and evaluation of the patient.

PROCEDURES
Dermabrasion

Dermabrasion, or mechanical skin resurfacing, was once viewed as the popular first-line technique in resurfacing and rejuvenation.[3] Although dermabrasion may have lost its popularity over the years with the advent of novel lasers and technologies, a superficial approach still remains a viable option for rejuvenation of the upper eyelid. The following 3 subtypes of dermabrasion are currently in use:

1. Manual
2. Motorized
3. Microdermabrasion

Of these, manual dermabrasion is ideal for the upper eyelid because it provides greater control of the depth of injury and the area treated. Manual dermabrasion methods use silicon carbide sandpaper, and with variation in the force and duration, or number of passes, of the procedure can provide superficial to deep resurfacing. This results in noticeable improvement in dyschromia and rhytids.

Motorized dermabrasion uses abrasive materials driven by a rotary power-driven motor, and is best suited for deeper lines and wrinkles. Generally, it is not used for the upper eyelid because of the bulky nature of the instrument, delicate nature of upper eyelid, and prolonged recovery time.

Microdermabrasion treatment uses either a motorized device that rapidly shoots and recaptures aluminum oxide or other crystals, or a crystal-free diamond tipped wand for the removal of the stratum corneum and superficial spinous layers. Although effective for mild dyschromia and texture enhancement, microdermabrasion is rarely used for upper eyelids.

Peels

Chemical peels remain a popular method for resurfacing because of their long history of safety, efficacy, relatively low cost, and the ability to tailor the depth of injury by choosing the appropriate agent, concentration, and technique.[4,5] This control is especially important when dealing with the thin skin of the upper eyelid. Chemical peels are generally subdivided into superficial, medium, and deep depth types, and have a broad range of indications including treatment for photoaging, wrinkles, scarring, and dyschromia.

Superficial peels
Like microdermabrasion, superficial chemical peels can be used for exfoliation to improve mild photoaging and epidermal dyschromia. They offer the advantage of use on all skin types with minimal risk of postinflammatory hyperpigmentation. Options for superficial chemical peels include 20% to 50% glycolic acid, 10% to 30% trichloroacetic acid (TCA), and Jessner solution (a combination of resorcinol, salicylic acid, and lactic acid in 95% EtOH), among others. Superficial chemical peels are generally performed as a series of treatments separated by several weeks. The major side effects associated with superficial chemical peels are local irritation, burning, and stinging sensations.

Before treatment with chemical peels and depending on the type and intended depth, prophylactic antiviral therapy, nonsteroidal anti-inflammatory drugs or even narcotics, as well as systemic glucocorticoids are administered.

Medium-depth peels
Medium-depth chemical peels include 35% TCA in combination with Jessner solution, 70% glycolic acid, solid carbon dioxide, or, less commonly, 40% to 50% TCA. These agents cause injury, inflammation, and subsequent neocollagenesis to the level of the superficial reticular dermis, inducing inflammation and allowing for treatment of moderate photoaging, mild wrinkling, and dyschromia.[6] Medium-depth peels can be used for both rejuvenation of the periorbital skin, and for improving the transition between the periorbital area and rest of the facial skin following resurfacing of the face. In general, a conservative approach should be taken when treating the upper eyelid, by the use of lower concentrations and avoiding overapplication, because of the sensitive nature of the cosmetic unit. In addition, particular attention must be used to

prevent exposure of the eye to the peeling agent. For this reason, TCA is usually avoided in treating the upper eyelid. After the procedure, medium-depth peels will lead to edema for 1 to 2 days, crust formation during days 4 through 8, and reepithelialization by 1 to 2 weeks.

Deep peels

Deep chemical peels include greater than 50% TCA, phenol, or, most commonly, occluded or unoccluded Baker-Gordon formula (3 mL of 88% phenol, 2 mL of tap water, 8 drops of Septisol, and 3 drops of croton oil).[7] Although they offer the advantage of treating moderate to severe photoaging and deep wrinkles, the ability of these agents to penetrate deep into the dermis poses a significant risk when used on the upper eyelid. If deep chemical peels are performed in the periorbital region, a modified Baker-Gordon formula should be used, using mineral oil in place of water (as water enhances penetration of phenol) and decreasing the drops of croton oil, and extreme caution should be used to avoid scarring. Cardiac arrhythmia is a major potential side effect of phenol, requiring preoperative evaluation and continuous cardiac monitoring. The risk of cardiac toxicity is even higher on the eyelid because the skin absorption of phenol is the greatest on the thin upper eyelid. The recovery process and wound-healing process is similar to that of the medium-depth peels, except that wound dressings and wound care are necessary because of more extensive dermal damage, with the end result leading to a more organized and compact dermis and rejuvenated epidermis. As with many of these procedures, care must be taken to avoid potential scarring.

Lasers, Light, and Other Energy Devices

Lasers are the currently the most popular method for resurfacing and rejuvenation because of their ability to selectively target specific components of the skin at specific depths. Laser resurfacing and rejuvenation of the upper eyelid and brow can be performed as an isolated procedure, when the entire cosmetic unit is treated and appropriate eye protection is in place. Alternatively, these areas are included as part of full-face resurfacing treatment. Ablative and nonablative, as well as fractional and nonfractional lasers can be successfully used for this purpose.[8–10]

Laser resurfacing for rejuvenation was first widely offered in the 1980s using ablative carbon dioxide (CO_2) lasers. Although these are the most aggressive and effective, they also possess the greatest side-effect profile and downtime. At the other end of the spectrum, the least invasive and least effective are the nonablative lasers. The

fractionation of some of these lasers allows for an improved side-effect profile, with more limited downtime, and in most cases still with considerable improvement from baseline. An ideal candidate for ablative laser resurfacing is healthy, lightly pigmented, and without prior history of scarring, radiation to the region, or recent isotretinoin use. As with any procedure, a lengthy discussion of the risks and benefits, associated downtime, the need for prophylaxis against infections, and realistic expectations must be undertaken before the procedure. For most of these laser procedures, as with some chemical peels, patients receive prophylactic antiviral and pain medication, as well as systemic corticosteroids. As mentioned previously, when treating areas on or near the eyelid, it is necessary to protect the eye with proper placement of an opaque stainless steel or plastic ocular shield.

In addition to treating rhytids, ablative lasers can offer tissue tightening, as upper eyelid dermatochalasis has been shown to significantly improve with CO_2 laser skin resurfacing.[11] Ablative and fractional ablative laser resurfacing can be performed using the CO_2 (10,600 nm) or Erbium:YAG (2900 nm) laser. Both result in destruction of the epidermis and part of the dermis by targeting water, leading to remodeling of healthy tissue via wound healing. Because the depth of tissue penetrance with the Erbium:YAG laser is less than that of the CO_2 laser, the ablation process can be controlled and titrated more precisely with the Erbium:YAG laser by altering the number of passes and the energy fluence. Additional advantages of the Erbium:YAG laser compared with CO_2 lasers include minimal thermal damage, decreased intensity and duration of erythema, faster recovery time, and decreased risk of scarring; however, there is a greater risk of dermal bleeding, lack of immediate collagen contracture, and decreased efficacy on deep wrinkles with the Erbium:YAG lasers compared with CO_2 lasers.

Side effects of ablative laser resurfacing include erythema lasting for several months, postinflammatory hyperpigmentation, relative hypopigmentation compared with untreated skin, delayed hypopigmentation, aceniform eruptions, irritant contact dermatitis, infection, and scarring. Many of these are mitigated with use of a fractionated device, and benefits have been reported in laxity and periorbital rhytids, as well as brow elevation using a fractional CO_2 device.[12]

Although ablative lasers provide excellent treatment for advanced aging of the upper eyelid, nonablative lasers have an excellent safety profile and treatments typically result in minimal to no downtime, making them a good option for younger patients seeking mild resurfacing. Nonablative lasers include the 532-nm pulsed KTP laser, and 585-nm pulsed dye, 1320-nm Nd:YAG, and 1450-nm diode lasers; however, these are not frequently used for skin rejuvenation. Several studies specific to the periorbital region have examined the role of these nonablative lasers in the treatment of photodamaged skin, with an overall finding of moderate benefit of mild to moderate wrinkles, with little to no improvement in severe wrinkles. Furthermore, the longevity of the benefits are poorly characterized. It is clear from these studies, however, that nonablative lasers have an excellent safety profile with the most common side effect being transient purpura or pigmentary changes. Efficacy of these lasers is further enhanced with fractionated nonablative lasers.

Photodynamic therapy (PDT) uses an exogenous photosensitizer, 5-aminolevulinic acid (ALA), that is applied to the treatment area and activated by a light source, usually blue or red light. This therapeutic option achieves improvement in fine lines, shallowness, and mottled pigmentation.[13] PDT is not routinely used around the eyes, however, given the possibility of conjunctival irritation secondary to the ALA.

Intense pulse light (IPL) therapy has became a popular method for achieving complete photorejuvination for mild to moderate photodamage because of its ability to target pigmented and vascular lesions and achieve improvement in textural skin changes, owing to its safety profile.[14] IPL uses a flashlamp to generate light consisting of wavelengths between 500 nm and 1200 nm, which is differentially filtered to achieve the desired effect. Most common side effects of IPL include transient pain, erythema, pigmentary changes, and superficial crusting. Although ocular protection is standard of care with IPL treatment, the upper eyelid can be treated; however, the practitioner must keep in mind that the pigmented iris absorbs light in the range of 400 nm to 750 nm, and is vulnerable to damage.[15]

At the time of publication, several new laser and energy devices were entering the therapeutic armamentarium for skin tightening and contouring, wrinkle reduction, and overall rejuvenation of the upper third of the face. These devices include, but are not limited to, the fractionated 1927-nm nonablative Thulium laser (Fraxel Re: store Dual, Solta Medical, Hayward, CA), which has a Food and Drug Administration (FDA) indication for treatment of actinic keratoses, and is also used in the treatment of photodamage, including dyspigmentation and fine lines, as well as those devices using focused ultrasound (Ulthera, Mesa, AZ) and bipolar and monopolar radiofrequency (ePrime, Candela, Wayland, MA; Thermage, Hayward, CA) technologies for skin tightening, contouring, and wrinkle reduction.

The fractionated 1927-nm nonablative Thulium laser uses fractional photothermolysis to create relatively superficial zones of thermal coagulation underneath an intact stratum corneum. This superficial depth of injury and the preservation of stratum corneum help to minimize the potential risk for scarring or infection more commonly seen with ablative and nonfractionated devices. Although ablative and nonablative lasers are successful in achieving thermally induced skin tightening, however, the depth of energy penetration and resultant dermal effect is limited by their respective wavelengths. The delivery of focused acoustic ultrasound energy can be used not only to image the area undergoing treatment but also to induce thermal injury of the mid to deep dermis without damaging more superficial layers. Monopolar and bipolar radiofrequency devices similarly increase penetration depth to the dermis and subcutaneous junction. These latter energy devices stimulate collagen synthesis and contraction, resulting in improved contour.

Neuromodulation

Botulinum toxin is highly versatile in the periorbital region. It is the treatment of choice for dynamic wrinkles and shaping of the eyebrow, and can be used with fillers to achieve excellent rejuvenation of the face, as well for shaping of the brow. Botulinum toxin is a naturally occurring heterodimeric neuromodulatory polypeptide, produced by *Clostridium botulinum*, that weakens or paralyzes the targeted muscle by inhibition of acetylcholine release at the neuromuscular junction, leading to degeneration of the neuromuscular junction. The effects of botulinum toxin are irreversible, but efficacy is eventually lost owing to generation of new axon terminals over 3 to 6 months. There is a great deal of variability in the type of botulinum toxin, concentration used, and injection technique applied by an individual physician. Before treatment, appropriate patient selection, education, and counseling must take place. Patients should be made aware of the excellent safety profile and efficacy of botulinum toxin, as well as its transient nature, requiring repeated treatments at regular intervals to maintain the desired effect (**Fig. 2**).

Side effects of neuromodulators

The most common side effects of botulinum toxin are injection-related local erythema, pain, bruising, and headache. A rare side effect of botulinum toxin use in the periorbital region is eyebrow and eyelid ptosis, owing to paralysis of the inferior frontalis muscle and levator palpebrae, respectively. The side effect of ptosis, upper eyelid and/or brow, should always be considered when treating

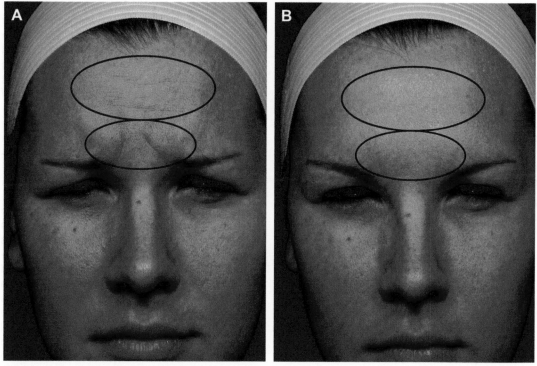

Fig. 2. (*A*) Horizontal and vertical ("eleven lines") dynamic rhytids before treatment with botulinum toxin (*B*) three weeks after treatment with botulinum toxin to frontalis, procerus and corrugator muscle. (*Courtesy of Laser & Skin Surgery Center of New York.*)

a patient with neuromodulation in the periocular region or the forehead or when evaluating the periorbital region of a patient who has recently has undergone cosmetic procedures (**Figs. 3** and **4**).

Brow ptosis results from a relatively greater degree of paresis of the brow elevators compared with the brow depressors during treatment of the forehead rhytids. The best way to avoid this side effect is conservative treatment of the inferior aspect of the frontalis muscles. It can sometimes be corrected by use of an additional neuromodulator to the lateral brow of the depressor fibers of

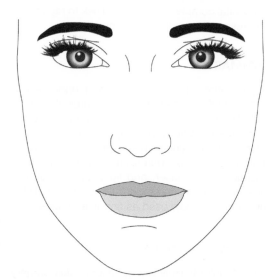

Fig. 3. Bilateral eyebrow ptosis.

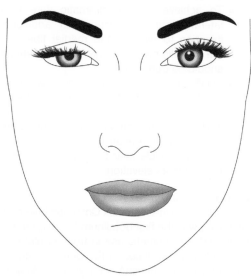

Fig. 4. Unilateral eyelid ptosis.

the orbicularis to achieve a better balance. Eyelid ptosis results from paresis or paralysis of the levator palpebrae muscle, which occurs if botulinum toxin inadvertently passes through the supraorbital foramen into the periocular muscles. The best way to avoid eyelid ptosis is to avoid injection in the midpupillary line, at the level of the eyebrow. Alpha-adrenergic agonists, such as apraclonidine, can be used to alleviate eyelid ptosis.[16] Usually bilateral, brow ptosis often results in patients complaining of "heaviness" in their forehead or difficulty putting on eye makeup. Fortunately, as botulinum toxin–induced paresis dissipates, this feeling quickly resolves.

Advanced techniques in using botulinum toxin

- An advanced technique using botulinum toxin is brow shaping by modulating the activity of the major eyebrow depressors, the corrugator, procerus, and depressor supercilii muscles, and eyebrow elevator, the frontalis. Strategic placement of small aliquots of neurotoxin allows practice with altering the shape of the brow, as previously discussed.
- Injection of both lateral and medical fibers of depressors will allow a uniform elevation of the eyebrow.
- Weakening the deep medial fibers of corrugators will permit an elevation of the medial eyebrow. Care must be taken to prevent paralysis of the superficially running frontalis muscle.
- Elevation of the lateral eyebrow can be approached by either combination of injecting a small amount of botulinum toxin into the lateral tail eyebrow to weaken the depressor without altering the frontalis muscle and by concomitant treatment of the crow's feet area.
- To achieve a more dramatic flare with lateral eyebrow elevation, an additional injection to weaken the medial fibers of the frontalis muscle in the central forehead should be performed.
- Finally, to generate an arched eyebrow, small amounts of botulinum toxin can be injected into the medial and central brow, while leaving the lateral eyebrow untreated. This results in a relative dominance of the frontalis muscle near the medial eyebrow, leading to its elevation.

Types of botulinum toxin

OnabotulinumtoxinA, or Botox Cosmetic (Allergan, Irvine, CA), was the first botulinum toxin approved by the FDA for cosmetic use in treating glabellar lines, and was introduced in the United States in 2002. AbobotulinumtoxinA, or Dysport (Medicis, Scottsdale, AZ), was approved and introduced in the United States in 2009 for cosmetic use in treatment of glabellar lines. IncobotulinumtoxinA, or Xeomin (Merz, Greensborough, NC), was approved by the FDA and introduced in the United States in 2011 for the treatment of glabellar lines. Of importance, Xeomin does not contain any additives, and therefore may decrease the risk of developing antibodies.

Dermal Fillers

Soft tissue fillers are an excellent treatment for correcting deep folds, static rhytids, and volume loss. Aging causes volume loss of the upper eyelid, resulting in hollowing as well as drooping of the eyebrow. Mild to moderate correction of this can be effectively achieved with the use of autologous fat or hyaluronic acid fillers for volume augmentation of the postseptal area, especially the lateral aspect.[17,18] The use of a small volume of filler in the upper eyelid will produce a youthful fullness to the upper eyelid while providing a mild brow elevation. As with fillers used elsewhere, local anesthesia or topical or local nerve blocks should be used to minimize pain. The most common side effects of fillers include local bruising, erythema, tenderness, and edema. Rare but serious side effects include injection site necrosis (most common in the glabellar region), arterial embolization, and occlusion of the ophthalmic artery. In addition, depending on the filler agent used, there is variable risk of hypersensitivity reaction, granuloma reactions, infections, and lumps and bumps. Details of these side effects and treatment options are discussed elsewhere.[19] With proper knowledge of anatomy, products, technique, and experience, fillers can be effectively used in the periorbital complex with minimal risk to rejuvenate and reshape the upper eyelid and brow.

SUMMARY

Rejuvenation of the eyebrow and upper eyelid once meant the need for invasive surgical options, including the isolated brow lift, blepharoplasty, or total face lift. With proper appreciation for facial anatomy and patient expectations, however, minimally invasive procedures, such as dermabrasion, chemical peels, laser, and light and energy devices, as well as neuromodulation and dermal filler injections, are now used as first-line treatments.

ACKNOWLEDGMENTS

We thank Mr Tony Rivas, Laser & Skin Surgery Center of New York, for his illustration work.

REFERENCES

1. Salasche SJ, Bernstein G, Senkarik M. Surgical anatomy of the skin. East Norwalk (CT): Appleton and Lange; 1988. p. 3–10,13–6, 54–6, 70–8, 163–74,183–97.
2. Alex JC. Aesthetic consideration in the elevation of the eyebrow. Facial Plast Surg 2004;20(3):193–8.
3. Patel U, Glaser DA. Enhancing the eyes: use of minimally invasive techniques for periorbital rejuvenation. J Drugs Dermatol 2010;9(8):118–28.
4. Rubin MG. Chemical peels. Philadelphia: Elsevier Saunders; 2005.
5. Burgess CM. Cosmetic dermatology. New York: Springer; 2005. p. 53–82.
6. Brodland DG, Cullimore KC, Roenigk RK, et al. Depths of chemoexfoliation induced by various concentrations and application techniquest of tricholoroacetic acid in a porcine model. J Dermatol Surg Oncol 1989;15(9):967–71.
7. Glogau RG, Matarasso SL. Chemical peels: trichloroacetic acid and phenol. Dermatol Clin 1995; 13(2):263–76.
8. Alexiades-Armenakas MR, Dover JS, Arndt KA. The spectrum of laser skin resurfacing: nonablative, fractional, and ablative laser resurfacing. J Am Acad Dermatol 2008;58(5):719–37 [quiz: 738–40].
9. Brightman LA, Brauer JA, Anolik R, et al. Ablative and fractional ablative lasers. Dermatol Clin 2009; 27(4):479–89.
10. Sukal SA, Chapas AM, Bernstein LJ, et al. Eyelid tightening and improved eyelid aperture through nonablative fractional resurfacing. Dermatol Surg 2008;34(11):1454–8.
11. Alster TS, Bellew SG. Improvement of dermatochalasis and periorbital rhytides with a high-energy pulsed CO2 laser. Dermatol Surg 2004; 30:483–7.
12. Ancona D, Katz BE. A prospective study of the improvement in periorbital wrinkles and eyebrow elevation with a novel fractional CO2 laser—the fractional eyelift. J Drugs Dermatol 2010;9(1):16–21.
13. Goldberg DJ. Photodynamic therapy in skin rejuvenation. Clin Dermatol 2008;26(6):608–13.
14. Goldman MP, Weiss RA, Weiss MA. Intense pulsed light as a nonablative approach to photoaging. Dermatol Surg 2005;31:1179–87.
15. Lee WW, Murdock J, Albini TA, et al. Ocular damage secondary to intense pulse light therapy to the face. Ophthal Plast Reconstr Surg 2011;27(4):263–5.
16. Wollina U, Konrad H. Managing adverse events associated with botulinum toxin type A: a focus on cosmetic procedures. Am J Clin Dermatol 2005; 6(3):141–50.
17. Finn JC, Cox S. Fillers in the periorbital complex. Facial Plast Surg Clin North Am 2007;15(11): 123–32.
18. Kranendonk S, Obagi S. Autologous fat transfer for periorbital rejuvenation: indications, technique, and complications. Dermatol Surg 2007;33(5):572–8.
19. Patel U, Fitzpatrick R. Facial shaping: beyond lines and folds with fillers. J Drugs Dermatol 2010;9(8): s129–37.

REFERENCES

The Varied Options in Brow Lifting

Farzad R. Nahai, MD

KEYWORDS

• Brow lift • Facial rejuvenation • Aging face • Surgical procedures

KEY POINTS

- Numerous options in brow lifting exist that can be broadly categorized as open and minimally invasive or endoscopic.
- Proper patient evaluation, procedural goals, and surgeon preference all play into procedure choice.
- There are common desirable traits of the esthetic brow. One must take into account sex differences when considering alteration of the brow.
- Multiple options exist for brow fixation.
- One must take into account 3 factors during brow lift: release of the brow, brow fixation after advancement, and depressor muscle release.
- A brow lift will affect the amount of excess upper lid skin and pretarsal lid show.

INTRODUCTION

Brow lifting is an integral part of facial rejuvenation, and in the past 20 years, the techniques used to achieve an aesthetic result have undergone a transformation based on 2 driving forces: (1) advances in technology available to perform the procedure and (2) a shift toward minimally invasive and minimal incision techniques.

Advances in surgical equipment (ie, scopes, cameras, and fixation devices) have allowed the surgery community to respond to the patient-driven interest in less-invasive procedures.

GOALS OF BROW LIFT

The pleasing brow in a woman is at or slightly above the orbital rim prominence and generally arches upwards as it sweeps laterally or has a break at about the two-thirds point (**Fig. 1**). The brows should be symmetric in shape and position. There is a natural and youthful fullness to the space between the lateral brow and the upper lid. This is the same space from which women pluck brow hair, because it is attractive and youthful to have this area without hair. There are limits, however, to brow height. Generally speaking, the medial aspect of the brow should be lower than the rest of the brow and the overall brow height should not exceed far beyond the orbital rim prominence. An elevated brow position in the presence of forehead rhytids (as seen with upper lid ptosis or dermatochalsis) is not esthetic and is an indicator of old age. The esthetic brow in a man is different: it should be flat and straight and at or slightly below the orbital rim. Brow configuration other than this in a man looks odd.

The distance between the brow and the hair bearing scalp must be taken into consideration during patient assessment and surgical planning. Typical youthful distances for forehead height are 4.5 to 5.5 cm,[1] although balance with the middle third and lower third of the face must also be considered. A high hairline contributes to an aged appearance. Some brow procedures raise the hairline (endoscopic and coronal brow lifts);

Paces Plastic Surgery, 3200 Downwood Circle, Suite 640, Atlanta, GA 30327, USA
E-mail address: frnahai@gmail.com

Clin Plastic Surg 40 (2013) 101–104
http://dx.doi.org/10.1016/j.cps.2012.08.007
0094-1298/13/$ – see front matter © 2013 Published by Elsevier Inc.

plasticsurgery.theclinics.com

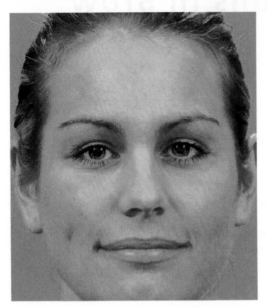

Fig. 1. A young woman with attractive brows.

some lower the hairline (pretrichial hairline advancement with concomitant brow lift); and some have no affect (direct brow and transblepharoplasty techniques).

ACCESS OPTIONS

There are numerous options for access to brow lifting: full open coronal, pretrichial hairline, direct mid-forehead, directly above the brow, transblepharoplasty, temporal brow, and endoscopic (**Fig. 2**). Each of the these options has its indications and its pros and cons in terms of access, resultant scar, potential for sensory changes, elevation of hairline, and degree of lift (**Table 1**).

FIXATION OPTIONS

Once the brow and forehead are mobilized and released, some sort of fixation must be used to maintain the desired brow position.

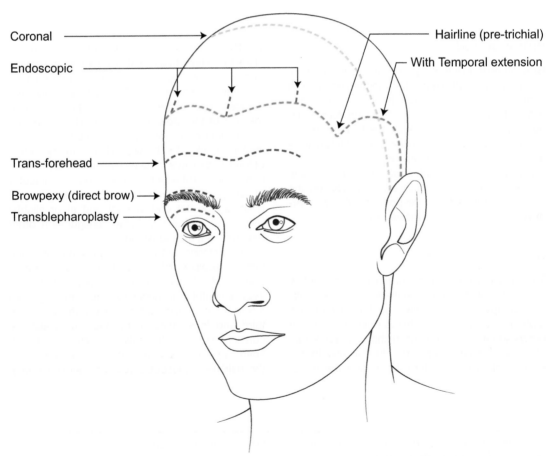

Fig. 2. Options for access to brow lifting: full open coronal, pretrichial hairline, direct mid-forehead, directly above the brow, transblepharoplasty, temporal brow, and endoscopic.

Surgical note: One of the keys to a successful and long-lasting browlift is to secure durable forehead tissues to each other.

The options in fixation are quite numerous, and no single method has been demonstrated superior to all others.[2] These are principally divided into suture techniques, device techniques, and others. The portion of the frontal bone between the temporal lines of fusion does not possess a ready durable layer of fascia to secure the galea; therefore, multiple techniques have been developed to use the bone as an anchoring point. Techniques include the following:

- Unicortical permanent screws that are removed later[3]
- Unicortical absorbable screws with an eyelet to pass a suture

- A tined plate that plugs into the outer cortex[4]
- A screw with Gortex (Gore Medical; Flagstaff, AZ) tab[5]
- A Mitek (DePuy; Raynham, MA) anchoring screw[6]

Other techniques that have been reported include, among many:

- Emory taping[7]
- T-to-V advancement[7]
- k-wires[8,9]
- Fibrin glue[10]
- Exterior bolster fixation[11]

One of the problems that can occur with excessive tension on the scalp, from either excision or fixation techniques, is alopecia. Techniques that have withstood the test time are those that are reliable, predictable, and safe; have a low complication rate; and do not incur excessive extra cost.

Table 1
The Varied Options in Brow Lifting

	Degree of Lift	Effect on Hairline	Favorable Scar	Potential for Sensory Changes	Access to Forehead Musculature
Coronal brow lift	✓✓✓✓	Raises	✓✓	✓✓✓	✓✓✓✓
Endoscopic brow lift	✓✓✓	Raises	✓✓✓	✓	✓✓✓✓
Pretricheal	✓✓✓✓	Can raise or lower	✓✓✓✓	✓✓✓	✓✓✓✓
Direct forehead	✓✓✓	No effect	✓✓	✓	✓
Direct brow	✓✓	No effect	✓✓	✓	✓
Transblepharoplasty	✓	No effect	✓✓✓✓	✓	✓✓✓

Choosing the Right Approach

	Coronal Brow Lift	Endo Brow Lift	Pretricheal	Direct Forehead	Direct Brow	Transblepharoplasty
Hairline						
High			✓	✓	✓	✓
Normal	✓	✓	✓	✓	✓	✓
Low	✓	✓	✓	✓		✓
Degree of brow ptosis						
Mild		✓	✓	✓	✓	✓
Moderate	✓	✓	✓	✓	✓	
Severe	✓	✓	✓			
Skin rhytids						
Mild	✓	✓	✓			✓
Moderate	✓	✓	✓		✓	✓
Severe	✓	✓	✓	✓	✓	✓

Values range from ✓ (*least favorable*) to ✓✓✓✓ (*most favorable*).

SUMMARY

There are multiple access incision and fixation options in brow lifting. Very good long-lasting results can be achieved with many different approaches. It is up to the surgeon to consider the physical findings and esthetic goals and to formulate an operative plan that can achieve them in a safe and effective manner.

REFERENCES

1. Farkas LG, Eiben OG, Sivkov S, et al. Anthropometric measurements of the facial framework in adulthood: age-related changes in eight age categories in 600 healthy white North Americans of European ancestry from 16 to 90 years of age. J Craniofac Surg 2004;15(2):288–98.
2. Rohrich RJ, Beran SJ. Evolving fixation methods in endoscopically assisted forehead rejuvenation: controversies and rationale. Plast Reconstr Surg 1997;100(6):1575–82 [discussion: 1583–4].
3. Ramirez O. Cosmetic follow-up: anchor subperiosteal forehead lift: from open to endoscopic. Plast Reconstr Surg 2001;107(3):868–71.
4. Berkowitz RL, Jacobs DI, Gorman PJ. Brow fixation with the endotine forehead device in endoscopic brow lift. Plast Reconstr Surg 2005;116(6):1761–7. http://dx.doi.org/10.1097/01.prs.0000187686.87209.5a.
5. Byrd H, Burt J. Cosmetic achieving aesthetic balance in the brow, eyelids, and midface. Plast Reconstr Surg 2002;110(3):926–33. http://dx.doi.org/10.1097/01.PRS.0000019877.41086.EB.
6. Fiala T, Owsley J. Use of the Mitek fixation device in endoscopic brow lifting. Plast Reconstr Surg 1998;101:1700.
7. Bostwick J III, Eaves FF III, Nahai F. Forehead lift and glabellar frown lines. In: Bostwick J III, Eaves FF III, Nahai F, editors. Endoscopic plastic surgery. St. Louis (MO): Quality Medical Publishing; 1995. p. 212–5.
8. Kim SK. Endoscopic forehead-scalp flap fixation with K-wire. Aesthetic Plast Surg 1996;20:217.
9. Chasan PE, Kupfer DM. Direct K-wire fixation technique during endoscopic brow lifts. Aesthetic Plast Surg 1998;22:338.
10. Marchac D, Ascherman J, Arnaud E. Fibrin glue fixation in forehead endoscopy: evaluation of our experience with 206 cases. Plast Reconstr Surg 1996;100:704.
11. Smith DS. A simple method for forehead fixation following endoscopy. Plast Reconstr Surg 1996;98:1117.

Technical Considerations in Endoscopic Brow Lift

Adam M. Terella, MD, Tom D. Wang, MD*

KEYWORDS

- Endoscopic • Brow lift • Surgical procedure • Plastic surgery • Aging face

KEY POINTS

- The goal of endoscopic brow lifting is stabilization of the brow at an aesthetically ideal height and orientation.
- The procedure results in reliable and reproducible surgical outcomes.
- A full understanding of the surgical anatomy, especially in the temporal dissection pockets, will help to prevent complications and optimize results.
- An understanding of brow aesthetics is necessary before beginning this procedure.
- There is debate as to the best method of brow fixation.
- A thorough understanding of the endoscopic brow-lift equipment enables a safe, efficient, and effective procedure.

INTRODUCTION

The breadth of human emotion is conveyed through our eyes; thus, the eyes must play a fundamental role in aesthetic surgery of the face. During the aging process, there is a gradual loss of tissue elasticity and forehead rhytids become more prominent. Descent of the brow may ensue and, in time, may contribute to lateral upper eyelid hooding and visual field deficits. This brow ptosis and lateral hooding may be misconstrued as fatigue, tiredness, and lethargy, despite good rest, energy, and health. An endoscopic brow lift, often in conjunction with blepharoplasty, rhytidectomy, and volume replacement, aims to restore a more youthful and rested appearance. (Terella AM, Wang TD. Debate on current topics in facial plastic surgery: upper face rejuvenation. *Facial Plastic Surgery Clinics of North America*. Submitted for publication, October, 2011.)

The goals of any brow-lifting procedure are to stabilize the brow at an aesthetically ideal height and orientation and provide reproducible and lasting results while concealing scars and avoiding the stigmata of a facial plastic surgery: hairline elevation, overelevated brows, or a quizzical appearance. (Terella AM, Wang TD. Debate on current topics in facial plastic surgery: upper face rejuvenation. *Facial Plastic Surgery Clinics of North America*. Submitted for publication, October, 2011.) The authors emphasize the concept of brow *stabilization* instead of brow *elevation*. Rather than raising the eyebrows, the goal is to fixate the brows to minimize progressive brow ptosis. These goals were the impetus for developing the endoscopic brow-lift technique.

Since first being described by Isse in 1992,[1] the endoscopic brow lift has become a technique capable of producing reliable and lasting brow restoration. This approach allows for correction of both brow ptosis and glabellar rhytids. As the authors discuss, meticulous surgical technique, adherence to anatomic dissection planes, and direct visualization used at key points in the

Division of Facial Plastic and Reconstructive Surgery, Department of Otolaryngology–Head and Neck Surgery, Oregon Health and Science University, 3181 Southwest Sam Jackson Park Road, Mail Code PVO1, Portland, OR 97239, USA
* Corresponding author.
E-mail address: wangt@ohsu.edu

Clin Plastic Surg 40 (2013) 105–115
http://dx.doi.org/10.1016/j.cps.2012.06.004
0094-1298/13/$ – see front matter © 2013 Elsevier Inc. All rights reserved.

procedure enables a safer, more-complete dissection and ultimately a better outcome.

ANATOMY

The ability to limit morbidity is the primary advantage of the endoscopic technique over more traditional coronal approaches. A detailed understanding of forehead, scalp, and temporal anatomy serves as the basis for a safe, efficient, and successful endoscopic procedure.

It is generally accepted that the supraorbital ridge separates the forehead and the midface, whereas the hairline separates the forehead from the scalp. It is effective to discuss the brow, forehead, and scalp anatomy in respect to layers. This region is commonly divided into 5 layers:

1. Skin
2. Subcutaneous tissue
3. Aponeurosis (galea)
4. Loose areolar tissue
5. Pericranium

A layer of thick skin overlies and is fixed to the subcutaneous tissue by fibrous septa traversing from the skin to the galea aponeurosis. The galea aponeurosis lies deep to the subcutaneous tissue and is a fibrous fascial layer that connects the frontalis and occipitalis muscles. It represents the continuation of the superficial musculoaponeurotic system (SMAS) layer of the forehead and scalp. The galea sits on top of loose areolar tissue, which separates the galea from the pericranium, and provides for relatively free movement of the galea over the pericranial layer. The pericranium densely adheres to the skull.

Brow Muscles

The brow musculature consists of the frontalis, procerus, and the paired corrugator muscles. Each of these muscles independently contributes to brow positioning, lateral eyelid hooding, and forehead/glabellar rhytids. In the discussion of brow lifting, it is useful to classify these muscles into *brow elevators* and *brow depressors.* The frontalis muscle is the primary brow elevator and is responsible for deep horizontal brow rhytids. It originates from the galea and inserts into the dermis via fibrous septa. The main depressors of the brow include the procerus muscle, the paired corrugator supercilii, and the paired orbicularis oculi musculature. The procerus originates from the nasal bones and upper lateral cartilages and inserts into the caudal border of the frontalis muscle. The contraction of this muscle results in the horizontal rhytids in the glabella region. The paired corrugator supercilii muscles originate from the nasal process of the frontal bone and attach in an interdigitating fashion to the frontalis and orbicularis oculi muscles. The contraction of the corrugators will medialize and depress the brow, thus creating vertical glabellar furrows. The orbicularis oculi serves the important role of palpebral sphincter and is a rather minor depressor of the brow (**Fig. 1**).[2,3]

Brow Innervation

The temporal branch of the facial nerves provides motor innervation to the brow musculature and the superior portion of the orbicularis oculi muscle. The nerve leaves the parotid gland deep to the SMAS and crosses the zygomatic arch over the middle third, traveling between the SMAS and periosteum. As the nerve travels above the zygomatic arch, it travels within the temporoparietal fascia (TPF) until inserting into the undersurface of the musculature. The muscular insertion point is on average 1 cm above the supraorbital rim.[4] The course of the nerve can be approximated by drawing a line spanning a point 0.5 cm anterior to the tragus and 1.5 cm lateral to the lateral taper of the brow.[5]

Afferent branches of the ophthalmic division of the trigeminal nerve, via the supraorbital and supratrochlear nerves, are responsible for sensation to the forehead and brow. It should be noted that after emerging from the supraorbital notch, the nerve travels in a supramuscular plane on the surface of the frontalis muscle. The lacrimal nerve supplies lateral brow innervation.

The forehead and brow enjoy a robust arterial blood supply from the internal and external carotid systems. The internal carotid terminally branches into the ophthalmic artery, which then branches distally into the supraorbital and supratrochlear arteries to provide for the central forehead and scalp. The external carotid terminally branches into the superficial temporal artery, which, through arborization, provides for the lateral forehead. The zygomaticotemporal artery branches off the superficial temporal artery to provide for the lateral brow.

The zygomaticotemporal venous drainage that receives branches bridging the surgical plane between the superficial temporal fascia and deep temporal fascia (DTF) deserves special mention. A large perforating vein in this system has been named the *sentinel vein* because it has been found to predictably fall within 2 mm of the temporal branch of the facial nerve. This vein is located approximately 1 cm lateral to the frontozygomatic suture line. Importantly, when more than one bridging vessel is encountered during the

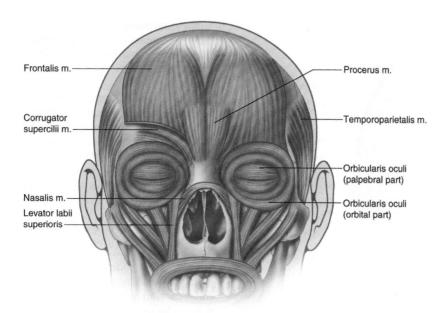

Fig. 1. Eyebrow musculature. Brow elevators include the frontalis. Brow depressors include the procerus, corrugator supercilii, and orbicularis muscles. (*From* Stallworth CL, Wang TD. Endoscopic and forehead rejuvenation. In: Massry GG, editors. Master techniques in blepharoplasty and periorbital rejuvenation. Springer; 2011; with kind permission from Springer Science and Business Media.)

dissection, there is often a corresponding temporal branch of the facial nerve in proximity. These vessels are located in close proximity and serve as a topographic marker for the frontal branch of the frontal nerve during endoscopic dissection.[6]

Of critical importance to endoscopic brow lifting is a comprehensive understanding of the fascial planes of the scalp, forehead, brow, and temporal regions. The SMAS envelops the mimetic musculature of the lower and midface. As the SMAS extends above the zygomatic arch, it becomes continuous with the TPF. Superiorly, in the region of the brow and scalp, the TPF/SMAS is in continuity with the galea aponeurosis. In the temporal region, the DTF lies beneath the TPF. The DTF envelops the temporalis muscle, thus splitting into a deep and superficial layer (**Fig. 2**). The superficial layer of the DTF and the deep layer of the DTF form a confluence with the frontoparietal periosteum to form the *temporal line*. The DTF and the lateral extent of the galea also fuse with the lateral orbital rim and medial zygomatic arch periosteum to form the *conjoined tendon*. The fusion of the galea and frontal periosteum at the supraorbital rim creates the arcus marginalis, which serves to anchor the brow and represents the peripheral attachment of the orbital septum and, thus, will limit ones ability to achieve brow mobilization if not completely released.

EVALUATION

An accurate evaluation of the upper face and brow necessitates a thorough understanding of forehead and brow aesthetics. The aesthetically ideal upper brow remains a source of debate. In women, the youthful brow should be arched and lie just above the supraorbital rim. In men, however, the youthful brow position and contour is flatter without the high-arching lateral component and should sit at or near the supraorbital rim.[5] It is generally accepted that in women, the brow should arch with an apex in line with the lateral limbus or the lateral canthus. The lateral brow should approximate an oblique line drawn from the nasal ala through the lateral canthus. A line vertically tangent to the lateral nasal ala should approximate the medial extent of the brow (**Fig. 3**). (Terella AM, Wang TD. Debate on current topics in facial plastic surgery: upper face rejuvenation. *Facial Plastic Surgery Clinics of North America.* Submitted for publication, October, 2011.)

Patient Expectations

As with any cosmetic surgical procedure, the patients' motivation and expectations for surgery must be understood. A thorough ophthalmologic history, including risk factors of bleeding diathesis or prior ophthalmologic trauma, should be elicited. A history of dry eyes or previous blepharoplasty

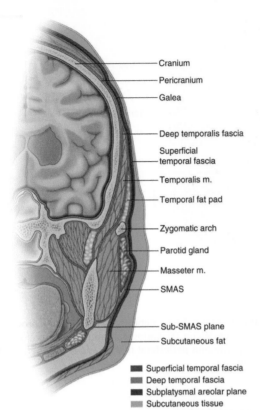

Cranium

Pericranium

Galea

Deep temporalis fascia

Superficial
temporal fascia

Temporalis m.

Temporal fat pad

Zygomatic arch

Parotid gland

Masseter m.

SMAS

Sub-SMAS plane

Subcutaneous fat

- Superficial temporal fascia
- Deep temporal fascia
- Subplatysmal areolar plane
- Subcutaneous tissue

Fig. 2. Fascial planes. The TPF is continuous with the SMAS in the midface. Above the zygomatic arch, the temporal branch of the facial nerve is within the TPF. The DTF envelopes the temporalis muscle. Superiorly, the fusion of deep and superficial layers of the DTF constitutes the temporal line. (*From* Stallworth CL, Wang TD. Endoscopic and forehead rejuvenation. In: Massry GG, editors. Master techniques in blepharoplasty and periorbital rejuvenation. New York: Springer; 2011; with kind permission from Springer Science and Business Media.)

must also be identified because of an increased risk for lagophthalmos in this patient population. (Terella AM, Wang TD. Debate on current topics in facial plastic surgery: upper face rejuvenation. *Facial Plastic Surgery Clinics of North America.* Submitted for publication, October, 2011.)

Overview Facial Assessment

The assessment proceeds with an overview of the face, brow, and eyes. Facial or brow asymmetries, eyelid ptosis, and lid laxity must be identified because they will influence surgical planning. The hairline is documented using the Norwood classification. Prominent frontal bossing has implications for an endoscopic brow-lift procedure and should be noted. Next, the relationship of the eyebrow to the supraorbital rim is evaluated.

The ideal patient for an endoscopic brow lift has been described as having medium to thin skin thickness, prominent glabellar rhytids, and relatively mild brow ptosis with minimal skin redundancy.[7]

Eyebrow volume also can be inspected. Despite the observation of volume wasting in the midface with the aging process, and orbital hollowing, the eyebrow volume may not actually decrease with age. The combined effect of a stable eyebrow volume and orbital hollowing is an accentuated impact of light reflections and shadows, creating a false impression of eyebrow ptosis.[8]

Identifying Relative Contraindications to Endoscopic Brow Lift

Relative contraindications exist for women with high hairlines, men with male pattern baldness, patients with thick adherent skin, and patients with extensive bone attachments.[9] In patients with male pattern baldness, difficulty can arise in attempting to place the access incisions posterior to the receding hairline. In this setting, the calvarium may prevent endoscopic visualization over the horizon. However, in the senior author's experience, with meticulous wound closure, the endoscopic brow-lift incisions heal with minimal visibility even in a non–hair-bearing scalp.

Patient Photographs

Lastly, preoperative photographs are obtained. Standardized photographic views are important for preoperative and postoperative assessments. They should include a 5-view head series, along with close-up views of the eyes (closed/open/upward gaze/lateral gaze). (Terella AM, Wang TD. Debate on current topics in facial plastic surgery: upper face rejuvenation. *Facial Plastic Surgery Clinics of North America.* Submitted for publication, October, 2011.)

PATIENT PERSPECTIVE

As with all facial plastic surgery, a successful outcome begins with a good rapport between patients and the surgeon. Both the patients and surgeon must share an understanding of the motivation for seeking this cosmetic change and must share realistic expectations.

In the authors' opinion, it is important for patients to develop an understanding of aging face physiology. Specifically, the authors discuss that, in the aging face, there is a loss of skin elasticity, decreased bulk of subcutaneous tissue, and increased skull bone resorption. Further, there is an inherent imbalance between the brow elevators

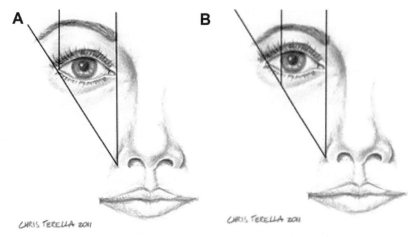

Fig. 3. Ideal brow position: (*A*) In women, the brow should rest slightly above the supraorbital rim. The brow should be lightly curved, with an apex in line with the lateral canthus or (*B*) at the lateral limbus.

and brow depressors, favoring the depressors in the lateral brow. Together these factors contribute to the development of forehead and eyebrow ptosis, most notably in the lateral eyebrow.[10] Emphasis is placed on illustrating that the upper eyelid may be affected by the eyebrow position. The lateral descent of the brow adds significant fullness and redundancy to the upper lateral eyelid. Empowering patients with this understanding helps to guide expectations and facilitates an appreciation of the utility of endoscopic brow lifting.

In discussing the specifics of the endoscopic brow-lift procedure, there has been an evolution in the authors' conceptualization of the lifting component of the procedure. As mentioned previously, the authors now approach the technique as a *stabilization* of the brow more so than a *lifting* procedure. As such, the procedure is described to patients as one to effectively resist the unopposed pull of the lateral brow depressors and minimize the continued descent of the brow. This consideration is of great importance for male patients in whom avoiding overelevation is critical.

Realistic expectations to provide patients include

1. Effective restoration and stabilization of the brow at a more youthful and aesthetically pleasing height
2. Resolution of brow ptosis
3. Improved lateral eyelid hooding caused by brow ptosis
4. Improved forehead and glabellar rhytids

Patients should seem more rested and revitalized. Their eyes should seem brighter and less tired. The authors emphasize that the changes are permanent but that the aging process will continue to occur. In this sense, the upper face will always seem more rejuvenated than if the brow lift had never been completed.

SURGICAL PROCEDURE FOR BROW LIFT
Instrumentation

Several companies offer endoscopic brow-lift instrumentation. The senior author uses instruments by Snowden-Pencer (Snowden-Pencer Inc, Tucker, Georgia) (**Table 1**).

Additionally, the authors use

- Endoscopy tower with telescopic input and video display

Table 1	
Endoscopic brow lift instrumentation	
Manufacturer	Description
Snowden Pencer	EndoForehead Ramirez curved dissector
	EndoForehead Ramirez spreader
	EndoForehead Ramirez parietal elevator
	Ramirez EndoForehead T dissector
	Ramirez EndoForehead A/M dissector
	Daniel EndoForehead nerve dissector

- Storz Hopkins II 30° Telescope, 7228 BA (Karl Storz Endoscopy-America Inc, El Segundo, California)
- Stryker TPS Drill (Stryker Craniomaxillofacial, Portage, Michigan)
- Synthes drill bit 1.5 × 4 mm with stop (Synthes Inc, West Chester, Pennsylvania)

Patient Positioning

Once the patient has been placed on the operating room table in the supine position, general anesthesia is induced by general endotracheal or laryngeal mask airway. The head of the bed is then rotated 90° from anesthesia, which enables the endoscopic tower to be placed at the foot of the bed and in easy line of sight of the operating surgeon. The bed is placed in 5° to 10° of reverse Trendelenburg position.

Incisions

Five access incisions, each approximately 1 cm in length, are typically planned.

- A midline incision is drawn 1.5 cm posterior to the hairline and oriented in a coronal plane.
- Two lateral incisions are planned just medial to the temporal line. These lateral incisions are oriented in a sagittal plane and planned to lie along the vector of maximal brow elevation.
- Lastly, the temporal access incisions are drawn in the temporal tuft of hair (1 cm behind the hairline) at the height of the lateral canthus in the coronal plane (**Fig. 4**).
- Next, the hair is parted directly over the planned incisions, twisted into small tufts, and secured with dental elastics.

Anesthesia

- The incisions are injected with an anesthetic mixture of 1% lidocaine and 0.5% bupivacaine, both with 1:100,000 epinephrine.
- A ring block around the forehead and brow is also completed.
- The local anesthetic is deposited in the anticipated plane of dissection, subperiosteal in the midline and deep to the TPF in the lateral temporal pockets.
- The patient is then prepped and draped in a standard sterile fashion.
- The eyes are left exposed in the surgical field and not draped.

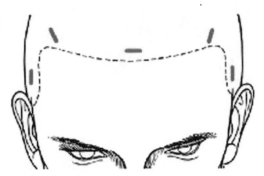

Fig. 4. Endoscopic brow lift access incisions. Five access incisions (*red dashes*), approximately 10 mm in length, are created. A midline coronal incision approximately 1.5 cm posterior to the hairline, 2 lateral sagittal incisions medial to the temporal line (approximating the desired position of greatest brow height), and bilateral temporal incisions in the temporal hair tufts at the level of the lateral canthus. (*From* Angelos PC, Stallworth CL, Wang TD. Forehead lifting: state of the art. Facial Plast Surg 2011;27(1):50–7; with permission.)

Preprocedure Assessment

- Before beginning the procedure, the brow is examined and the brow mobility is assessed.
- The point of maximum brow elevation is planned according to aesthetic ideals and functional needs.
- The brow is elevated manually to help assess the anchoring effect of the intact arcus marginalis; when intact, the arcus marginalis will hold the upper eyelids in repose.
- Once adequately released, manual elevation of the brow will significantly improve lateral eyelid hooding, dermatochalasis, and brow ptosis.

Subcutaneous Tissue Exposure

- The senior author prefers to begin the procedure with an incision at the left temporal access port and then continuing left to right, completing all incisions. The depth of these incisions is through the dermis only.
- A surgical assistant uses a narrow double skin hook to expose the subcutaneous tissue.
- A tenotomy, Metzenbaum, or other blunt-tip scissor is used to bluntly separate the subcutaneous tissue. The use of electrocautery is avoided in the subcutaneous tissue in an attempt to limit injury to the hair follicles and prevent alopecia.

- A similar blunt dissection technique is used in the temporal tuft to avoid injury to the superficial temporal artery and vein, which travel within the TPF. The depths of each dissection are critical.
- The 3 central access points are carried down to the pericranium, which is then cauterized to enable a subpericranial dissection.
- The 2 lateral temporal access points are carried down to the superficial layer of the DTF.

Dissection of Central Optical Pockets

- Next the dissection of the central optical pockets performed. A curved periosteal elevator is used for this dissection. The surgeon's dominant hand completes the dissection while the nondominant hand secures the endoscope.
- The first assistant attempts to stabilize the head by grasping the nasal root.
- The central pocket is dissected first and developed to communicate with the 2 temporoparietal access ports. Extreme care is taken to maintain a subperiosteal dissection plane. Violation of the periosteum will create bloodied optical pockets, making further endoscopic dissection challenging.
- The central optical pocket is developed laterally up to, but not through, the temporal line.
- As the dissection is carried anteriorly, the curvature of the forehead will limit further dissection. The senior author prefers using an instrument with increased angulation to carry the optical pocket further toward the orbital rim.
- This part of the dissection proceeds without endoscopic visualization. Instead, the surgeon relies on tactile feedback to ensure the dissection remains on bone and deep to the periosteum. The inferior extent of the dissection is carried to the arcus marginalis and laterally to the conjoint tendon. The supraorbital notch is palpated and protected by placing a thumb directly over this location. Dissection proceeds preserving a 1-cm radius of tissue around the neurovascular bundle.
- At this point, the temporal optical pockets are elevated through the temporal tuft incisions.
- The spatula-shaped dissector is used to develop the plane between the TPF and the superficial layer of the DTF.

- The elevator is used in a lifting motion, to elevate the TPF from the underlying DTF. The elevator is not pushed blindly forward but instead passively advanced as the fascial layers are separated. This technique lessens the chance of inadvertently crossing fascial planes during the dissection.
- As the dissection continues medially, the temporal line is encountered and the dissector is used to postage stamp through into the subperiosteal plane of the central optical pocket.
- This dissection process is repeated until the temporal and central optical pockets are joined.
- This technique is continued until the pocket is open from the lateral canthal height to the zygomaticofrontal buttress and the conjoined tendon.
- Assuming the proper dissection planes have been maintained, the temporal branch of the facial nerve should remain undisturbed in the TPF.
- The same dissection is then completed on the right side.
- It should be noted that the area of flap elevation is confined to the tissues anterior to the incisions. No posterior elevation is performed. This practice helps to minimize undesired elevation of the hairline.

Release of Arcus Marginalis and Conjoined Tendon

- With the temporal and central optical cavities connected, release of the arcus marginalis and conjoined tendon is performed.
- The elevator is used to release the arcus and conjoined tendon from the superior orbital rim.
- As this release is performed, the elevator will be seen transitioning from the thicker brow tissue to the thinner, soft, upper eyelid tissue.
- This dissection can begin without endoscopic visualization but quickly transitions to the 30° endoscope. The endoscope, with a sheath, is inserted into the left temporal pocket and the dissector is inserted into the left temporoparietal port.
- Using endoscopic visualization, remaining attachments of the temporal line and conjoined tendon are examined and released.
- As the TPF is elevated laterally, the sentinel vein is encountered. This vessel is a branch

of the zygomaticotemporal vein, identified in the deep temporal fat approximately at the level of the frontozygomatic suture.[6] This vein serves as a reliable marker for the temporal branch of the facial nerve (**Fig. 5**). The authors prefer to preserve this vein because sacrifice of this vessel has occasionally resulted in unsightly postoperative temporal varicosities caused by venous engorgement.

- The elevation continues until the level of the lateral canthus is reached.[9]
- Through the endoscopic view, the arcus marginalis is a fascial line paralleling the superior orbital rim (**Fig. 6**). A back elevator dissector is necessary to achieve full release of this fascial condensation. This release begins from the lateral two-thirds of the orbital margin and proceeds medially but does not continue medial to the neurovascular bundles. Limiting the dissection lateral to the supraorbital neurovascular bundle limits undesirable medial brow elevation.
- Full release of the arcus is confirmed when manual elevation of the forehead draws the brow *and* upper lid superiorly as a single unit. Further, the underlying retro-orbicularis oculi fat is visualized inferior to the arcus line (see **Fig. 6**). (Terella AM, Wang TD. Debate on current topics in facial plastic surgery: upper face rejuvenation. *Facial Plastic Surgery Clinics of North America.* Submitted for publication, October, 2011.)

Corrugator and Procerus Muscle Sectioning

- With the arcus marginalis release complete, the corrugator and procerus muscle fibers are identified and sectioned.

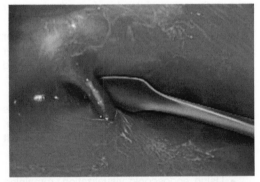

Fig. 5. Identification of the sentinel vein. The vein should be preserved during the dissection. (*From* Stallworth CL, Wang TD. Endoscopic and forehead rejuvenation. In: Massry GG, editor. Master techniques in blepharoplasty and periorbital rejuvenation. Springer Science1Business Media, LLC; 2011; with permission.)

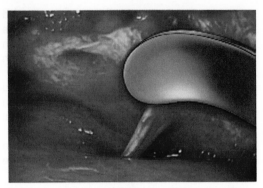

Fig. 6. To achieve stabilization of the upper brow, complete release of the arcus marginalis is necessary. Here, the supraorbital neurovascular bundle is identified and the arcus marginalis is being elevated above the supraorbital rim. (*From* Stallworth CL, Wang TD. Endoscopic and forehead rejuvenation. In: Massry GG, editor. Master techniques in blepharoplasty and periorbital rejuvenation. Springer Science1Business Media, LLC; 2011; with permission.)

- The corrugators are typically sectioned and teased apart with a small endoscopic elevator. On occasion, the fibers are more robust in men and may be sectioned with endoscopic electrocautery forceps.

Some surgeons argue that corrugator sectioning results in an undesirable lateralization of the brow. The authors think that the brows become drawn together over time, so slight widening is actually preferable. Additionally, some surgeons cauterize the frontalis in attempts to reduce horizontal forehead wrinkles; however, the senior author does not.

Fixation Techniques in Brow Lift

Several methods have been described, and there is much debate about fixation techniques in endoscopic brow lifting. These techniques include the use of fibrin glue, external bolsters, screws, miniplates, the Endotine® MicroAire, Charlottesville, VA system, and an absorbable suture anchored to a bone bridge. The criticism with many of these techniques is the failure to provide long-term results and the risk of alopecia. Kim and colleagues[11] showed, in an animal model, that periosteal readhesion of the scalp periosteum after elevation approaches preoperative strength 12 days postoperatively. This analysis helps in understanding the duration of fixation required to ensure a lasting cosmetic result.

- External bolsters have the negative effect of occasionally resulting in alopecia. It is hypothesized that this effect is caused by applying pull to the skin as opposed to the galea.

- Multiple screw techniques have been described that involve placing the hardware in the outer cortex of the skull. Many of these techniques leave patients with hardware protruding through the wound, necessitate removal in the clinic, and have a documented risk of alopecia surrounding the screw sites.
- The Endotine system, fabricated of polylactic acid, has the benefit of being bioabsorbable.

Multiple-tine fixation is predicted to reduce the tension in the periosteum fixation and, thus, prevent loosening and release of the scalp over time; however, this device is associated with increased costs. The senior author prefers to use a 2-0 Vicryl (Ethicon, INC. Somerville, NJ) suture secured to a free-hand drilled bone bridge in the outer calvarium. In the authors' opinion, this is technically the easiest and most secure method of fixation.

- An assistant facilitates the creation of the bone bridge by exposing the skull deep to the temporoparietal access ports.
- A Stryker (Kalamazoo, MI) TPS drill with a 1.5- × 4.0-mm bit, with stop, is used to drill the bone bridge. The bridge should be oriented parallel to the vector of brow elevation. It is critical that the 2 limbs of the tunnel communicate beneath an approximately 2-mm × 2-mm bone bridge.
- A 26-gauge wire, folded onto itself and bent into a *J* configuration is passed retrograde, beneath the bone bridge.
- The 2-0 Vicryl suture is threaded through the wire and then drawn beneath the bone bridge.
- The suture is placed buried in the dermis, galea, and periosteum approximately 3 cm inferior to the extent of the incision. This location places the fixation point anterior to the hairline, minimizing undesirable hairline elevation.
- The authors find it easiest to pass the suture completely through all layers and then reentering through the exit site, pass the needle back through all layers, burying the stitch below the epidermis. This technique facilitates a substantial tissue purchase.
- Both left and right suspension sutures are placed before tying.
- To aid in suspension, an assistant manually elevates the brow as the knots are tied.
- A smooth Webster needle driver is used to clasp the first knot and helps prevent recoil caused by tension.

- Once tied, dimpling of the overlying forehead skin is expected.
- The temporal suspension sutures are placed last. These sutures are placed in a buried fashion, using a 2-0 Vicryl suture, obtaining a robust scalp bite, and then anchoring it posteriorly to the DTF.
- The superficial temporal vessels travel in close proximity to the anchor site and should be avoided.
- All skin incisions are closed with a 5-0 Vicryl Rapide (Ethicon, INC. Somerville, NJ.) suture. The skin incisions are dressed with Vaseline (Unilever, London, United Kingdom) and a head wrap of Kerlix (Covidien, Mansfield, MA.) gauze is applied to help lessen the risk of hematoma formation.

Overcorrection of Brow

In general, the authors do not overcorrect the brow. The senior author thinks this helps avoid overelevation of the lateral brow, which may produce a more-feminized appearance in male patients, and avoid overelevation of the medial brow, which can produce a disappointed or quizzical expression.

Concurrent Blepharoplasty with Endoscopic Brow Lift

Concurrent upper blepharoplasty is commonly performed with an endoscopic brow lift. If planned, the blepharoplasty and lid skin pinch excision is completed after the brow lift. Once the arcus marginalis has been completely released, the forehead and brow can move as a single unit and secondarily elevate the upper eyelids. In this way, the brow lift decreases upper eyelid skin redundancy and reduces the amount of skin excised during blepharoplasty. (Terella AM, Wang TD. Debate on current topics in facial plastic surgery: upper face rejuvenation. *Facial Plastic Surgery Clinics of North America*. Submitted for publication, October, 2011.)

BROW-LIFT AFTER CARE

All patients having undergone an endoscopic brow lift are given adequate pain medications and, if completed in conjunction with rhytidectomy, are given a 5-day course of oral antibiotics. The authors routinely see patients on the first postoperative day to remove their head dressing, assess all wounds, and complete a hair wash. Showering is allowed following the removal of the head dressing. The authors recommend using an ice pack around the eyes for the first 24 hours and sleeping with the head elevated for 1 week to minimize bruising and swelling. Thereafter, patients are asked to return at 1 week, 1 month, 3 months, 6 months, and 1 year. Photographic documentation should occur at the 3-month and 12-month visits. The authors recommend the avoidance of vigorous activity for approximately 2 weeks after the operation.

COMPLICATIONS IN ENDOSCOPIC BROW LIFT

The surgical technique for endoscopic brow lifting is significantly less invasive than the coronal approach. Short incisions limit scarring, and direct endoscopic visualization, used at key points in the procedure, enables a safer and more complete dissection.

Despite these advantages, there remain complications inherent to endoscopic brow lifting:

- Bleeding and hematoma
- Lagophthalmos
- Alopecia
- Temporary hypesthesia of forehead
- Permanent anesthesia of forehead
- Brow paresis

The risk of *bleeding and hematoma* is low but present and seems to be related to the extent of dissection and elevation. In a large review of 538 consecutive patients undergoing endoscopic brow lift, Jones and Colleagues[12] observed no hematomas. This finding is consistent with the senior author's experience. As previously described, to lessen the risk of hematoma, the authors routinely perform injection of local anesthetic with epinephrine in a ring-block pattern as well as in the planes of dissection. When bleeding occurs, the superficial temporal and/or zygomaticotemporal vessels are often the source. Maintaining the dissection in the appropriate anatomic planes should help inadvertent injury to this vasculature. A head wrap with Kerlix, placed for the first 24 hours, helps eliminate dead space within the optical pockets.

Lagophthalmos must be considered a risk of brow lifting. Once complete release of the arcus marginalis has been achieved, considerable elevation of the upper eyelid will occur with brow elevation. Patients who have undergone a previous upper blepharoplasty are most at risk. The authors attempt to limit this risk by performing the brow lift procedure *before* performing the upper blepharoplasty. Further, the authors typically limit the upper eyelid blepharoplasty to a skin resection with a conservative muscle strip.

The risk of *alopecia* is significantly less with the endoscopic technique than in the coronal-approach brow lifting. However, hair follicle

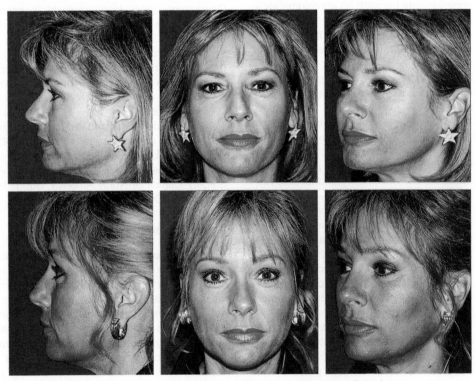

Fig. 7. One year after endoscopic brow lift; illustrating effective stabilization of the brow.

damage can occur at any of the 5 incision sites, resulting in transient or permanent alopecia. To prevent this, the atraumatic soft tissue technique is important. In addition, the use of cautery must be limited in the subcutaneous layer where the follicle resides.

There is inherent risk of *temporary hypesthesia* or even *permanent anesthesia* of the forehead. The authors think that the temporary hypesthesia commonly seen after an endoscopic brow lift is likely secondary to a traction neuropraxia of the supratrochlear and supraorbital neurovascular bundles that occurs during elevation and release of the arcus marginalis. In the senior author's experience, this deficit has always been temporary. A discussion with patients regarding the possibility of hypesthesia should always occur before surgery and helps curb concerns postoperatively.

Lastly, injury to the temporal branch should not occur during endoscopic brow lifting to avoid *brow paresis.* With a thorough understanding of the facial nerve's course through the fascial compartments of the temporal area and forehead, and meticulous attention to maintaining correct dissection planes, the temporal branch of the facial nerve should remain undisturbed. In his review, Jones[12] reported that 1 out of 538 patients experienced a brow paresis, which spontaneously resolved at 4 months. If paresis is noted in the immediate postoperative period, one must consider the possible temporary effect of local anesthetic. However, if paralysis has remained for several weeks, without evidence of improvement, nerve conduction studies can be considered.

SUMMARY

Comprehensive management for upper facial rejuvenation must consider the brow and eyelid complex. The ideal brow lift procedure would

1. Stabilize the brow at an aesthetically ideal height and orientation
2. Provide reproducible and lasting results
3. Conceal scars
4. Preserve forehead sensation[5]
5. Avoid unfavorable hairline displacement

The endoscopic brow lift has become the approach of choice for patients and surgeons alike. Armed with a comprehensive understanding of scalp, forehead, brow, temporal anatomy, and the appropriate endoscopic instrumentation, the endoscopic brow-lift procedure produces reproducible, consistent, safe, and lasting restoration to the upper brow (**Fig. 7**).

REFERENCES

1. Isse NG. Endoscopic forehead lift. In: Presented at the annual meeting of the Los Angeles County Society of Plastic Surgeons, Los Angeles (CA), September 12, 1992.
2. Knize DM. Anatomic concepts for brow lift procedures. Plast Reconstr Surg 2009;124:2118–26.
3. Ridgway JM, Larrabee WF. Anatomy for blepharoplasty and brow-lift. Facial Plast Surg 2010;26: 177–85.
4. Keller GS, Hutcherson RW. Brow lift: a facial plastic surgeon's perspective, Chap. 14. In: Thomas Romo III, Arthur L, Millman, editors. Aesthetic facial plastic surgery – a multidisciplinary approach. New York: Thieme; 2000. p. 226–35.
5. Friedman O, Wang TD, Cook TA. Management of the aging periorbital area, Chap. 32. In: Cummings CW, Flint PW, Harker LA, et al, editors. Cummings otolaryngology – head and neck surgery. Philadelphia: Mosby; 2005. p. 764–89.
6. Sabini P, Wayne I, Quatela VC. Anatomical guides to precisely localize the frontal branch of the facial nerve. Arch Facial Plast Surg 2003;5:150–2.
7. Angelos PC, Stallworth CL, Wang TD. Forehead lifting: state of the art. Facial Plast Surg 2011;27(1): 50–7 [Epub 2011 Jan 18]. Review.
8. Papageorgiou KI, Mancini R, Garneau HC, et al. A three-dimensional construct of the aging eyebrow: the illusion of volume loss. Aesthet Surg J 2012; 32(1):46–57.
9. Stallworth CL, Wang TD. Endoscopic and forehead rejuvenation. In: Massry GG, Murphy MR, Azizzadeh B, et al, editors. Master techniques in blepharoplasty and periorbital rejuvenation. ©Springer Science+Business Media, LLC; 2011. http://dx.doi.org/10.1007/978-1-4614-0067-7_7. 69.
10. Adamson PA, Brunner E, Pearson DC. The aging forehead, Chap. 179. In: Bailey BJ, Johnson JT, Newlands SD, editors. Bailey's head and neck surgery – otolaryngology. 4th edition. Philadelphia: Lippincot Williams & Wilkins; 2006. p. 2663–83.
11. Kim JC, Crawford Downs J, Azuola ME, et al. Time scale for periosteal readhesion after brow lift [Erratum appears in Laryngoscope 2004;114:788]. Laryngoscope 2004;114:50–5.
12. Jones BM, Grover R. Endoscopic brow lift: a personal review of 538 patients and comparison of fixation techniques. Plast Reconstr Surg 2004; 113(4):1242–50 [discussion: 1251–2].

The Open Brow Lift

Joseph D. Walrath, MD*, Clinton D. McCord, MD

KEYWORDS

- Plastic surgery • Brow lift • Aging face • Surgical techniques • Facial rejuvenation

KEY POINTS

- The vast array of open brow lift techniques provides a durable correction to brow ptosis.
- Some open techniques are more powerful than others, with incisions closer to the brow (direct brow lift) offering a greater correction in brow height.
- The pretrichial open brow lift is the procedure of choice for brow elevation and treatment of forehead rhytids in patients with a high hairline or long forehead.
- With meticulous wound closure and proper patient selection, there is high postprocedure patient acceptance of the incisional scar after pretrichial open brow lift, mid-forehead brow lift, and direct brow lift.
- Direct brow lifting rarely results in sensory disturbances, provided that the depth of the excision remains above the frontalis medially.

INTRODUCTION

Open brow lifting has been performed for nearly a century[1,2] and is a widely performed cosmetic procedure today. Open brow lifting encompasses a range of techniques including coronal hair-bearing approaches, frontal pretrichial approaches with or without temporal hair-bearing incisions, temporal hair-bearing approaches for lateral brow ptosis, mid-forehead approaches, and direct brow supraciliary approaches. Combined with small-incisional endoscopic brow elevation, transpalpebral brow elevation, and various forms of browpexy, a palette of options must be considered jointly by the surgeon and patient in determination of the appropriate procedure for each individual patient.

There is an ebb and flow in the approach to treatment of various surgical problems, cosmetic or otherwise. This trend is certainly present in oculoplastics, where today there are, for example, regional differences in the preferred surgical treatment of blepharoptosis. In the strongly consumer-driven markets of cosmetic surgery, these fluctuations can be massive. Some of this fluctuation is media driven, some patient driven, some surgeon driven,

and some technology driven. Attaching words like endoscopic or laser-assisted to any procedure generally makes that procedure appealing to patients, as it implies that the procedure is somehow less invasive, less risky, or has less down time. It also implies that the surgeon is current in his or her skills and is at the forefront of the field, whether or not there is any merit to this assumption. How else can one explain laser-assisted blepharoplasty? This phenomenon likely contributed to the wide adoption of endoscopic small-incision brow lifting procedures in the 1990s. Vasconez[3] and Isse[4] first presented the small-incision endoscopic approach to brow lifting in 1992. Initial indications for endoscopic brow lifting were essentially the same as for open techniques, and the requisite small incisions were easily accepted by patients. After an initial upswell in endoscopic brow lifting, the technique is not performed as often today, although clearly in the proper patient with the proper technique, the results can be excellent. The reasons for the shift back to open techniques relate to durability, prevention of hairline elevation (or designed lowering of the hairline), and a desire for less dependence on technology.

Paces Plastic Surgery, 3200 Downwood Circle, Suite 640, Atlanta, GA 30327, USA
* Corresponding author.
E-mail address: jdwalrath@gmail.com

Clin Plastic Surg 40 (2013) 117–124
http://dx.doi.org/10.1016/j.cps.2012.06.002

plasticsurgery.theclinics.com

PATIENT EVALUATION FOR BROW LIFT

The first branch point in the brow lift decision-making process is determined by the patient's goals. In the oculoplastic practice, where many patients are referred from general ophthalmologists, often the primary goal of treating brow ptosis and dermatochalasis is to improve vision, with the secondary goal being minimal out-of-pocket expense. In these patients, extended dissection in the region of the frontal branch of the facial nerve makes little sense, so the direct supraciliary brow lift and mid-forehead lift are the only surgeries offered. It is important in this functional population to assess eyelid position while the brow is at rest; it is not uncommon for true blepharoptosis to accompany dermatochalasis and brow ptosis. After performing a brow lift, the central drive to elevate tissue out of the visual axis is reduced, and a true blepharoptosis is unmasked (**Fig. 1**).

Once the patient has indicated that cosmetic considerations predominate, the evaluation focuses on determining the most effective technique for brow lifting and forehead rhytidectomy that is consistent with the most acceptable risk profile for that particular individual. The clinical examination (**Table 1**) focuses on the position and stability of the brow, the distance from the top of the brow to the pupil, the length of the forehead, the presence of baldness or anterior hairline thinning, the presence of "widow's peaks" and other contour irregularities of the hairline, the quality of the forehead skin and depth and prominence of rhytids, heaviness of the tissue about the brow, and the thickness of the brow cilia.

As a rough guide, it has been suggested that a brow-to-pupil distance of 2.5 cm (measured from the top of the brow cilia; **Fig. 2**) indicates that no further brow lifting be considered. A forehead height of approximately 5 cm (measured at the midline, the distance from the line connecting the top of the brow cilia to the frontal hairline) is considered average,[5] and a forehead length of greater than approximately 6 cm[6] has been used as a criterion in the decision to perform pretrichial open brow procedures instead of endoscopic or coronal procedures. For some surgeons, including the senior author, the pretrichial and coronal hair-bearing open approaches are the procedures of choice, with the pretrichial procedures far outweighing the coronal procedures in frequency. Occasionally a combined pretrichial and hair-bearing approach is indicated to reduce hairline contour abnormalities. In these instances, the path of the incision can span hair-bearing and pretrichial scalp to even out hairline irregularities such as the widow's peak.

The brow configuration is a central consideration. In younger patients, early lateral hooding can be addressed with an isolated hair-bearing temporal lift. In these patients, it may not even be necessary to disrupt the temporal fusion line with this procedure. The temporal brow and lateral canthal region also need to be considered in the context of the other procedures that the surgeon is going to perform. For example, if a midface lift is part of the operative prescription, a temporal lift is often required to redistribute the excess tissue that normally would accumulate at the superolateral leading edge of the midface lift.

The ophthalmic history and physical examination focuses on the presence or absence of lagophthalmos, lid position at rest, and ocular surface disorders including dry-eye disorder. A history of refractive procedures, some of which can lead to temporary denervation of portions of cornea, is noted. If warranted, a slit-lamp examination of the ocular surface is performed. As noted earlier, subconscious brow elevation is often part of a compensatory mechanism for blepharoptosis. Therefore, eyelid position with the brow at rest must be documented, and an appropriate ptosis repair procedure may need to be included in the operative plan.

SURGICAL ANATOMY

The anatomy relevant to forehead lifting has been well described,[7] particularly with respect to the facial nerve and supraorbital bundle. The most feared complication of brow lifting remains palsy of the temporal branch of the facial nerve. Above the zygomatic arch, the branch lies along the deep aspect of superficial temporal fascia (superficial to the deep temporal fascia). As dissection

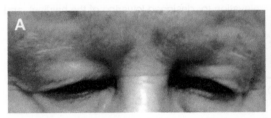
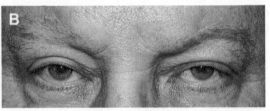

Fig. 1. (*A*) A patient with severe brow ptosis preoperatively. (*B*) Postoperatively, after direct brow elevation, true blepharoptosis is appreciated.

Table 1
Targeted elements of the examination that help to determine the technique chosen for brow lifting

Hairline	Brow/Forehead	Periocular
Presence of thinning or male pattern baldness Presence of "widow's peak" or other contour irregularities	Height of forehead from superior brow border to anterior hairline Quality of forehead skin: thick and sebaceous? Severity of forehead rhytids Thickness of brow cilia	Height of brow from superior cilia to center of the pupil Medial versus lateral brow ptosis Blepharoptosis? Lagophthalmos? Ocular surface disease?

moves inferiorly, deep temporal fascia proper splits into two layers:

1. Intermediate temporal fascia, inserting on the anterior aspect of the arch
2. Deep temporal fascia, inserting on the posterior aspect of the arch

Dissection remains along the intermediate deep temporal fascia to avoid injury to the overlying temporal branch. As is widely appreciated, the temporal branch runs in a supermedial direction approximately 1 fingerbreadth above the lateral aspect of the brow.[8]

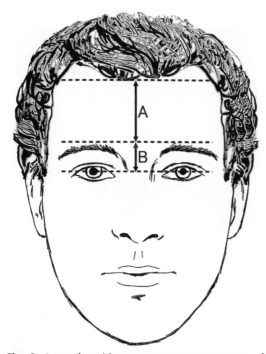

Fig. 2. A rough guide to average measurements of forehead and brow height. Line segment A averages about 5 cm in length; if line segment B is approximately equal to 2.5 cm, lifting the central brow is not appropriate. (*Adapted from* McKinney P, Mossie RD, Zukowski ML. Criteria for forehead lift. Aesth Plast Surg 1991;15:141–7; with permission.)

The sentinel vein, where it perforates the temporalis fascia, is in close proximity to the temporal branch of the facial nerve. It passes from the subcutaneous plane through superficial temporalis fascia and then through the deep temporalis fascia, at the outer aspect of the superolateral orbital rim, near the tail of the nonptotic brow.[9] Exercising the standard cautions during dissection in this region is prudent:

1. Remain along the deep temporal fascia proper.
2. Avoid aggressive flap elevation near the tail of the brow to avoid tractional injury to the facial nerve.
3. Penetrate the temporal line of fusion from lateral to medial to avoid inadvertently choosing a plane that is too superficial, placing the nerve at risk.

PATIENT PERSPECTIVE

Large incisional surgery is occasionally met with some resistance from patients at the outset. However, most patients also recognize and have distaste for the high forehead that can result from using a small-incision endoscopic technique in the wrong patient, or the high forehead that exists naturally or in association with hairline recession (**Fig. 3**). Review of postoperative photos from patients who have undergone pretrichial forehead lifting can help to reassure the patients about the minimal impact on the incisional scar on their appearance (**Fig. 4**). Patients are counseled that they may not be able to wear their hair in certain styles at least temporarily, or possibly permanently, because of scar visibility although, in general, problems related to the incision have not been the experience of the authors.

PREOPERATIVE AND POSTOPERATIVE ROUTINE

In addition to the usual suspension of antiplatelet and anticoagulant agents, the patients are instructed to perform Hibiclens scrubs and shampooing for several days before the procedure. The usual postoperative precautions on activity, care of the incision, and icing apply. There are no

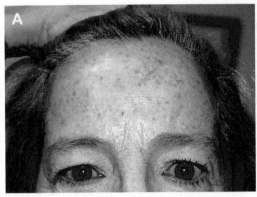
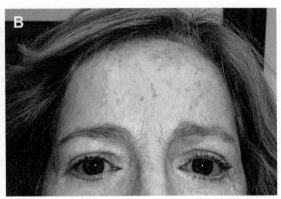

Fig. 3. (*A*) Preoperative photo of a patient before undergoing open pretrichial brow elevation. (*B*) Postoperatively, she has a faint pretrichial scar. The brows are elevated by 0.5 cm bilaterally, and the forehead is reduced in length by approximately 16%. The hairline contour is improved.

elaborate forehead wraps applied, and the patients return for suture removal at 1 week.

SURGICAL TECHNIQUE FOR OPEN BROW LIFT
Pretrichial Coronal Forehead Lift with Hair-Bearing Temporal Lift

Preparation

- Lidocaine 2% with epinephrine is injected about the proposed incision line, and along the corrugators and superior orbital rim: the "vascular tourniquet."
- Lidocaine 0.25% with epinephrine is injected throughout the forehead at the level of the periosteum to provide hemostasis and to provide some hydrodissection.
- The hair is rinsed with a chlorhexidine solution.
- If incisions are to be performed in the temporal hair-bearing region, the hair in this region is parted and stapled out of the way of the proposed incision site.

If a temporal lift is to be performed, that portion is performed first.

- An approximately 5- to 6-cm incision is marked 2 to 3 cm posterior to the hairline temporally (**Fig. 5**), beveled so as to remain parallel to hair follicles.

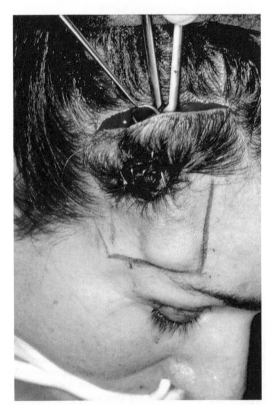

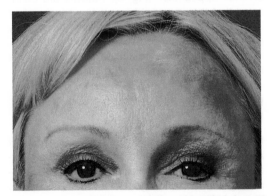

Fig. 4. Long-term follow-up after pretrichial frontal incision for a forehead-lowering procedure.

Fig. 5. A typical incision used for open hair-bearing temporal brow lifting.

- Dissection is carried down to the deep temporal fascia with monopolar cautery. It is helpful to staple a 4 × 4 sponge to the posterior aspect of the incision to keep hair out of the field.
- Blunt dissection is then performed down to the level of the superolateral orbital rim.
- Dissection is performed blindly until approaching within approximately 2 cm of the rim. At this point, a lighted Aufrecht retractor or endoscope can be used to aid in the identification and preservation of the sentinel vein.

Surgical Pearl: Care is taken to avoid aggressive elevation of the overlying tissue at this point so as to avoid tractional injury to the temporal branch of the facial nerve.

- The central forehead pretrichial incision is made with a 15 blade, is not beveled, and generally spans the arc from temporal fusion line to temporal fusion line (**Fig. 6**A).
- The subgaleal plane is entered with sharp iris scissors.
- A subgaleal blunt dissection using a peanut is performed (**Fig. 6**B); this often naturally becomes subperiosteal as the dissection continues inferiorly.
- The dissection is extended down to the root of the nose without direct visualization (**Fig. 6**C), but in the region of the medial brow, it stops short of the supraorbital notch by approximately 2 cm.
- At this point, a lighted Aufrecht retractor or endoscope can be used to assist in the dissection around the supraorbital bundle.
- The periosteum along the rim is released with a combination of blunt and sharp dissection, and the corrugators are disrupted.
- At this point, the temporal pocket can be connected up with the central pocket by releasing the temporal fusion line from the lateral direction.

Closure of the pretrichial incision

- With the central forehead flap on traction with Alice (or similar) clamps, a central pilot cut is made to aid in the determination of the amount of tissue to remove.
- When making this assessment, the assistant pushes the tissue along the superior aspect of the incision inferiorly, and the amount of tissue overlap is noted.

- The ellipse of tissue is then marked for the excision; it typically ranges between 1 and 2 cm of tissue. Additional pilot cuts laterally are useful in developing the elliptical excision (**Fig. 6**D).
- The deep aspect (galea) is then closed with 2-0 polydioxanone (PDS) buried sutures (**Fig. 6**E).
- Subcutaneous closure is performed with many 5-0 Vicryl horizontal mattress sutures.
- The skin is closed meticulously with 6-0 nylon running locking vertical mattress sutures (**Fig. 6**F).

Closure for hair-bearing temporal incision

- Closure of the deep aspect of the temporal incision is layered, with the deep aspect of the temporal flap secured to the deep temporal fascia with 2-0 PDS.
- The number of buried 5-0 Vicryl horizontal mattress sutures placed in the subcutaneous layer is limited, so as to prevent alopecia.
- Skin staples are used for the skin closure.

Aftercare

No head wrapping is performed. A 5-day course of oral antibiotics and rest is prescribed. Follow-up is in 1 week.

Mid-Forehead Lift

Men with deep rhytids, heavy brows, and thick sebaceous skin often require an open lift that is more proximal to the brows. Central forehead rhytids can be used for access, if they are prominent. The excision can span 2 prominent rhytids, or alternatively the excision can be constructed as an ellipse centered on the most prominent rhytid (**Fig. 7**). The technique is relatively simple and involves a full-thickness excision centrally, tapering to skin-only temporally. Corrugator and procerus muscles can be addressed. Sensory loss is generally more of a problem with this approach. Scarring can be minimized by a meticulous layered closure (**Fig. 8**).

Direct Incisional Brow Lift

The incision in direct brow lifting is placed above the brow cilia for the full extent of the brow.

- An elliptical incision is marked about with the peak over the central brow, or just lateral to this, depending on the brow configuration.
- Beveling the incision does not seem particularly helpful in this region, as it may compromise the ability to achieve the

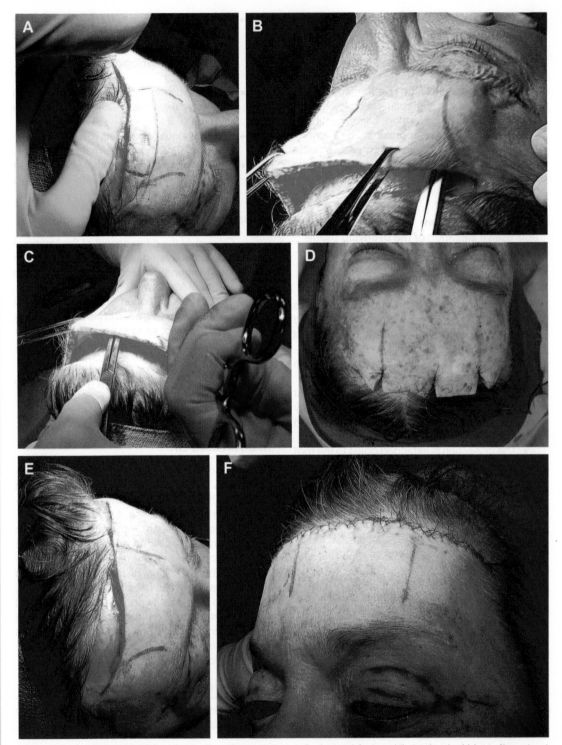

Fig. 6. (*A*) A typical pretrichial incision spanning both lines of temporal fusion. (*B*) A subgaleal blunt dissection is performed with a peanut. (*C*) Blunt dissection is carried down toward the root of the nose blindly. (*D*) Pilot cuts are useful in determining the amount of skin to excise. (*E*) Deep closure is performed in layers: the galea is secured with 2-0 polydioxanone suture and the subcutaneous aspect is secured with multiple 5-0 Vicryl horizontal mattress sutures. (*F*) Meticulous skin closure is critical.

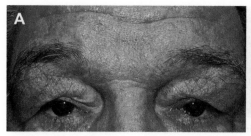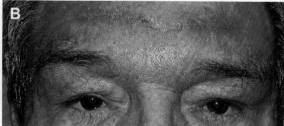

Fig. 7. (*A*) Preoperative brow ptosis and blepharoptosis in a patient with a complaint of decreased peripheral vision laterally. Note the very heavy brows and the deep central rhytid. (*B*) Postoperative photo at 1 week demonstrating segmental mid-forehead open brow lift and lateral temporal direct brow lift.

most accurate wound closure and scar minimization.

- Medially and laterally, the incision depth is through skin only, to protect the supraorbital nerves and the temporal branch, respectively.
- Closure does not incorporate the periosteum, unless extra support is clinically indicated, as in facial palsy (**Fig. 9**).

Coronal Brow Lift

Although the open brow lift is considered the gold standard in brow lifting and longevity of the lift, it has fallen out of favor because of its long scalp incision, somewhat overdone appearance, and tendency to elongate the forehead. In clinical situations where the forehead is short and the brow needs significant repositioning, an incision can be made several centimeters behind the hairline from just above one ear to the other ear. Straight incisions are easier to see, so a trick to better conceal the scalp incision is to corrugate the incision so that when the hair lays down it is more difficult to see.

- The dissection is done deep to galea and superficial or deep to the periosteum, depending on surgeon preference.

- Once the brow is mobilized the scalp flap is advanced back, the redundant portion is resected, and a 2-layer closure is performed, being sure to include the galea.
- Occasionally the periosteum or galea associated with the medial brow can be left intact to avoid an overdone appearance or overly elevated medial brow.

COMPLICATIONS IN BROW LIFT

The unique feature of pretrichial, mid-forehead, or direct brow lifting is the requirement for an incision in a non–hair-bearing location. The presence of this scar needs to be discussed with the patient. This discussion emphasizes that the scar will be prominent initially, but that it will fade and not remain problematic. Meticulous layered closure of the incisions is critical. Performance of a precise closure has led to very high patient satisfaction; to date, the senior author has never had to revise a pretrichial scar. Other than the incision, the risk profile is similar to other brow lifting procedures.

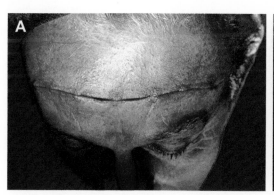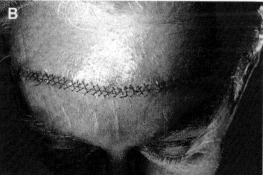

Fig. 8. (*A*) Subcutaneous closure approximating wound edges after mid-forehead excision. (*B*) Meticulous closure to minimize scarring after open mid-forehead lift.

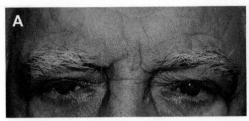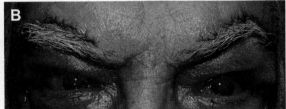

Fig. 9. (*A*) Preoperative brow ptosis in a patient who had direct incisional brow lift. (*B*) Closure does not incorporate the periosteum.

SUMMARY

Open brow lifting techniques are durable and well tolerated procedures that can address brow ptosis and forehead rhytids, while maintaining appropriate forehead heights and pleasing aesthetic appearances. Pretrichial forehead lifting (often the authors' procedure of choice) is appropriate in most women and many men. Mid-forehead and direct supraciliary brow lifting are essential components of the operative plan in men with deep rhytids or very heavy brows.

REFERENCES

1. Hunt HL. Plastic surgery of the head, face, and neck. Philadelphia: Lea & Febiger; 1926.
2. Paul MD. The evolution of the brow lift in aesthetic plastic surgery. Plast Reconstr Surg 2001;108:1409.
3. Vasconez LO. The use of the endoscope in brow lifting. A video presentation at the Annual Meeting of the American Society of Plastic and Reconstructive Surgeons. Washington, DC, September 25, 1992.
4. Isse NG. Endoscopic forehead lift. Presented at the Annual Meeting of the Los Angeles County Society of Plastic Surgeons. Los Angeles (CA), September 12, 1992.
5. McKinney P, Mossie RD, Zukowski ML. Criteria for forehead lift. Aesthetic Plast Surg 1991;15:141–7.
6. Mottura AA. Open frontal lift: a conservative approach. Aesthetic Plast Surg 2006;30:381–9.
7. Knize DM. Galea aponeurotica and temporal fascias. In: Knize DM, editor. Forehead and temporal fossa: anatomy and technique. Philadelphia: Lippincott Williams & Wilkins; 2001. p. 45.
8. Knize DM. Anatomic concepts for brow lift procedures. Plast Reconstr Surg 2009;124:2118.
9. Trinei F, Januskiewicz J, Nahai F. The sentinel vein: an important reference point for surgery in the temporal region. Plast Reconstr Surg 1998;101(1):27–32.

Surgical Manipulation of the Periorbital Musculature

Phillip R. Langsdon, MD[a,b,*], Parker A. Velargo, MD[a],
David W. Rodwell III, MD[a]

KEYWORDS

- Blepharoplasty • Brow • Periorbital • Surgical technique • Transblepharoplasty • Plastic surgery

KEY POINTS

- Brow position has a great impact on facial aesthetics and emotional portrayal.
- The corrugator supercilii, depressor supercilii, procerus, and orbicularis oculi muscles all contribute to brow depression as the aging process progresses.
- The gender of the patient, position of the hairline, presence of forehead tissue redundancy, and patient preference determine the approach to the brow and periorbital musculature.
- Many patients present with the false notion that eyelid surgery elevates the brow. It is important to demonstrate and discuss the influence of brow position on the outcome of upper blepharoplasty surgery.
- A transblepharoplasty brow lift in combination with brow depressor myotomy and extensive subgaleal forehead undermining can provide mild to moderate brow elevation in carefully selected patients.

INTRODUCTION

The position of the brow has an impact on the apparent state of facial aging, general facial aesthetics, and the status of human emotion. Achieving a youthful result with brow-lifting procedures, while maintaining a natural appearance and facial dynamics, may be challenging no matter which surgical approach is selected. When tissue redundancy or a heavy brow is not present, stand-alone weakening of the brow depressor muscles may yield a satisfactory elevation. In this scenario, a transblepharoplasty approach to the periorbital musculature can provide excellent exposure and produce natural-looking results.[1,2]

ANATOMY OF THE UPPER FACE

The upper third of the face is defined by the boundaries of the forehead—from the hairline to the glabella. A forehead with a gentle convexity on profile is most aesthetically ideal. The ideal nasofrontal angle is from 115° to 135°.[3,4]

Brow

In both men and women, the medial brow head lies along a tangent with the medial canthus and nasal ala, whereas the lateral brow head lies along an oblique line drawn from the nasal ala through the lateral canthus (**Fig. 1**). In women, the ideal shape displays the highest point of the brow arch above lateral limbus or lateral canthus, with the brow lying just above the supraorbital rim. In men, the ideal brow has little to no arching and sits at the supraorbital rim.[3,4]

Orbit

The orbit is located in the lower third of the upper face and the upper third of the midface. The width

Disclosures: No commercial or financial disclosures or conflicts of interest for any of the authors.
[a] Division of Facial Plastic and Reconstructive Surgery, Department of Otolaryngology–Head and Neck Surgery, University of Tennessee Health Science Center, 910 Madison Avenue, Suite 429, Memphis, TN 38163, USA; [b] The Langsdon Clinic, 7499 Poplar Pike, Germantown, TN 38138, USA
* Corresponding author.
E-mail address: langsdon@bellsouth.net

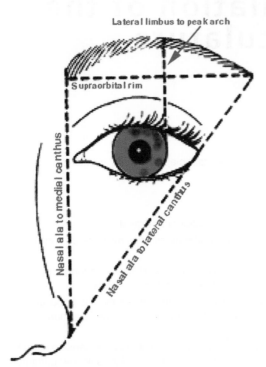

Lateral limbus to peak arch

Supraorbital rim

Nasal ala to medial canthus

Nasal ala to lateral canthus

Fig. 1. Ideal brow position.

of one eye from medial to lateral canthus ideally measures one-fifth of the facial width and the inter-canthal distance equals the width of one eye. Average intercanthal distances are[4] for women, 25.5 mm to 37.5 mm, and for men, 26.5 mm to 38.7 mm.

Eye and Lid

The ideal eye is almond-shaped with the lateral canthus positioned slightly higher than the medial canthus. The palpebral opening averages 10 mm to 12 mm in height and 28 mm to 30 mm in width.[4] The upper lid crease averages approximately 11 mm from the lash line but can vary between 7 mm and 15 mm.[4] Although the upper eyelid normally covers a small portion of the iris, it does not cover the pupil. The lower eyelid lies on 1 mm to 2 mm of the iris on neutral gaze, without scleral show below the iris margin.[3,4]

Corrugator Supercilii, Depressor Supercilii, Procerus, and Orbicularis Oculi

The corrugator supercilii, depressor supercilii, procerus, and orbicularis oculi muscles all play a role in brow depression as the aging process progresses.[1,2,5–7] The procerus muscle originates from the nasal bone (where it is a continuation of the frontalis muscle) and inserts on the skin medial to the brow. The procerus acts to draw the brow inferiorly, producing horizontal wrinkles across the nasal bridge. The corrugator supercilli muscle originates from the medial portion of the supercilli-ary arch, orbital portion of the orbicularis occuli muscle, and lateral portion of the nasal bone. It inserts into the skin of the medial half of the brow and serves to draw the eyebrow in an inferomedial direction, producing vertical wrinkles across the nasal bridge and forehead. Lastly, the orbicularis occuli muscle, which has 3 distinct portions, serves as a brow depressor as well. The orbital portion is responsible for both medial and lateral brow depression. The orbital portion of the orbicullaris occuli muscle originates from the medial orbital margin and the medial palpebral ligament and inserts on the skin of the upper lateral cheek. Other portions of this muscle include the palpebral and lacrimal segments, which have minimal bearing on brow depression. With brow depression, the frontalis muscle tone increases to compensate for the brow depression. With aging, this compensatory frontalis tone results in horizontal forehead rhytids.

EVALUATION OF THE BROW

With aging, the loss of skin elasticity, subcutaneous tissue atrophy, and increased skull bone resorption along with extrinsic factors, such as genetics, facial expression habits, skin type, sun exposure, and smoking history, all play a role in the development of forehead and eyebrow ptosis.[4] A heavy and depressed brow may make a person appear angry, tired, or sad. Brow ptosis is typically associated with tissue redundancy, an overactive depressor muscle action, or both.

When planning brow-repositioning surgery, along with an appropriate history, physical, and eye examination, patient expectations are addressed and asymmetries are pointed out. Particular attention is paid to the position of the hairline, the position of the brow in relation to the superior orbital rim, and lid laxity. The gender of the patient and the position of the hairline influence the decision on approach to the brow and periorbital musculature. If tissue redundancy is present, an open brow or endoscopic approach can be selected. If brow depression is mostly due to depressor muscle action, then neuromodulation and/or myotomy may be indicated. When muscle modulation is all that is necessary, the approach to myotomy need not necessarily be approached through a coronal, pretricheal, direct brow, or endoscopic access. In this situation, a transblepharoplasty brow approach can be considered.

A demonstration and discussion of the dynamic nature of brow position, as well as the impact of the change in brow position related to the differences seen between the upright or recumbent position, is stressed. Adequate preoperative and postoperative photographs are obtained in all patients under conditions of total forehead muscular complex relaxation.

PATIENT PERSPECTIVE

Many patients notice excess upper eyelid tissue bunching and a lack of a lid fold, but few understand the contribution to the problem from a ptotic brow. Patients also often have a false notion that eyelid surgery elevates the brow. Demonstration and discussion of the impact of brow position on the fullness of the upper eyelids can help each patient understand the limitations of upper eyelid blepharoplasty and, in appropriate situations, the potential need for brow elevation.

SURGICAL OPTIONS FOR BROW AND PERIORBITAL AREA

Many techniques for brow elevation and periorbital musculature manipulation have been described, including coronal or pretricheal incisions, direct incision of the suprabrow or forehead, endoscopic techniques, use of absorbable fixation devices, transblepharoplasty brow lift with concurrent corrugator/procerus myotomy, and chemical paralysis of the brow depressors.[8–10]

Brow Depressors

Tissue redundancy and/or contracture of the brow depressors are the main contributing factors in brow ptosis. When tissue redundancy is not severe, addressing the corrugator, procerus, and lateral orbicularis muscles can improve brow depression. It is the authors' belief that the contraction of the brow depressors has more of an impact on brow depression than is usually recognized. Furthermore, almost any approach that weakens the depressors can aid in brow elevation. For example, the brow depressors can be treated with neurotoxins to obtain a significant elevation in many patients who do not present with heavy brow tissue redundancy. Direct surgical myotomy, no matter what exposure technique is used, has the potential to allow a separation of the musculature and provide a relief on the natural downward pull on the brows. When tissue redundancy is significant, however, a coronal, pretricheal, or direct brow lift may be indicated. The authors' procedure choice depends on several factors: gender, hairline, presence of excess skin, and patient preference. In many cases, the brow depressor muscles need to be addressed.

Men with Mild to Moderate Brow Ptosis

In male patients with mild to moderate brow ptosis and minimal tissue redundancy, more can be accomplished in terms of reducing brow depression by performing an upper eyelid transblepharoplasty corrugator and procerus myotomy. If the tail of the brow is low, the authors may perform a division and separation of the lateral orbicularis. If, however, the medial brow is not low, the authors may forego a division of the corrugator and procerus muscles and concentrate on lateral release and stabilization.

Muscular division weakens the impact of muscular contraction, but myoneural connections remain intact unless a complete or near-complete muscular avulsion is performed. Therefore, neuromodulation is an excellent adjunct to the myotomy or partial muscle removal. In addition to myotomy and neuromodulation, the authors may perform a lateral brow stabilization technique if indicated to allow the elevated forehead tissues the opportunity to heal in a superior position.

Men with Severe Brow Ptosis

In cases of severe brow ptosis with excessive redundant forehead skin in a male patient, a direct brow lift may be necessary in addition to the myotomy. As an alternative, the authors have previously described a transblepharoplasty brow lift in combination with brow depressor myotomy and extensive subgaleal forehead undermining, which can provide good results and satisfaction ratings in many patients.[1,2]

Women with Mild to Moderate Brow Ptosis

In general, the authors' female patients are more accepting of brow-altering surgery and the typical pattern of female hair broadens the options. In limited female brow ptosis, the authors may recommend neurotoxin relaxation of the brow depressor muscles, as in male patients. For mild to moderate brow ptosis, however, the authors may recommend either a transblepharoplasty myotomy and brow elevation or a lateral temporal pretricheal subcutaneous brow elevation along with a division of the brow depressors. For even more significant brow ptosis, the authors may perform a coronal forehead lift (in cases of a low hairline) or a pretricheal coronal forehead lift (in cases of a high hairline). In a female patient with thinning hair, the authors may use a transblepharoplasty brow depressor myotomy with stabilization (as described previously for male patients).

Endoscopic Brow Lift

The senior author finds that an endoscope has no advantage over a transblepharoplasty approach for brow lifting and/or corrugator and procerus myotomy because there is ample exposure under direct visualization. Currently, the senior author's only indication for an endoscopic approach is when there is no need for an upper lid blepharoplasty or if a patient refuses an upper eyelid incision. In cases where the transblepharoplasty approach is used and parietal scalp mobilization is necessary, a small scalp incision can be used to blindly extend the frontal scalp elevation into the parietal region. In patients with unusually high hairlines, the pretricheal approach may be an excellent option. One recent systematic review indicated that there was no clear evidence to indicate that open methods of brow surgery are inferior to endoscopic approaches.[8]

SURGICAL DESCRIPTIONS

Coronal, pretricheal, endoscopic, and direct approaches are discussed elsewhere in this issue by Terella and Wang and by Walrath and McCord. The transblepharoplasty approach can be simple and provide easy access to the brow depressor muscles. A simple stepwise approach can be used (**Box 1**).

Box 1
Simplified approach to transblepharoplasty brow lift

1. Standard upper eyelid blepharoplasty incision.

2. Develop suborbicularis skin/muscle flap in lateral two-thirds of upper eyelid.

3. Enter subgaleal plane just above the supra-orbital rim.

4. Undermine the forehead laterally, then medially.

5. Proceed with medial dissection to expose the brow depressors.

6. Cauterize and divide the corrugators and procerus muscles.

7. Consider lateral division of the orbital portion of the orbicularis oculi muscle if additional lateral elevation is needed.

8. Suspend the brow using suture or an absorbable implant.

9. Obtain hemostasis and close with 6-0 fast-absorbing plain gut.

10. Use tape to support the forehead elevation.

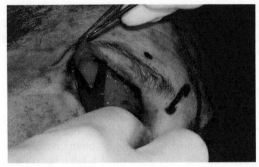

Fig. 2. Lateral development of the suborbicularis skin/muscle flap. (© *Phillip R. Langsdon*.)

The transblepharoplasty brow lift with corrugator and procerus myotomy is performed through a standard upper eyelid blepharoplasty incision.[6]

- After upper eyelid cutaneous and muscle strip excision, a superiorly based suborbicularis skin-muscle flap is raised by blunt spreading-scissor dissection in the region of the lateral two-thirds of the upper eyelid (**Fig. 2**).
- The flap dissection is carried superiorly to a point just above the superior orbital rim.
- Spreading-scissor dissection is then directed toward the supraorbital bone until the subgaleal plane is reached. The depth of dissection remains superficial to the pericranium (**Fig. 3**).
- The lateral temporal line is incised if increased lateral mobility is necessary.
- The dissection is also performed medially, remaining superior to the supraorbital neurovascular bundle.
- The medial portion of the upper eyelid is elevated in the suborbicularis plane, isolating and remaining medial to the supraorbital neurovascular bundle.
- The dissection is continued medially (**Fig. 4**).

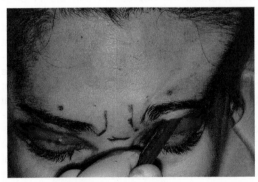

Fig. 3. Development of frontal elevation in the subgaleal plane. (© *Phillip R. Langsdon*.)

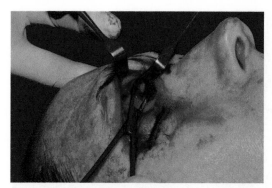

Fig. 4. Medial dissection and exposure of the brow depressors. (© *Phillip R. Langsdon.*)

- The medial dissection exposes the corrugator and depressor supercilii muscles. To obtain medial elevation of the brow, these muscles are cauterized and then incrementally divided with eyelid scissors (see **Fig. 4**). The usual abundant blood supply in the corrugator requires careful hemostasis.
- Once divided, scissor dissection is continued medially until the procerus is encountered and divided in a similar manner.
- If a lateral elevation of the brow is needed, the orbital portion of the orbicularis oculi is divided in the lateral one-third point of the eyelid (**Fig. 5**).
- Because the orbicularis oculi muscle is much thinner than the medial depressors, careful and light cautery is performed over the planned muscular division site, followed by an incremental scissor division of the muscle that extends from the blepharoplasty incision inferiorly to the inferior extent of the eyebrow superiorly.
- Once divided, the orbicularis is spread in a medial-to-lateral direction with scissors.

If lateral brow stabilization is considered, 2 options exist:

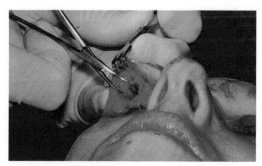

Fig. 5. The orbicularis oculi can be divided for additional lateral elevation. (© *Phillip R. Langsdon.*)

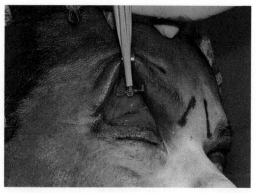

Fig. 6. Placement of an absorbable L-polylactic acid implant for brow suspension above the lateral limbus. (© *Phillip R. Langsdon.*)

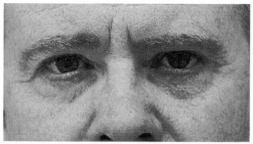

Fig. 7. Preoperative view of a male patient demonstrating vertical glabellar rhytids from corrugator muscle contraction, dermatochalasis of the upper lids, and depression of the brows. Note the slight asymmetry in brow position. This patient had prior blepharoplasty by another doctor before coming to the authors' clinic. (© *Phillip R. Langsdon.*)

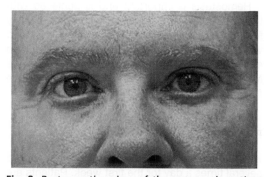

Fig. 8. Postoperative view of the same male patient after transblepharoplasty corrugators, procerus, and lateral orbicularis myotomy. No neuromodulation was used in this photograph. Note the tremendous improvement in brow positioning as well as the lack of vertical glabellar rhytids. (© *Phillip R. Langsdon.*)

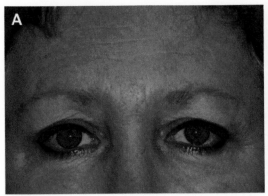
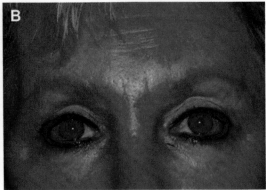

Fig. 9. (*A*) Preoperative and (*B*) 44-month postoperative views of a 54-year-old woman who had upper eyelid blepharoplasty with transblepharoplasty brow lift using an absorbable fixation device. (© *Phillip R. Langsdon*.)

1. Placement of an absorbable fixation device
2. Suture suspension
   a. An absorbable L-polylactic acid anchor can be placed approximately 10 mm above the orbital rim, near a vertical line from the lateral limbus of the eye after first drilling a bone anchor site.
   b. The brow is then redraped over the device and secured with pressure onto the tines (**Fig. 6**). Alternatively, suture suspension can be used for suspension (nylon, prolene, or polydioxanone). Suture suspension of the lateral aspect of the orbicularis oculi muscle relies on the presence of supra-brow periosteum.

Brow stabilization has the added benefit of creating more lateral elevation of the brow, which can be aesthetically pleasing, especially in female patients. Some investigators have also proposed suture suspension of the lateral brow tissue to the temporal fascia for added lateral elevation and support.[11]

Hemostasis is important and is achieved with the use of bipolar cautery with guarded cautery forceps and a headlight. The incision is closed with 6-0 fast-absorbing plain gut suture. If the entire forehead has been elevated, benzoin and Micropore tape is used to partially stabilize the forehead for 2 weeks.

POSTOPERATIVE CARE

Hydrogen peroxide and petroleum jelly are applied several times a day for the first week. Patients are asked to sleep in an upright position to decrease the inevitable swelling. Remaining sutures are removed at 1 week. The tape is removed in 2 weeks. Hypesthesia is expected for several months, and patients should be appropriately counseled regarding this. Puckering of the eyelid may occur but usually resolves without any treatment.

COMPLICATIONS WITH TRANSBLEPHAROPLASTY APPROACH

- Bruising and swelling are normal.
- Frontal branch paralysis of the facial nerve is possible but uncommon. The authors have not seen this occur in their practice.
- Early loss of suspension support is possible. Avoidance of this potential complication is possible with careful intraoperative technique and appropriate aftercare, including the use of supportive tape (as described previously).
- Full excision of the corrugator and procerus muscles, although effective in eliminating brow depression, may cause unsightly divots to the overlying skin. Muscle or fat can be placed if necessary at the time of surgery, or injectable fillers can be used several months postoperatively.

SUMMARY

The transblepharoplasty approach to division of the brow depressor muscles is an expedient way to release the brows for elevation. Patient and surgeon satisfaction rates are consistently high without significant complications (see **Fig. 6**; **Figs. 7–9**).[6] The normal contraction of the frontalis muscle with decreased opposition of the brow depressor muscles can provide a nice elevation. Tissue redundancy may require additional surgical maneuvers if brow ptosis is not the sole result of muscular depression. Transblepharoplasty muscle division may be combined with other forehead procedures to reduce tissue redundancy. Small parietal incisions may also be used to blindly elevate the parietal scalp. Tissue may also be stabilized from this position.

REFERENCES

1. Langsdon PR. Transblepharoplasty brow suspension: an expanded role. Ann Plast Surg 2008;60(1): 2–5.
2. Langsdon PR. Transblepharoplasty brow suspension with a biodegradable fixation device. Aesthet Surg J 2010;30(6):802–9.
3. Carruthers JD, Glogau RG, Blitzer A, Facial Aesthetics Consensus Group Faculty. Advances in facial rejuvenation: botulinum toxin type a, hyaluronic acid dermal fillers, and combination therapies—consensus recommendations. Plast Reconstr Surg 2008;121(Suppl 5):5S–30S [quiz: 31S–6S].
4. Nassif PS. Management of the aging brow and forehead, Ch. 31. Bailey's head and neck surgery—otolaryngology. 4th edition. Philadelphia: Lippincot Williams & Wilkins; 2006.
5. Ahn MS, Catten M, Maas CS. Temporal brow lift using botulinum toxin A. Plast Reconstr Surg 2000; 105(3):1129–35 [discussion: 1136–9].
6. Knize DM. Muscles that act on glabellar skin: a closer look. Plast Reconstr Surg 2000;105:350–61.
7. Knize DM. An anatomically based study of the mechanism of eyebrow ptosis. Plast Reconstr Surg 1996;97:1321–33.
8. Rohrich RJ. Brow lift in facial rejuvenation. Plast Reconstr Surg 2011;128(4):335–41.
9. Angelos PC, Stallworth CL, Wang TD. Forehead lifting: state of the art. Facial Plast Surg 2011;27(1): 50–7 [Epub 2011 Jan 18]. Review.
10. Stevens WG. The endotine: a new biodegradable fixation device for endoscopic forehead lifts. Aesthet Surg J 2003;23(2):103–7.
11. Ramirez OM. Transblepharoplasty forehead lift and upper face rejuvenation. Ann Plast Surg 1996; 37(6):577–84.

Upper Blepharoplasty
The Aesthetic Ideal

Jon-Paul Pepper, MD*, Jeffrey S. Moyer, MD, FACS

KEYWORDS

• Blepharoplasty • Aesthetics • Upper eyelid anatomy • Aging face • Plastic surgery

KEY POINTS

- Upper lid aging is characterized by changes in the curvature of the upper lid and the position of the lateral canthus. Periorbital volume loss and skin elasticity changes result in the characteristic dermatochalsis and smaller visible palpebral aperture associated with the aging upper lid.
- Accurate preoperative assessment of the anatomic problem is critical.
- Precise incision marking will in large part determine a successful upper lid blepharoplasty.
- Fat-sparing techniques are most commonly used to avoid a hollow upper lid and excessive pretarsal show.

INTRODUCTION

Upper lid blepharoplasty was first described by the Hindu surgeon Susruta in approximately the second century AD, in the *Susruta Samhita*.[1] Eyelid surgery was largely forgotten for centuries but experienced a revival in the eighteenth and nineteenth centuries via the work of Beer and Von Graafe.[2] Slowly there evolved a more detailed understanding of upper lid anatomy and the correction of age-related changes. Early approaches focused on the excision of redundant soft tissue.[3] It was not until recently that surgeons gained an appreciation of the esthetic benefits of conservation of periorbital fat.[3] In the past 15 years, many authors have decried the skeletonized and hollow upper lid as the stigmata of overaggressive fat resection during upper lid blepharoplasty.[4]

ANATOMY AND AGE-RELATED CHANGES IN THE UPPER EYELID

Perhaps the most critical component to performing consistently successful upper lid blepharoplasty is accurate facial analysis during the presurgical consultation. As is widely known, the upper lid is analyzed simultaneously with the brow and the entire periorbital region. As such, the eyebrows should be at or above the orbital rim, with the medial brow at a vertical line drawn through the alar-facial sulcus and the medial canthus. The lateral margin terminates at a line drawn from the ala, through the lateral canthus (**Fig. 1**). The lateral canthus should be 2 mm cephalad to the medial canthus, creating a positive canthal tilt of 3° to 4° in the women and 1° to 2° in the men.[5]

Supratarsal Crease

The essential landmark of upper lid blepharoplasty is the supratarsal crease. The supratarsal crease is commonly 7 to 10 mm from the palpebral margin, usually 8 to 9 mm above the lid margin in women and 7 to 8 mm in men. It is thought that the supratarsal crease is created by the fusion of the levator aponeurosis with the orbital septum and the insertion of the fascia of the orbicularis oculi into the dermis.[3] Recent anatomic studies reveal that the levator aponeurosis has 2 distinct layers.[6] The anterior layer reflects upward and inserts on the orbital septum. The posterior layer inserts

Division of Facial Plastic and Reconstructive Surgery, Department of Otolaryngology–Head and Neck Surgery, Center for Facial Cosmetic Surgery, University of Michigan, Livonia, MI, USA
* Corresponding author.
E-mail address: jonpaul@med.umich.edu

Clin Plastic Surg 40 (2013) 133–138
http://dx.doi.org/10.1016/j.cps.2012.07.001
0094-1298/13/$ – see front matter © 2013 Elsevier Inc. All rights reserved.

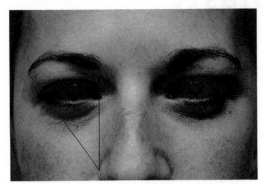

Fig. 1. Example of youthful periorbital anatomy. Note the relationship of the medial and lateral ends of the brow with respect to lines drawn through the alar-facial sulcus and medial canthus as well as the alar-facial sulcus and lateral canthus, respectively.

onto the tarsal plate and the subcutaneous tissue superficial to the tarsal plate's lower third.

Age-Related Changes in the Periorbital Area

The tarsal portion of the orbicularis is thought to be particularly susceptible to age-related changes, and the involution of the pretarsal soft tissue causes a concomitant elevation in height in the supratarsal fold and increased skin laxity in this location. As attachments to the thin dermis at the supratarsal crease are lost, the soft tissue herniates inferiorly, creating the characteristic dermatochalasis of the aged upper lid (**Fig. 2**).

The orbital fat of the upper lid is thought to comprise the medial (nasal) and preaponeurotic ("prelevator") fat pads. Anteriorly, there is a relative demarcation between the 2, whereas posteriorly the fat pads comingle with little distinguishing features.[7] The preaponeurotic fat traverses the lateral portion of the superior periorbita, curling behind the posterior aspect of the lacrimal gland. There is a clear demarcation between the preaponeurotic and medial fat pads. The medial horn of the levator aponeurosis and the lateral fascia on the superior oblique muscle both serve to separate the central compartment from the medial compartment. The medial compartment is pale yellow or white due to a greater percentage of connective tissue, thereby imbuing this tissue with paler hues.[3] The central/preaponeurotic fat has a higher concentration of carotenoids, which gives this fat a yellow hue, in contrast to the pale medial compartment fat.[8]

General loss of skin elasticity and loss of soft tissue volume combine to increase upper lid skin redundancy.[4] Oh and Colleagues[9] demonstrate a relative *increase* in the subjective volume of the *nasal* fat pad during the aging process. The central

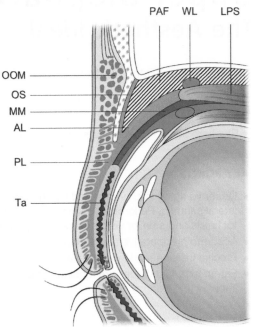

Fig. 2. Sagittal section of the periorbital region and upper lid. Note the connections between the posterior layer of the levator aponeurosis and the pretarsal skin. *Abbreviations:* AL, anterior layer of levator aponeurosis; LPS, levator palpebrae superioris muscle; MM, mullers muscle; OOM, orbicularis oculi; OS, orbital septum; PAF, preaponeurotic fat; PL, posterior layer of levator aponeurosis; Ta, tarsus; WL, Whitnall's ligament.

fat pad, in contrast, seems to diminish in terms of its apparent volume as patients age. This is the driving factor in the skeletonized or hallowed look of the superior periorbital region. The supratarsal crease often migrates cephalad as the eye ages; it is thought that relative volume loss may either cause or exacerbate this cephalad repositioning of the supratarsal crease (**Fig. 3**).

As summarized by Lambros, the 2 key stigmata of periorbital aging include[10]:

1. Upper lid "arc shift" from medial to lateral
2. Apparent decrease in size of palpebral fissure

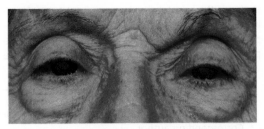

Fig. 3. Aged periorbital region. Note the elevation of the supratarsal fold in combination with asymmetric blepharoptosis.

The arc of the upper lid has its peak on the medial aspect of the lid in the youthful face in both men and women (see **Fig. 1**; **Fig. 4**).[10] As patients age, the peak of the upper lid's arc migrates to a more lateral position. Depending on the method of study, it has been assumed that the periorbital retaining ligaments lose elasticity as patients age,[11] which may contribute to migration of the lateral canthal angle.[10] This is a matter of some debate. A cross-sectional study of 320 patients found little to no migration of the lateral canthal angle with respect to other lid photogrammetric landmarks.[12] Contrary to conventional assumption, the lateral canthal angle did not descend inferiorly with age with respect to the pupil and lid surface reference landmarks. Instead, the lateral canthus was found to be migrating anteriorly with respect to the anterior corneal surface on lateral view. The end sum of this migration is the perception of a smaller palpebral aperture and a smaller surface area of conjunctiva in the aging eye, which seems to be a point of consensus in the literature.[10] It is worth noting that the medial canthal angle, by contrast, is thought to be relatively stable throughout the aging process. Also, the globe itself does not change size as patients age, nor is globe descent a prominent part of the aging process.[10]

Although many anthropometric analyses are beginning to scratch the surface of the myriad age-associated changes of upper lid anatomy, there are several additional considerations that directly impact surgical esthetic goals. Particularly, gender- and ethnicity-related influences exert independent effects on the aging process of the periorbital region. Furthermore, there may be significant a priori differences between genders and races in terms of the esthetic goals with regard to upper lid surgery. For instance, lower eyelid

sagging is often more pronounced in men and may therefore be of higher concern to male patients seeking periorbital rejuvenation.[12] Both genders experience more superior placement of the supratarsal crease as they age, as well as eyebrow elevation.[13] This is a burgeoning area of research, and nearly all preliminary data show significant differences between different genders and different ethnic groups that exert an influence on the periorbital aging process.[12–14]

As a whole, these studies have begun to establish an understanding of the normative anatomy of the periorbital region as it varies by race and age. Although this certainly impacts the esthetic ideal, it by no means defines it. Future investigations will, we hope, elucidate to what extent gender and ethnicity may affect a patient's assessment of surgical outcome as well as their goals when initially seeking blepharoplasty.

EVALUATION FOR UPPER LID BLEPHAROPLASTY

The most critical aspect of successful upper lid blepharoplasty is the preoperative office evaluation, which enables accurate preoperative incision planning. The presurgical consultation must include an examination of visual acuity as well as visual field testing. The Snellen chart is the standard for monocular visual acuity. A thorough visual field examination is critical, particularly if the patient seeks blepharoplasty for functional reasons and may be covered by his or her insurer.

Dry Eye

All patients must be queried regarding dry eye symptoms, and this is an important consideration given the high prevalence of dry eye complaints in patients seeking upper eyelid surgery (up to 15%).[15] A Schirmer's test is no longer considered the standard of care for the diagnosis of dry eye syndrome.[15] There is a well-documented association between dry eye symptoms and autoimmune disease, and therefore patients with suspected undiagnosed autoimmune disease are referred to a rheumatologist for further evaluation. Other relevant aspects of the past medical history include glaucoma, hypertension (the patient's blood pressure is measured), anticoagulation (including low-dose aspirin), renal failure, and edema of the extremities.

Patients are specifically asked if they have recently undergone laser vision correction surgery. Current guidelines recommend that patients wait at least 6 months before undergoing blepharoplasty due to temporary dysfunction in tear film

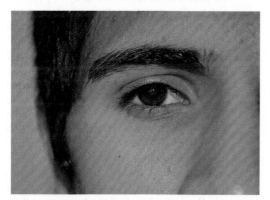

Fig. 4. Youthful periorbital region in a male patient. As in the photograph of a female patient (see **Fig. 1**), there is an arc that is highest laterally and a superolateral fullness of the upper lid.

production and corneal sensation that may occur after laser vision surgery.[16]

Facial Nerve Function, Lagophthalmos, Bell's Phenomenon, Ectropion, Blepharochalasis

The role of the lid in corneal protection is paramount; therefore, careful evaluation of facial nerve function and determination of the presence or absence of lagophthalmos, Bell's phenomenon, and ectropion are critical. During the evaluation of the upper lid, blepharochalasis is ruled out. Blephrochalasis is an IgE-mediated condition marked by recurrent swelling and erythema.[3] It is likely to recur and these patients are poor candidates for blepharoplasty.

Dermatochalasis

Dermatochalasis may result in compensatory frontalis contraction and this should be pointed out during the patient consultation and evaluation. Once the dermatochalasis is surgically corrected, the compensatory contraction may cease. This may result in the brow soft tissue to slide inferiorly, thereby minimizing the impact of the blepharoplasty. Tonic, subconscious compensatory frontalis contraction is common. Mild scarring forces after upper lid blepharoplasty may further exacerbate undiagnosed brow ptosis.

Ptosis

Both bilateral and unilateral blepharoptosis can have important ramifications for presurgical planning before upper lid blepharoplasty. Ptosis can be most accurately assessed via an anterior view photograph, by comparing the margin to corneal light reflex distance of the upper and lower lids. Note that unilateral ptosis is often accompanied by compensatory brow elevation. Ptosis should be suspected in any patient with more than 2 to 3 mm of lid overlap of the upper limbus of the iris. In the patient with a high supratarsal crease and unilateral ptosis, the surgeon should suspect levator palpebrae superioris dehiscence. This may be addressed simultaneously with upper lid blepharoplasty but should be evaluated by an ophthalmologist before surgery.

INCISION PLANNING

The patient is positioned upright, as analysis and marking while supine can cause any medial pseudoherniation to seem less severe due to the effect of gravity. Also, the brow and lid are pulled superiorly by the scalp when the patient lies supine.

- The brow is elevated with the surgeon's nondominant hand so as to minimize the confounding effect of the brow soft tissues on true upper lid dermatochalasis. Failure to suspend the brow soft tissue may result in overresection and a supratarsal crease that is more superior than originally intended. Given that elevated supratarsal crease position is associated with the aged eye, this is a complication that should be avoided.
- The usual location of the supratarsal crease is 8 to 9 mm above the lid margin in women and 7 to 8 mm in men. A fine-tipped skin marker is used, with alcohol pads available for remarking as needed. It may be easier to identify the crease by having the patient look downward.
- The inferior incision line is marked first. For a patient with a supratarsal crease that is 9 mm above the lid margin, the inferior mark is begun 1 to 2 mm inferior to the actual crease.
- Medially, the planned incisions slope downward toward the medial canthus, approximately 7 to 8 mm.
- The incision is stopped at the superior lacrimal punctum. This is thought to lessen the chance of forming a medial canthal web.
- The lateral extent of the inferior limb incision drops inferiorly to within approximately 5 mm of the lateral canthus.
- The incision is then brought back superiorly into a natural skin crease. We avoid extending the lateral incisions beyond the orbital rim if possible due to the unfavorable scar that may result, particularly in the patient with few lateral periorbital rhytids. However, the presence of lateral hooding may require a lateral extension of the incision with a gentle curve upward past the lateral canthus.
- Higher placement of the inferior incision will result in more pretarsal show. This may also create the illusion that the upper lid margin has a more caudal resting position and therefore can be used to the surgeon's advantage if there is any preoperative asymmetry with respect to the resting position of the upper lid margin.
- The superior incision is marked based on the degree of soft tissue redundancy. We use Green fixation forceps to grasp redundant soft tissue, placing them sequentially in the medial, central, and lateral portions of the lid to determine the width of the

excised tissue. This width determines the location of the superior incision.

- Care is taken to preserve at least 15 mm of skin between the superior incision and the lower margin of the brow and 8 to 10 mm of eyelid skin between the incision and the eyelid margin. The total amount removed is variable but is greater in older patients with more lax tissues. Overaggressive resection places the patient at risk of postoperative lagophthalmos.

- Not all patients have a supratarsal crease that is the classic 8 to 9 mm from the ciliary margin of the upper lid. If the crease is caudal, such as in the lid of Caucasian male patients, the entire inferior incision line should be adjusted to accommodate the difference and avoid the creation of a double crease. Additionally, larger amounts of dermatochalasis may demand more aggressive resection of the medial skin. A W-plasty may be helpful in these instances to keep the medial incision from extending beyond the lacrimal punctum.

A detailed description of the surgical technique is made elsewhere in this issue. Briefly, following sharp elevation and excision of the thin skin flap as described above, the surgeon is faced with the decision to either incise the orbicularis oculi muscle or perform plication of the muscle. The surgeon must keep in mind that the orbicularis is the main depressor muscle of the upper lid. Incision through the muscle may denervate distal pretarsal fibers, thereby allowing more unopposed levator palpebrae superioris function and, therefore, an elevation in the resting position of the lower lid. This is a favorable result for most blepharoplasty procedures. This should be considered carefully, however, if the surgeon is performing an orbicularis plication alone without resection and limited fat cautery versus resection. Notably, some authors believe that preservation of orbicularis in the upper lid allows for an "accordion" effect of bunching the muscle fibers and thereby providing more fullness to the upper lid.[4] The esthetic principle is to preserve or restore a convex contour to the lid brow junction in addition to resecting redundant tissue.

PATIENT PERSPECTIVE

During the preoperative counseling session, patients are counseled about the attendant risks of blepharoplasty. On average, upper lid blepharoplasty is a well-tolerated procedure with a high rate of satisfaction for both patient and surgeon. However, a recent prospective study of patient satisfaction following blepharoplasty demonstrated that patients may underestimate the amount of postoperative swelling and pain and the degree to which their recovery affects their ability to function in their daily activities.[17] It seems, then, that despite the long track record of success, there may still be room for more accurate preparation of patients, particularly for the early stages of surgical recovery.

In the senior author's view, both male and female patients are in search of a more youthful upper lid. It is commonly presumed that male patients seeking blepharoplasty more frequently do so for functional reasons (ie, restriction of the temporal visual fields).[18] However, this is tempered by an individualized approach that takes into account the patient's age, ethnicity, and gender.

AFTERCARE

Immediately on skin closure, ice packs are applied and replaced every half hour once the patient is in the recovery room. Ophthalmic bacitracin ointment is used on the incision line. We ask that patients apply ice packs every hour after leaving the recovery room. Patients are counseled to avoid the use of alcohol and anticoagulant medications if feasible, based on their medical history and comorbidities. Patients are asked to avoid significant physical activity for 1 week to limit postoperative edema and ecchymosis. The patient is seen in clinic for postoperative evaluation 5 to 7 days after surgery, at which time the sutures are removed and any concerns are addressed.

SUMMARY

Upper lid blepharoplasty is a surgical procedure with a high level of patient and surgeon satisfaction. Keys to successful results and reproducible technique depend greatly on accurate preoperative assessment of the anatomic problem and precise marking of the soft tissues in the presurgical suite. The anatomy of this region is complex, and our understanding of the periorbital aging process is a work in progress. First and foremost, our ability to more precisely understand the age-related changes of the upper lid will drive future surgical (and nonsurgical) innovation. Last, our grasp of the efficacy of the existing surgical techniques will improve as more evidence-based outcomes studies are performed.

REFERENCES

1. Dalwi DM. The Hindu origins of modern medicine. New Sci 1984;26:43.

2. Dupuis C, Rees TD. Historical notes on blepharoplasty. Plast Reconstr Surg 1971;47:246–51.
3. Rohrich RJ, Coberly DM, Fagien S, et al. Current concepts in aesthetic upper blepharoplasty. Plast Reconstr Surg 2004;113:32e–42e.
4. Fagien S. The role of the orbicularis oculi muscle and the eyelid crease in optimizing results in aesthetic upper blepharoplasty: an new look at the surgical treatment of mild upper eyelid fissure and fold asymmetries. Plast Reconstr Surg 2010; 125:653–66.
5. Wolfort FG, Gee F, Pan D, et al. Nuances of aesthetic blepharoplasty. Ann Plast Surg 1997;38:257–62.
6. Jones LT. The anatomy of the upper eyelid and its relation to ptosis surgery. Am J Ophthalmol 1964; 57:943–59.
7. Sires BS, Lemke BN, Dortzbach RK, et al. Characterization of human orbital fat and connective tissue. Ophthal Plast Reconstr Surg 1998;14:403–14.
8. Kakizaki H, Malhotra R, Selva D. Upper eyelid anatomy: an update. Ann Plast Surg 2009;63(3): 336–43.
9. Oh SR, Chokthaweesak W, Annunziata CC, et al. Analysis of eyelid fat pad changes with aging. Ophthal Plast Reconstr Surg 2011;27(5):348–51.
10. Lambros V. Observations on periorbital and midface aging. Plast Reconstr Surg 2007;120(5):1367–76 [discussion: 1377].
11. Pelletier AT, Few JW. Eyebrow and eyelid dimensions: an anthropometric analysis of African Americans and Caucasians. Plast Reconstr Surg 2010; 125(4):1293–4.
12. van den Bosch WA, Leenders I, Mulder P. Topographic anatomy of the eyelids, and the effects of sex and age. Br J Ophthalmol 1999;83(3):347–52.
13. Price KM, Gupta PK, Woodward JA, et al. Eyebrow and eyelid dimensions: an anthropometric analysis of African Americans and Caucasians. Plast Reconstr Surg 2009;124(2):615–23.
14. Kunjur J, Sabesan T, Ilankovan V. Anthropometric analysis of eyebrows and eyelids: an inter-racial study. Br J Oral Maxillofac Surg 2006;44(2):89–93 [Epub 2005 Jun 4].
15. Friedland JA, Lalonde DH, Rohrich RJ. An evidence-based approach to blepharoplasty. Plast Reconstr Surg 2010;126(6):2222–9.
16. Lee WB, McCord CD Jr, Somia N, et al. Optimizing blepharoplasty outcomes in patients with previous laser vision correction. Plast Reconstr Surg 2008; 122(2):587–94.
17. Parbhu KC, Hawthorne KM, McGwin G Jr, et al. Patient experience with blepharoplasty. Ophthal Plast Reconstr Surg 2011;27(3):152–4.
18. Flowers RS. Periorbital aesthetic surgery for men. Eyelids and related structures. Clin Plast Surg 1991;18(4):689–729.

Esthetic Enhancements in Upper Blepharoplasty

Judy W. Lee, MD*, Shan R. Baker, MD

KEYWORDS

- Blepharoplasty • Upper periorbital aging • Periorbital volume • Esthetic outcomes

KEY POINTS

- Similar to recent trends in lower blepharoplasty toward volume conservation and repositioning, improved understanding of upper periorbital aging has allowed surgeons to develop new or modified techniques to improve esthetic outcomes in upper blepharoplasty.
- Repositioning the more robust nasal fat compartment laterally toward the central preaponeurotic fat can improve medial redundancy without compromising central upper eyelid volume.
- With little to no morphologic or functional change in orbicularis oculi with aging, muscle preservation during upper blepharoplasty may prevent unnecessary complications or scarring in selected patients with dermatochalasis as the primary concern.
- Volume loss in the lateral third of the upper eyelid can be restored with pedicled fat flaps or free fat grafts in conjunction with orbicularis oculi imbrication.
- The upper blepharoplasty incision allows direct access to the brow and orbital structures that may aggravate upper eyelid crowding and fullness. Internal brow elevation and sculpting and resuspension of a prolapsed lacrimal gland can be performed through the upper blepharoplasty incision.

INTRODUCTION

Upper blepharoplasty is one of the most frequent facial cosmetic surgical procedures for periorbital rejuvenation. The natural esthetic and youthful appearance of the periorbital region is characterized by soft tissue fullness framing the eye, whereas the aging eye is typically hollowed and surrounded by a deep upper lid sulcus with variable amounts of upper lid skin laxity with or without pseudoherniation of periorbital fat. When considering upper eyelid rejuvenation, it is imperative to consider all factors that may contribute to the aging upper eyelids. Standard treatments for upper lid dermatochalasis have focused on resection of redundant tissue, including skin, muscle, and fat from the upper eyelid. This may lead to hollowing of the upper lid sulcus from overresection

of soft tissue, resulting in an unfavorable appearance.

In recent years, the concept of periorbital volume restoration and augmentation, instead of reduction, has gained increasing popularity among cosmetic surgeons. Improved understanding of periorbital physiology from aging has led to modified techniques using fat conservation and repositioning, orbicularis oculi muscle preservation, and increasing lateral upper eyelid fullness to achieve esthetic enhancements in upper blepharoplasty.[1–9] These concepts in conjunction with adjunctive procedures, including internal brow elevation, lacrimal gland resuspension, and glabellar myectomy performed through an upper blepharoplasty approach, can provide a myriad of esthetic enhancements to standard upper blepharoplasty.[10–12]

Center for Facial Cosmetic Surgery, University of Michigan Department of Otolaryngology, 19900 Haggerty Road, Suite 103, Livonia, MI 48152, USA
* Corresponding author.
E-mail address: judy.lee@nyumc.org

Clin Plastic Surg 40 (2013) 139–146
http://dx.doi.org/10.1016/j.cps.2012.08.008

ANATOMY

The upper eyelid crease is located approximately 8 to 10 mm from the palpebral margin in the typical Caucasian eye. Loss of fascial attachments of the orbicularis oculi, levator aponeurosis, and orbital septum into the dermis can contribute to skin laxity and displacement of the crease inferiorly. In the brow, the frontalis muscle interdigitates with the procerus muscle medially, orbicularis oculi muscle laterally, and corrugator and orbicularis oculi muscles in the central portion of the brow. The galeal layer that gives rise to the fascia overlying these muscles contributes to brow height, symmetry, and shape.[13]

Upper Eyelid Fat

The upper eyelid fat is divided into nasal (medial) and preaponeurotic (central) fat pads divided by the superior oblique muscle tendon and is found posterior to the orbital septum. The nasal fat pad is usually pale yellow or white, whereas the lateral fat pad is more yellow. This difference is suggested to be caused by a greater amount of connective tissue and vascularity in the nasal fat and a greater amount of carotenoids in the lateral fat.[1] The retro-orbicularis oculi fat (ROOF) lies deep to the orbicularis oculi muscle but above and anterior to the orbital septum and should not be confused with the preaponeurotic fat pad, which lies deep to the orbital septum.[13,14] The ROOF is contiguous superiorly with the lateral brow fat pad, which lies beneath the orbicularis oculi and frontalis muscular layer. The ROOF is more fibrofatty than the preaponeurotic eyelid fat and provides fullness to the temporal eyelid and brow, which can persist after upper blepharoplasty if left unaddressed. The lateral brow fat should be distinguished from a prolapsed lacrimal gland, which can present with excessive lateral upper eyelid fullness caused mainly by relaxation of suspensory ligaments. The gland is firmer in texture than the surrounding fat and is tan.[12]

Orbicularis Oculi Muscle

Traditional upper blepharoplasty often includes an en bloc excision of skin and orbicularis oculi muscle. The palpebral portion of the muscle is limited to the eyelid and is divided into pretarsal and preseptal components. The functions of this muscle are primarily for eyelid closure, compression of tears, and dilation of the lacrimal sac. Although the skin and subcutaneous tissue layer undergo significant changes with aging, the orbicularis oculi muscle remains anatomically and physiologically intact and is not affected by advancing age, as described in a recent study by Pottier and colleagues.[2] Their histologic study showed that orbicularis oculi muscle fibers remained intact with the same bulk of fibers through the aging process. However, the loss of skin elastic fibers and skin laxity were significant and paralleled the advancement of age. Additionally, electromyographic analysis showed that age did not have a significant effect on motor unit action potentials and the force of muscle contraction. A similar histologic study by Lee and colleagues[3] showed that the orbicularis oculi muscle remained morphologically intact with advancing age in the Asian population. The authors concluded that a minimally invasive approach with muscle sparing in upper blepharoplasty in selected patients who desire volume preservation of the youthful convexity of the upper eyelid–brow junction could yield positive esthetic results and retain excellent eyelid function while minimizing postoperative complications.

Upper Eyelid Aging

Recent studies on anatomic, chemical, and biologic characteristics of the upper eyelid have shown that the central fat pad seems to diminish in volume with aging, whereas the nasal fat pad increases in volume with advancing age (**Figs. 1** and **2**).[4] This disparity seems to begin in the early fourth decade of age, with the most significant change after age 70 years. This disparity may be explained by differences in vascularity and connective tissue composition. The nasal fat pad is similar in composition to intraconal orbital fat, whereas the more yellow central fat pad is similar to adipose tissue found elsewhere throughout the body. Korn and colleagues[5] reported that there was a 2-fold increase in the number of adult stem cells derived from human orbital adipose tissue in the nasal fat pad compared with the central fat pad. The authors suggest that the relative abundance in progenitor stem cells in the nasal fat may explain the relative increase in nasal fat pad volume during an individual's lifetime.

EVALUATION

When determining a surgical treatment plan for a patient who presents with excess periorbital tissue and heaviness in the upper eyelids, it is important to consider all of the factors that may contribute to the redundancy of the upper eyelids. The surgeon must evaluate the patient's individual periocular features, both in the present and in his or her past youthful state. The gradual loss of skin elasticity, with or without pseudoherniation of periorbital fat, is primarily responsible for the

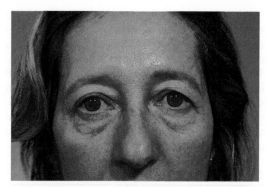

Fig. 1. Preoperative view of a patient who presented for periorbital rejuvenation. Note the redundancy of the nasal fat compartment and significant lateral hooding from excess skin laxity and lateral brow ptosis.

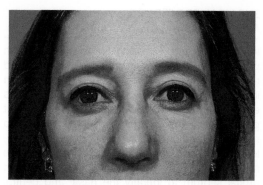

Fig. 2. Postoperative view of the same patient 2 years after upper blepharoplasty with conservative nasal and central fat excision and bilateral subcutaneous temporal lift.

aging look of the upper eyelid. Dermatochalasis in the older population can impair peripheral vision as a result of an excessive fold of upper eyelid skin. Preoperative ophthalmologic consultation is recommended for documentation of visual field impairment in this patient population.

It is also important to consider less common etiologies for upper eyelid redundancy when evaluating a patient for upper blepharoplasty. Excessive bulging in the lateral third of the upper eyelid may be caused by a prolapsed lacrimal gland, which can be identified preoperatively with manual compression over the globe, which may show a slightly movable defined mass in the lacrimal fossa.[12] A prolapsed gland can be observed in approximately 10% of patients at the time of surgery.[11,12] Unintentional resection of the lacrimal gland as a result of erroneously mistaking the gland for periorbital fat can lead to disruption of lacrimal secretory function. Another condition that can present with upper eyelid heaviness is blepharochalasis, a recurrent inflammatory condition resulting in intermittent edema and erythema of the upper eyelid skin because of an increased histamine and immunoglobulin E response.[15] Unlike dermatochalasis, blepharochalasis is often difficult to correct.

A complete evaluation of the upper eyelid includes an assessment of the brow shape and its position relative to the eye. Upper blepharoplasty performed alone in the presence of significant brow ptosis can result in further lowering of brow position. It may also lead to excessive skin excision, which can overly narrow the space between the palpebral margin and the brow.[10,14] Additionally, this may introduce the heavier thick brow skin into the upper eyelid, potentially worsening brow ptosis and lid function. Medial brow ptosis may be associated with deep glabellar

rhytids, particularly as a result of the strong depressor action of the corrugator and depressor supercilii muscles.

A thorough medical and ophthalmologic history must be obtained from the patient, including a history of diabetes, hypertension, cardiac disease, thyroid disease, bleeding disorders, problems with dry eyes or excessive tearing, and prior periorbital or ocular surgery. Old photographs of patients in their youth are particularly helpful in determining the approach to upper eyelid rejuvenation. These photographs enable the surgeon to evaluate eyelid crease height, palpebral fissure size, periorbital asymmetries, brow position, and brow shape in the patient's youthful state. All of these factors must be considered before selecting the surgical plan that best suits the patient's needs.

PATIENT PERSPECTIVE

When evaluating a patient for upper blepharoplasty, it is imperative to assess the individual patient's esthetic goals. Old photographs showing youthful brow position and upper eyelid crease height can be helpful in pointing out preoperative brow and facial asymmetry to give patients reasonable expectations of the improvements that can be made. Central and lateral eyelid volume that is present in the youthful eye should be pointed out to avoid unnecessary postoperative patient dissatisfaction. It is also important to discuss both brow contour and eyelid shape, which are features often overlooked by the patient. Once the patient's expectations and goals have been properly addressed, the surgical treatment plan can be tailored to the individual's aging characteristics for effective esthetic periorbital rejuvenation.

SURGICAL PROCEDURE
Nasal Fat Repositioning

In recent years, increasing emphasis has been placed on volume preservation in upper eyelid rejuvenation. Massry has described a modification in traditional upper blepharoplasty that moves excess nasal fat based on a freely mobile fat pedicle into the central fat compartment to restore volume and to prevent postoperative hollowing of the upper lid sulcus.[6] Incisions are made through the orbicularis oculi muscle and orbital septum to identify the nasal and central fat compartments. A portion of the nasal fat is then isolated and freed from all connective tissue adhesions. The mobilized segment of fat remains attached medially and is draped over the central levator aponeurosis and secured to the orbital septum or arcus marginalis, with care taken to avoid any tension on the levator aponeurosis (**Fig. 3**). In younger patients in whom there is typically less nasal fat, the fat is secured as far laterally as possible to provide continuity with the central fat pad. No patients in this study reported residual upper lid fullness or were found to have excessive fat pseudoherniation on examination at 1-year follow-up. Additionally, there were no cases of postoperative superior sulcus hollowing. The author suggests that translocating the nasal fat, which remains more robust than the central compartment fat during the aging process, replenishes the often volume-depleted central upper eyelid and can be an adjunctive tool in upper eyelid rejuvenation.

Orbicularis Oculi Preservation

Traditional upper blepharoplasty typically includes the excision of excessive upper eyelid skin and variable amounts of orbicularis oculi muscle. Muscle is commonly excised at the inferior extent of the skin excision to induce a more defined upper eyelid crease from scarring between the levator aponeurosis and overlying eyelid skin. It may be argued that this may disrupt aponeurotic and orbital septal attachments to the tarsus, resulting in scarring of the pretarsal skin. With recent studies showing little to no change in orbicularis oculi

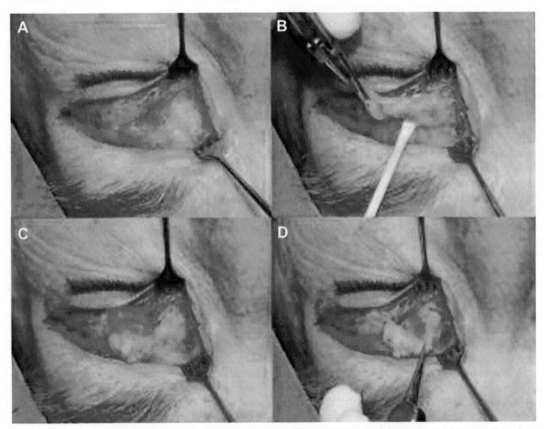

Fig. 3. The nasal fat (A) is mobilized (B) and transposed over the central levator aponeurosis (C) to restore volume (D). (*From* Massry GG. Nasal fat preservation in upper eyelid blepharoplasty. Ophthal Plast Reconstr Surg 2011;27(5):352–5; with permission.)

histology and function with aging, some authors have suggested preserving orbicularis oculi to maintain volume of the upper eyelid.[2,3,7,16] Fagien has suggested plicating the muscle centrally or laterally to predictably increase volume in a depleted-appearing upper eyelid.[7] This can be done in conjunction with spot cauterization to tighten the muscle and create a smooth pretarsal surface.

A recent randomized, double-blinded, left-right split study reported by Damasceno and colleagues[17] further examined the effect of orbicularis oculi resection on cosmetic outcomes in upper blepharoplasty. The authors reported that the side that underwent skin and orbicularis oculi resection had more postoperative discomfort compared with the contralateral eye that underwent skin resection only. At 3-month follow-up, there was no difference in final esthetic outcome as analyzed by 3 masked oculoplastic surgeons. The authors have suggested the orbicularis oculi muscle should be preserved in upper blepharoplasty for dermatochalasis without significant orbital fat prolapse.

Increasing Lateral Upper Eyelid Fullness

The youthful eye is characterized by fullness of the lateral upper eyelid from the eyebrow to the eyelid crease. Recent techniques for restoring volume in this area have mainly focused on fat grafting, which can be associated with resorption and contour irregularities. Sozer and colleagues[8] describe use of a pedicled fat flap from the central compartment to augment the lateral upper eyelid during upper blepharoplasty. The central fat flap is transposed laterally and deep to the orbicularis oculi muscle and secured to the periosteum of the superior orbital rim. When performing this technique, it is important to avoid excessive depletion of the central fat compartment to avoid hollowing of the central superior sulcus.

Another technique to enhance volume in the lateral upper eyelid is to transfer excised fat from the nasal compartment to the lateral eyelid deep to the orbicularis oculi muscle with imbrication of the overlying muscle.[9] The excised fat from the nasal compartment is divided into small pieces and arranged in the crease from lateral to medial, described by Gulyas as a "string-of-beads." The orbicularis oculi muscle is then imbricated vertically over the implanted fat beads to enhance lateral fullness while shortening the muscle in its vertical axis. At 6-month follow-up, the author reported no complications in any of the patients, and the implanted fat graft was not palpable or visible in any of the cases.

Lacrimal Gland Resuspension

If there is persistent fullness of the lateral third of the upper eyelid after upper blepharoplasty with the usual resection of palpebral fat pads, lacrimal gland prolapse should be suspected.[11,12] Partial resection of the orbital portion of the gland may be considered, but the surgeon should be aware of the potential risk of postoperative lacrimal secretory dysfunction and dry eye syndrome. In recent years, lacrimal gland resuspension, instead of resection, has gained increasing popularity as treatment of a prolapsed gland. Through the upper blepharoplasty incision, the orbital septum is opened to gain access to the fat compartments and the lacrimal gland. The gland is typically tan and firmer than the surrounding orbital fat. The anterior or inferior part of the lacrimal gland capsule is sutured to the periosteum inside the lacrimal fossa (**Fig. 4**). Care should be taken to avoid passing sutures directly through the gland parenchyma, as this may cause bleeding and postoperative dacroadenitis.[11]

Internal Brow Elevation and Glabellar Myectomy

Mild brow ptosis that aggravates upper eyelid heaviness can be addressed during upper blepharoplasty by internal brow elevation and excision of glabellar depressor muscles to improve the brow shape and position.[10,11] In contrast to typical transblepharoplasty techniques, which recommend periosteal fixation and can restrict brow movement, the lateral and central brow can be released from its retaining ligaments to immediately elevate the brow without affecting brow mobility. The technique described by Georgescu and colleagues[11] includes orbicularis oculi excision, followed by retraction of the muscle superiorly. Sharp scissor dissection is performed to incise brow retaining ligaments. The anterior layer

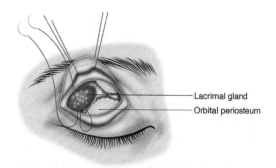

Fig. 4. A ptotic lacrimal gland may be resuspended to the orbital periosteum to reduce fullness of the lateral eyelid.

of the deep galea and orbital ligament are grasped with forceps at the lateral orbital rim and incised across the superior orbital rim to gain access to the brow fat pad laterally and depressor muscles medially. The brow fat pad is then suspended superiorly to the periosteum 1 to 2 cm above the lateral orbital rim. Burroughs and colleagues[10] described a similar technique in which the orbital ligament is grasped at the lateral orbital rim and transected at its inferior most extent between the lateral canthal tendon and zygomaticofrontal suture. Scissors are used to release the periosteal attachments of the anterior layer of the deep galea along the superolateral orbital rim. The underlying brow fat can be sculpted to further improve brow elevation.

Once the deep galeal attachments are released, the glabellar depressor muscles can be accessed through an extended medial dissection to excise the corrugator and depressor supercilii muscles and to weaken the procerus muscles. The galeal incision is carried medially using scissors with care taken to remain just above the bony orbital rim to avoid damage to the supraorbital and supra-trochlear neurovascular bundles.[10,11,18] This allows exposure of the corrugator muscle, which can be carefully excised by grasping the muscle belly in an anterosuperior direction over the supra-orbital notch to avoid injury to the underlying neu-rovascular bundles (**Fig. 5**). The muscle is excised en bloc to its medial attachments on the frontal bone.[11] Further dissection medially will allow access to the depressor supercilii muscles, which can be dissected from underneath the orbicularis oculi muscle at the medial canthus and excised sharply. Blunt scissor dissection under the thick glabellar skin can also be performed to undermine the procerus muscle and to free it from its deep bony attachments (**Fig. 6**). This release results in the immediate elevation of the medial brow.

AFTERCARE

Postoperative care following upper blepharoplasty should include cool compresses for 24 to 48 hours. Postoperative vision and ocular motility should be documented before discharge from the recovery room. Ophthalmic lubricating oint-ment can be applied while sutures are in place. If done appropriately, the postoperative recovery following upper blepharoplasty with the adjunctive esthetic techniques mentioned earlier should remain similar to that following upper blepharo-plasty alone. Increased postoperative upper eyelid edema may be seen in cases in which extensive muscle dissection or imbrication is performed. When all edema has subsided, the surgeon should

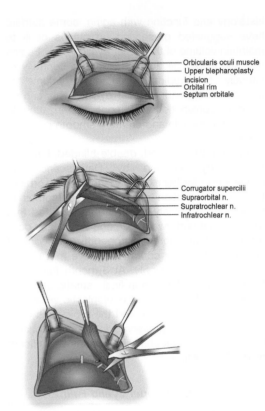

Fig. 5. The corrugator muscle is excised through an upper blepharoplasty incision deep to the orbicularis oculi muscle to elevate the medial brow.

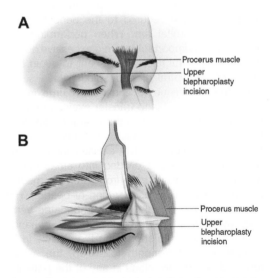

Fig. 6. The procerus muscle is released and may be transected through the upper blepharoplasty incision.

examine the upper eyelid shape and contour and identify nonoptimal results such as lid and brow asymmetry, crease irregularities, and webs.

COMPLICATIONS

Serious complications following upper blepharoplasty are rare but include bleeding, infection, and visual disturbance. Meticulous hemostasis during surgery is essential to help prevent hematoma formation. Retrobulbar hemorrhage resulting in visual loss is the most feared complication but remains extremely rare.[15,19] Infections after upper blepharoplasty are unusual because of the rich vascularity of the upper eyelids, and postoperative antibiotics are typically unnecessary. Dacroadenitis of the lacrimal gland can occur if the gland parenchyma is injured during resuspension of a prolapsed lacrimal gland. Diplopia from restricted ocular motility can occur from traction or compression of the superior oblique muscle during fat excision or repositioning. It is important to avoid placing any tension on the superior oblique muscle during nasal fat repositioning. Inadvertent levator aponeurosis injury during upper central fat excision or repositioning can result in iatrogenic blepharoptosis. Meticulous and conservative surgical technique when performing adjunctive procedures should be used to help prevent suboptimal esthetic results, such as upper eyelid crease asymmetry, brow asymmetry, superior sulcus hollowing from excessive fat excision, and upper eyelid contour irregularities.

SUMMARY

Traditional concepts in esthetic upper blepharoplasty are evolving with increasing understanding of the mechanisms responsible for upper periorbital aging. Modifications of well-established methods are gaining popularity among cosmetic surgeons, and several new or adjunctive techniques to enhance the esthetic result of upper blepharoplasty have emerged in recent years. Careful preoperative identification of all contributing factors to upper eyelid aging, including those less common, is essential to tailor the surgical plan to the needs and goals of the individual patient. With emphasis on upper periorbital volume restoration and preservation, instead of depletion, interest in adjunctive esthetic procedures that address the challenges of volume loss will likely continue to grow among surgeons.

REFERENCES

1. Sires BS, Lemke BN, Dortzbach RK, et al. Characteristics of human orbital fat and connective tissue. Ophthal Plast Reconstr Surg 1998;14:403–14.

2. Pottier F, El-Shazly NZ, El-Shazly AE. Aging of orbicularis oculi:Anatomophysiologic consideration in upper blepharoplasty. Arch Facial Plast Surg 2008; 10(5):346–9.

3. Lee H, Park M, Lee J, et al. Histopathologic findings of the orbicularis oculi in upper eyelid aging. Arch Facial Plast Surg 2012;14(4):253–7.

4. Oh SR, Chokthaweesak W, Annunziata CC, et al. Analysis of eyelid fat pad changes with aging. Ophthal Plast Reconstr Surg 2011;27:348–51.

5. Korn BS, Kikkawa DO, Hicok KC. Identification and characterization of adult stem cells from human orbital adipose tissue. Ophthal Plast Reconstr Surg 2009;25:27–32.

6. Massry GG. Nasal fat preservation in upper eyelid blepharoplasty. Ophthal Plast Reconstr Surg 2011; 27(5):352–5.

7. Fagien S. Advanced rejuvenative upper blepharoplasty: enhancing aesthetics of the upper periorbita. Plast Reconstr Surg 2002;110:278–91.

8. Sozer SO, Agullo FJ, Palladino H, et al. Pedicled fat flap to increase lateral fullness in upper blepharoplasty. Aesthet Surg J 2010;30(2):161–5.

9. Gulyas G. Improving the lateral fullness of the upper eyelid. Aesthetic Plast Surg 2006;30:641–8.

10. Burroughs JR, Bearden WH, Anderson RL, et al. Internal brow elevation at blepharoplasty. Arch Facial Plast Surg 2006;8:36–41.

11. Georgescu D, Belsare G, McCann JD, et al. Adjunctive procedures in upper eyelid blepharoplasty: internal brow fat sculpting and elevation, glabellar myectomy, and lacrimal gland repositioning. In: Massry GG, Murphy MR, Azizzadeh B, et al, editors. Master techniques in blepharoplasty and periorbital rejuvenation. New York: Springer Science+Business Media; 2011. p. 101–8.

12. Friedhofer H, Orel M, Saito FL, et al. Lacrimal gland prolapsed: management during aesthetic blepharoplasty: review of the literature and case reports. Aesthetic Plast Surg 2009;33:647–53.

13. Knize DM. An anatomically based study of the mechanism of eyebrow ptosis. Plast Reconstr Surg 1996;97(7):1321–33.

14. Presti P, Yalamanchili H, Honrado CP. Rejuvenation of the aging upper third of the face. Facial Plast Surg 2006;22(2):91–6.

15. Rohrich RJ, Coberly DM, Fagien S, et al. Current concepts in aesthetic upper blepharoplasty. Plast Reconstr Surg 2004;113:32e–42e.

16. Fagien S. The role of orbicularis oculi muscle and the eyelid crease in optimizing results in aesthetic upper blepharoplasty: a new look at the surgical treatment of mild upper eyelid fissure and fold asymmetries. Plast Reconstr Surg 2010;125:653–66.

17. Damasceno RW, Cariello AJ, Cardoso EB, et al. Upper blepharoplasty with or without resection of the orbicularis oculi muscle: a randomized

double-blind left-right study. Ophthal Plast Reconstr Surg 2011;27(3):195–7.

18. Knize DM. Transpalpebral approach to the corrugator supercilii and procerus muscles. Plast Reconstr Surg 1995;95(1):52–60.

19. Morrison CM, Langevin CJ, Zins JE. Eyelid and periorbital aesthetic surgery. In: Siemionow MZ, Eisenmann-Klein M, editors. Plastic and reconstructive surgery. London: Springer-Verlag; 2010. p. 297–311.

Ideal Female Brow Aesthetics

Garrett R. Griffin, MD[a],*, Jennifer C. Kim, MD[b]

KEYWORDS

- Brow lift • Forehead lift • Aesthetic surgery • Browplasty • Photography • Beauty • Fashion

KEY POINTS

- The ideal modern female brow aesthetic is becoming lower, flatter, and with a more lateral peak.
- There is likely an interaction between a woman's age and the perceived ideal brow position.
- volumizing the brow upper lid complex will likely supplant many of the traditional open brow lifting techniques.

The computer can't tell you the emotional story. It can give you the exact mathematical design, but what's missing is the eyebrows.
—*Frank Zappa*

http://www.brainyquote.com/quotes/keywords/eyebrows.html

INTRODUCTION

Few facial features are as powerful as the eyebrows. Sclafani[1] recently called them "the superior aesthetic frame of the eyes." This statement is significant because vision-tracking studies have shown that when viewing a face, people spend the most time looking at the periocular region.[2] The eyebrow can express wide-ranging and subtle emotions, even when the rest of the face is neutral. Elevated brows suggest surprise and, when lowered, they express fatigue and aging. Medially angled brows indicate anger, whereas laterally angled brows connote sadness.[3]

Given their importance in facial aesthetics and emotional expression, it is not surprising that women have sought ways to change the appearance of their eyebrows to better project youth, beauty, and energy. Plucking and dying can achieve modest changes, but more permanent and impressive alterations require surgical intervention. Browplasty was initially described nearly a century ago and became significantly more popular recently because of more effective and less invasive techniques. There are several potential indications for aesthetic forehead surgery, including the reduction of forehead rhytids and the repositioning of skin and soft tissue in the upper lid–brow complex[4]; however, it is difficult to perform significant forehead surgery without changing the location of the eyebrows. Most women undergoing aesthetic forehead surgery simply want to look younger and more alert. It will be difficult for them to more specifically articulate a goalresting brow position. Hence, it is important for the surgeon to possess an understanding of the ideal youthful female eyebrow.

THE IDEAL FEMALE BROW

Beauty is an evolving concept specific to a particular time and population. Contemporary ideas about the ideal female brow (in North America) originated with makeup artists like Westmore in the 1970s.[5] His formulation placed the medial and lateral brow at the orbital rim, with the peak located above the lateral limbus (LL) approximately 1 cm

The authors have no disclosures.
[a] Division of Facial Plastic & Reconstructive Surgery, Keck School of Medicine at USC, Los Angeles, CA, USA;
[b] Division of Facial Plastic and Reconstructive Surgery, Department of Otolaryngology – Head and Neck Surgery, University of Michigan Health System, 1904 Taubman Center, Reception A, 1500 East Medical Center Drive, Ann Arbor, MI 48109, USA
* Corresponding author. Center for Advanced Facial Plastic Surgery, 8665 Burton Way, #303, Los Angeles, CA 90048, USA.
E-mail address: griffin.fpsurgery@gmail.com

above the bony rim. Over the past 40 years, investigators have proposed several changes to Westmore's model.

Ellenbogen[3] stated that the inferior aspect of the medial eyebrow margin should start 1 cm above the supraorbital rim. Whitaker and colleagues[6] thought the brow peak should be at the junction of the middle and lateral thirds. This idea was supported by Byrd, who added that this point corresponded to the intersection of the brow with a line connecting the nasal ala and LL. Byrd also recommended that the peak should be 8 to 10 mm superior to the medial brow.[7] As far back as 1989, Cook and colleagues[8] stated that the peak of the eyebrow should be above the lateral *canthus* (LC) not the LL because a more medial peak yielded a surprised look. Several investigators have proposed even more strict numerical guidelines for the brow position. Connell and colleagues[9] recommended 1.5 cm between the eyebrow and the upper-lid skin crease. McKinney and colleagues[10] evaluated 50 young women and found an average of 2.5 cm from the midpupil to the superior brow. They concluded that a brow *less* than 2.5 cm from the midpupil was ptotic and sought to raise the brow to 2.5 to 2.8 cm above the pupil with a forehead lift. Matarasso and Terino[4] essentially reiterated the values proposed by Ellenbogen, Connell, and McKinney. These values were all based on extensive personal experience but remained largely subjective.

OBJECTIVE ANALYSIS

Objectively defining an ideal female eyebrow position is challenging, even beyond the fact that aesthetic trends are constantly changing. Who determines what is ideal when there is no gold standard? In such instances, it is helpful to analyze a problem from many different perspectives.

Observer Scored

Several investigators have used a group of observers to evaluate the brow position of women in photographs. Schreiber and colleagues[11] asked 100 individuals to rank 21 female and 6 male photographs for attractiveness on a 10-point scale (10 = most attractive). The photographs that were given a score greater than 7 were then analyzed for various eyebrow dimensions. Their measurements were all in relation to eye width to allow comparison between photographs. They measured medial canthus to medial brow, LC to lateral brow, and the location of the eyebrow peak in relation to the eye width. Observers preferred the brow peak at 71% of the distance across the eye width, which is roughly at the LL. A strength of this study

was its large number of raters. One weakness is that only a few photographs (fewer than 10) were analyzed for the ideal female eyebrow characteristics.[11]

Freund and Nolan[12] used Adobe Photoshop (Adobe Systems, Inc, San Jose, California) to alter the eyebrow characteristics in photographs of young Hispanic, Anglo-Saxon, and Slavic women. Two sets of images were generated. In the first set of images, the eyebrow shape was kept constant, but the medial brow was placed at, below, or above the supraorbital rim. In the second set, the eyebrow peak was placed medial or lateral to the LL, or the eyebrow was made completely flat without a clear peak. The altered photographs were then scored for attractiveness by 11 plastic surgeons and 9 established cosmetologists. Surgeons and aestheticians preferred a medial brow at or below the supraorbital rim; medial brows above the rim were considered unattractive. In the second set of images, both groups of raters preferred laterally peaked brows, then flat brows, then eyebrows with a medial apex.[12]

Baker and colleagues[13] used Adobe Photoshop to create 4 facial shapes (round, square, oval, and long) for 5 different models. They erased the eyebrows and asked a modern makeup artist to draw new appropriate eyebrows on each face. In a second set of images, they used eyebrows using Westmore's original criteria. They then asked 78 individuals to compare the makeup artist's and Westmore's eyebrow position for each of the 20 face/shape combinations. In the oval and round faces, the two eyebrow locations were each preferred by essentially 50% of the participants. However, 58% and 62% of participants preferred the makeup artist's brow in the long and square faces, respectively. The makeup artist altered the height, severity, and location of the peak to better complement the long and square faces.

Biller and Kim[14] photographed 4 women (a 30-year-old Caucasian, a 30-year-old Asian, a 60-year-old Caucasian, and a 60-year-old Asian) and used the Mirror Suite (Canfield Scientific, Fairfield, New Jersey) to alter brow position, nasal tip width, and nasolabial angle. Five unique eyebrow shapes were created for each model, with the eyebrow apex at a different location: midpupillary line, LL, halfway between limbus and canthus (HF), LC, and the lateral brow margin (LM). The images were rated by 171 observers. Each brow position, except LM, was ranked very similarly, with a nonstatistically significant trend toward preferring more lateral brow positions in the two younger models (highest ranking for HF) compared with the two older models (highest ranking for LL).[14]

Self-Evaluated

Only one study has asked people to try to create their own sense of a perfect eyebrow position. Sclafani and Jung[1] asked 23 women and 7 men to place their eyebrows in the optimal position and then took measurements. Patients had a ruler taped to their nose so actual measurements could be performed on the photographs. They found that women preferred their brow peak 13 mm (SD: ± 4 mm) above the medial brow height. There was no measurement taken of the brow peak in relation to the eye width, the LL, or the LC, which makes it difficult to compare this study with others.[1] It is difficult to know how accurate self-positioning the brow is, particularly when there is a ruler taped to the nose, which alters the sense of facial proportion.

The Ideal Female Brow as Portrayed in the Media

The studies discussed earlier used patients or observers to determine the characteristics of an attractive female eyebrow. A completely different approach is to analyze the eyebrow dimensions of models and actresses—women who are widely thought to be attractive.

Gunter and Antrobus[15] compared eyebrow characteristics between a group of models photographed in popular fashion magazines and a group of women seeking aesthetic facial surgery in Dallas, Texas. They did not report how many photographs were examined, and there was no report of an objective or statistical analysis. They concluded that fashion models' eyebrows tend to be low medially and ascended in a relatively straight line to a peak near the LC. In contrast, eyebrows of women in the patient group were often more curved and peaked closer to the LL.[15] The article does include an excellent discussion of how to tailor aesthetic forehead surgery to multiple eye types (deep set, and so forth).

Roth and Metzinger[16] performed the best analysis of eyebrow dimensions in fashion models to date. They analyzed the left eyebrow in full-frontal photographs of 100 women portrayed in magazines published in 2001. This group was compared with full-frontal photographs of 105 women aged 21 to 61 years. They calculated 5 measures for each photograph: the height of the lateral brow in relation to the medial brow; the relation of the medial brow to a vertical line through the nasal ala and medial canthus; the relation of the lateral brow to a line connecting the nasal ala and LC; how far across the eye width (medial to LC) the LL falls; and where the eyebrow peak was located in relation to the eye width. In both groups, the LL fell 75% (± 2%) of the way across

the eye width at neutral gaze. In fashion models, the lateral brow ended superior to the height of the medial brow; however, the medial and lateral brow were most commonly at the same level in the group of random women. The medial brow fell medial to the alar-medial canthal line in more than half of the models but was most commonly even with this line in the group of random women. The lateral brow in models typically ended right at the alar-lateral canthal line versus lateral to this line in the other group. The brow peak fell slightly more lateral in the group of models (98% vs 93% of the distance across the eye). In both groups, the brow peak was much closer to the LC than the LL.[16]

THE EVOLUTION OF THE PERFECT EYEBROW

Some investigators have suggested that the peak of the ideal female eyebrow has been moving more laterally. Roth and Metzinger's findings, as discussed earlier, certainly support a modern ideal brow peak very close to the LC, as opposed to Westmore's classic location at the LL. One of Roth and Metzinger's interesting findings was that in the random women older than 50 years, the eyebrow peak fell at only 87% of the distance across the palpebral fissure or more medial as compared with the distance in the 20- to 29-year-old age group (95%). This finding resonates with the findings of Biller and Kim in which observers preferred a brow peak at the LL in older women but at the LC in younger women.[14]

A person's preferences for music, movies, and clothing are primarily determined during young adulthood. The authors wondered if the interaction between age and ideal brow characteristics could be caused by changes in the media portrayal of the perfect female eyebrow over time. For example, if models in the 1960s portrayed a different eyebrow than they do now, it could account for some of the differences in the concept of the optimal eyebrow

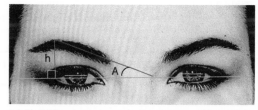

Fig. 1. Method of photographic analysis. A horizontal line (*green*) was drawn connecting the LC. The height (h) of the superior brow above the LC (*blue*) in millimeters was calculated by averaging the width of the irises (*yellow*) and setting this value equal to 11.8 mm. The takeoff angle (A) was calculated by drawing a line from the brow peak through the center of the medial brow segment (*red*).

Table 1
Location of the brow peak in relation to the LL and LC

Time	Photos	Eyebrows	Right Eyebrow				Left Eyebrow			
			LC	CLC	CLL	LL	LC	CLC	CLL	LL
1946–1955	25	50	36% (9)	28% (7)	12% (3)	24% (6)	48% (12)	16% (4)	16% (4)	20% (5)
1956–1965	27	52	50% (13)	31% (8)	4% (1)	18% (4)	31% (8)	35% (9)	27% (7)	7% (2)
1966–1970	25	50	24% (6)	24% (6)	24% (6)	28% (7)	20% (5)	32% (8)	16% (4)	32% (8)
1971–1980	22	43	27% (6)	23% (5)	27% (6)	23% (5)	38% (8)	24% (5)	33% (7)	5% (1)
1981–1990	27	54	37% (10)	22% (6)	19% (5)	22% (6)	52% (14)	26% (7)	11% (3)	11% (3)
1991–2000	24	47	22% (5)	43% (10)	22% (5)	13% (3)	46% (11)	38% (9)	8% (2)	8% (2)
2001–2011	24	45	41% (9)	41% (9)	9% (2)	9% (2)	10 (43%)	26% (6)	9% (2)	22% (5)

Abbreviations: LC, lateral canthus; CLC, brow peak closer to the LC than LL; CLL, brow peak closer to the limbus than canthus; LL, lateral limbus.

between young and old age groups today. The authors analyzed photographs from fashion magazines over the past 65 years. To their knowledge, there has never been an objective historical analysis of optimal female eyebrow characteristics as presented in the media.

METHODS

Microfilm versions of fashion magazines printed between 1946 and 2011 were examined for full-frontal photographs of models or actresses taken in the Frankfort plane. This position is important because even a relatively minimal head turn or tilt will change the apparent eyebrow characteristics. Images were excluded if eyes were closed, squinting, or there was any visible forehead rhytids (representing forehead muscle firing). Appropriate photographs were digitally captured from the microfilm, enlarged as needed in Microsoft Power-Point (Microsoft, Redmond, Washington), and printed. They were broken into 7 blocks of time for analysis: 1946-1955, 1956-1965, 1966-1970

(the hippie era), 1971-1980, 1981-1990, 1991-2000, and 2001-2011. A line was drawn between the LC to set a true horizontal (**Fig. 1**). This line usually crossed the inferior pupil. A digital caliper was then used to draw a line 90° perpendicular to this (a true vertical) up to the eyebrow peak. The position of the brow peak in relation to the palpebral fissure was recorded as falling at one of 4 locations: at or lateral to the LC; closer to the LC than the LL; closer to the LL than the canthus; and at the LL or medial to this point. A line was then drawn from the superior brow at the brow peak along the vector of the medial brow segment. The brow takeoff angle between the true horizontal and this vector was measured using the digital caliper. Finally, the height of the brow above the LC was calculated in millimeters. First, the width of both irises was measured in millimeters using a metric ruler, averaged, and set equal to the actual width of the human iris (11.8 mm).[17] This method yielded a multiplier that could be used to transform the height of the brow in the photograph into an actual measurement in millimeters.

Table 2
Brow height at the LC and takeoff angle of the medial brow segment

Time	Right Eyebrow		Left Eyebrow	
	Angle in Degrees (SD)	Height at LC (mm) (SD)	Angle in Degrees (SD)	Height at LC (mm) (SD)
1946–1955	21.3 (5.1)	21.9 (4.1)	19.4 (4.0)	22.2 (4.0)
1956–1965	21.0 (4.7)	23.9 (3.2)	19.1 (3.5)	24.1 (3.3)
1966–1970	19.1 (4.1)	21.4 (3.2)	19.0 (3.6)	21.6 (2.9)
1971–1980	20.6 (3.7)	21.9 (2.1)	19.5 (4.2)	22.2 (2.8)
1981–1990	19.9 (5.0)	21.1 (2.7)	17.8 (4.4)	21.1 (2.9)
1991–2000	18.8 (3.4)	19.6 (2.4)	17.2 (3.1)	20.1 (2.6)
2001–2011	19.7 (3.1)	21.2 (3.0)	17.1 (2.8)	21.0 (2.9)

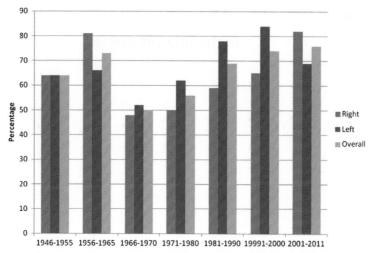

Fig. 2. The percentage of eyes when the brow peak fell closer to the LC than the LL versus time.

RESULTS

Tables 1 and **2** summarize the data for the brow peak location and the takeoff angle and brow height, respectively. Between 22 and 27 photographs were analyzed for each time period. This number is fewer than the goal, but very few fashion photographs are both full frontal and in a perfect Frankfort plane. Thus, quantity was sacrificed for quality. Occasionally, only one of the eyebrows was visible in an otherwise acceptable picture, which is why the total number of eyebrows analyzed is not always equal to exactly twice the number of photographs (see **Table 1**).

Fig. 2 shows the percentage of left, right, and overall eyebrows that are closer to the LC than the LL (CLC) (LC+CLC/total) versus time. Interestingly, there was a sudden medial shift in the location of the brow peak during the 1966-1970 period, with gradual lateral migration of the brow peak ever since. A review of these photographs shows that during the 1966-1970 timespan, eyebrows were closest to Westmore's ideal, with a very arched, rainbowlike configuration (**Fig. 3**A) as opposed to more recent periods (see **Fig. 3**B).

Eyebrow height at the LC and the takeoff angle has slowly decreased over time. Means are displayed in **Table 2** and expanded as box-and-whisker plots in **Figs. 4** and **5**. The average takeoff angle is lower for the left brow compared with the right for every time period. This finding likely has to do with a slight bias related to the fact that most people (including makeup artists and the author that performed the analysis of the photographs) are right-handed.

DISCUSSION

Aesthetic forehead surgery can help create facial balance after mid- and lower-face rejuvenation and can augment or obviate upper blepharoplasty depending on a patient's anatomy. In some cases, significant brow ptosis creates a pseudoexcess of upper-lid tissue that is completely eliminated once the brows are returned to a more appropriate location. All aesthetic forehead surgery has the potential to alter the location of eyebrows, even when this is not intended. Thus, the aesthetic forehead surgeon needs to have a concept of the ideal female eyebrow position.

Eyebrow Position and Dimension

The authors analyzed the eyebrow position of models and actresses as portrayed in the Western print media over the past 65 years to identify eyebrow dimensions that are considered beautiful

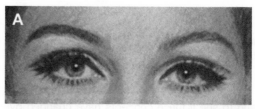
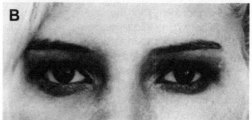

Fig. 3. Comparison of female brows as depicted in fashion magazines over time. (*A*) Example of brows from 1966 to 1970. (*B*) Example of brows from 2001 to 2010.

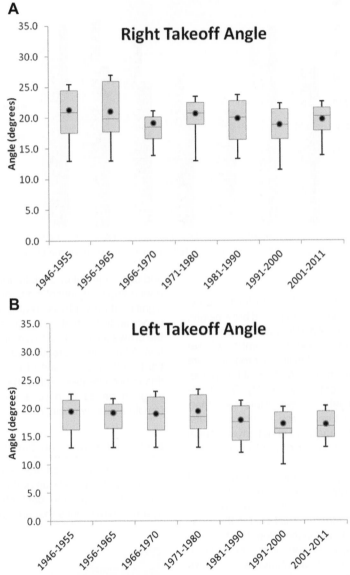

Fig. 4. Box-and-whisker plot of takeoff angle of the medial brow segment versus time. (*A*) Right brow. (*B*) Left brow.

and to see if these concepts have changed over time. It does seem that the location of the brow peak has been continuously and gradually migrating from the LL toward the LC since 1970. The brow peak was most medial during the 1966-1970 period, which was prospectively analyzed separately (vs the other groups which were 10-year blocks) because this corresponded to the hippie movement that challenged traditional gender roles and sexual mores. Westmore first presented his concept of the female eyebrow in the mid-1970s, and so his ideas may have simply been a summary of fashion trends at that time.

Height of Brow Peak

The authors also decided to analyze the height of the brow peak above a line connecting the LC as well as the takeoff angle that the medial brow makes with a true horizontal. These mean values have been more constant over time, although there has been a very gradual decreasing trend for both values (see **Figs. 4** and **5**). The mean height of the brow peak has been between 20 and 21 mm above the LC (central 50% range 15.4–21.6 mm), whereas the takeoff angle has averaged 17° to 20° (central 50% range 17.7°–22.4°), over the past 20 years.

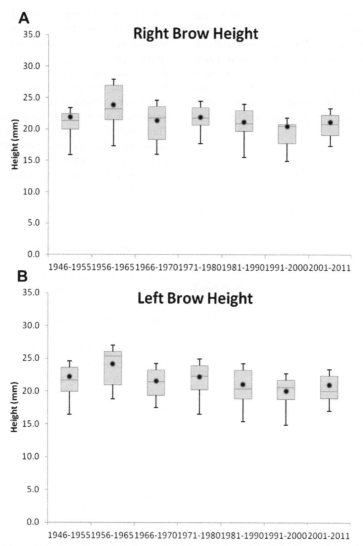

A

Right Brow Height

B

Left Brow Height

Fig. 5. Box-and-whisker plot of the brow height at the LC over time. (*A*) Right brow. (*B*) Left brow.

These values provide the aesthetic forehead surgeon with some guidelines that are relatively easy to measure intraoperatively, if desired. This data suggest that the ideal youthful female eyebrow has been getting lower, flatter, and less arched over time, with a more lateral peak and a lower takeoff angle of the medial brow segment (see **Fig. 3**B).

Some studies have found that the youthful female medial brow should be at or below the bony supraorbital rim.[12] The authors did not analyze the medial brow edge in this study because the supraorbital rim could not be reliably identified in most photographs. One of the more interesting and important findings over the past 10 years is that the medial extent of the female eyebrow frequently *rises* with age, instead of descending like most other facial features.[18,19] For many years,

investigators have cautioned against placing the female eyebrow peak too medial, which can create a surprised look.[8] The recent findings regarding female medial brow ascent with age call into question the concept of the brow-lift procedure. It would seem that, in many cases, the medial brow might actually need to be *lowered* to create a more youthful appearance. These findings also suggest that the location of the paramedian fixation points in an endoscopic brow lift should be moved more laterally. Traditionally, they were placed through an incision above the supratrochlear nerve bundle or pupil. This essentially guarantees that when the forehead soft tissues are elevated and fixated, the medial brow will be raised and the point of highest elevation will be medial to the LL. These effects are both undesired. A paramedian incision and fixation point superior to the LC should place the brow peak at the desired lateral canthal location and should also limit the elevation of the medial brow. This more lateral location may make it more difficult to dissect in the midline, which can be solved with a midline vertical scalp incision for instrument access.[20,21] In younger patients with predominantly lateral brow ptosis, deep temporal fixation only, without any paramedian fixation, may be adequate.[22]

Interaction Among Facial Shape, Eye Position, and Ideal Brow

As Baker and colleagues[13] and others have identified, there is an interaction between facial shape, eye position, and the ideal brow characteristics. Women with long faces should have lower and straighter eyebrows to prevent adding to the impression of an already long face. For square faces, typically heralded by a broad, angular jawline, the brow peak should be very gradual and the lateral brow segment should point more inferiorly, which softens the otherwise angular face. Close-set eyes can be made to seem farther apart by starting the medial brow lateral to the medial canthus, whereas wide-set eyes can be counteracted by starting the medial brow medial to the medial canthus. Some of these subtle alterations, particularly of the medial and lateral extent, are achievable with plucking and dying alone. However, women typically do not pluck the superior aspect of the brow (to lower it) and cannot easily add hairs to the superior eyebrow. Hence, the surgeon should concentrate his or her attention on the height and shape of the superior brow margin, with particular attention on the location of the brow peak.

Knize recently stated that "debate over just how far the eyebrows should be elevated or…shaped is not warranted. A (woman will be pleased if) the lateral eyebrow segments (are) visibly higher than the medial segments…"[23] The authors agree that, given the wide variation in facial and eye dimensions, there is no mathematical solution to determine a universally beautiful female eyebrow. That said, it can be argued that there are multiple types of data (summarized earlier) that together yield an updated concept of the female brow that can be used during aesthetic forehead surgery (**Box 1**).

SUMMARY

According to fashion magazines, the ideal youthful female eyebrow is gradually becoming lower and flatter than it used to be, making it less different than the male eyebrow. The authors surmise that this is, in part, a response to the increasing parity between men and women in the workplace. With the eyebrow shape alone less able to convey femininity, the fullness or luminance of the female brow may become increasingly important. Some investigators have started using changes in the volume or luminance of facial regions following aesthetic and reconstructive surgery as an objective outcome.[24,25] Lambros[26] and others have demonstrated that augmenting the volume of the upper lid *below* the brow to obscure the orbital rim and bring the tarsal crease closer to the lash line is incredibly effective at making the eye seem more youthful. In the future, adding volume to the upper lid–brow complex with injectable fillers, autologous fat, or fat transposition will augment and possibly supplant many of the traditional open and endoscopic brow-lift procedures.

REFERENCES

1. Sclafani AP, Jung M. Desired position, shape and dynamic range of the normal adult eyebrow. Arch Facial Plast Surg 2010;12(2):123–7.
2. Chelnokova O, Laeng B. Three-dimensional information in face recognition: an eye-tracking study. J Vis 2011;11(13):27.
3. Ellenbogen R. Transcoronal eyebrow lift with concomitant upper blepharoplasty. Plast Reconstr Surg 1983;71(4):490–9.
4. Matarasso A, Terino EO. Forehead-brow rhytidoplasty: reassessing the goals. Plast Reconstr Surg 1994;93:1378–89.
5. Westmore MG. Facial cosmetics in conjunction with surgery. Course presented at the Aesthetic Plastic Surgery Society Meeting. Vancouver (BC): British Columbia; 1975.

Box 1
Characteristics of the ideal youthful female eyebrow

- The medial limit is located at or below the orbital rim.
- There is a straight medial brow segment with a takeoff angle of 15° to 25°.
- The brow peak is located at the LC for younger women. The older the patient, the more medial the brow peak can be.
- The superior brow should be 20 to 25 mm above the LC.
- Plucking can subtly shape the brow to complement different eye and facial characteristics.

6. Whitaker LA, Morales L Jr, Farkas LG. Aesthetic surgery of the supraorbital ridge and forehead structures. Plast Reconstr Surg 1986;78:23–32.

7. Byrd HS. The extended browlift. Clin Plast Surg 1997;24(2):233–46.

8. Cook TA, Brownrigg PJ, Wang TD, et al. The versatile midforehead browlift. Arch Otolaryngol Head Neck Surg 1989;115:163–8.

9. Connell BF, Lambros VS, Neurohr GH. The forehead lift: techniques to avoid complications and produce optimal results. Aesthetic Plast Surg 1989;13:217–37.

10. McKinney P, Mossie RD, Zukowksi ML. Criteria for the forehead lift. Aesthetic Plast Surg 1991;15:141–7.

11. Schreiber JE, Singh NK, Klatsky SA. Beauty lies in the "eyebrow" of the beholder: a public survey of eyebrow aesthetics. Aesthet Surg J 2005;25:348–52.

12. Freund RM, Nolan WB. Correlation between brow life outcomes and aesthetic ideals for eyebrow height and shape. Plast Reconstr Surg 1996;97(7):1343–8.

13. Baker SB, Dayan JH, Crane A, et al. The influence of brow shape on the perception of facial form and brow aesthetics. Plast Reconstr Surg 2007;119:2240–7.

14. Biller JA, Kim DW. A contemporary assessment of facial aesthetic preferences. Arch Facial Plast Surg 2009;11(2):91–7.

15. Gunter JP, Antrobus SD. Aesthetic analysis of the eyebrows. Plast Reconstr Surg 1997;99(7):1808–16.

16. Roth JM, Metzinger SE. Quantifying the arch position of the female eyebrow. Arch Facial Plast Surg 2003;5:235–9.

17. Bray D, Henstrom DK, Cheney ML, et al. Assessing outcomes in facial reanimation: evaluation and validation of the SMILE system for measuring lip excursion during smiling. Arch Facial Plast Surg 2010; 12(5):352–4.

18. Matros E, Garcia JA, Yaremchuk MJ. Changes in eyebrow position and shape with aging. Plast Reconstr Surg 2009;124:1296–301.

19. Lambros V. Observations on periorbital and midface aging. Plast Reconstr Surg 2007;120:1367–76.

20. Angelos PC, Stallworth CL, Wang TD. Forehead lifting: state of the art. Facial Plast Surg 2011;27(1):50–7.

21. Romo T, Zoumalan RA, Rafii BY. Current concepts in the management of the aging forehead in facial plastic surgery. Curr Opin Otolaryngol Head Neck Surg 2010;18:272–7.

22. Nassif PS. Evolution in techniques for endoscopic brow lift with deep temporal fixation only and lower blepharoplasty-transconjunctival fat repositioning. Facial Plast Surg 2007;23(1):27–42.

23. Knize DM. Anatomic concepts for brow lift procedures. Plast Reconstr Surg 2009;124:2118–26.

24. Meier JD, Glasgold RA, Glasgold MJ. Autologous fat grafting: long-term evidence of its efficacy in midfacial rejuvenation. Arch Facial Plast Surg 2009;11(1):24–8.

25. Meier-Gallati V, Scriba H, Fisch U. Objective scaling of facial nerve function based on area analysis (OSCAR). Otolaryngol Head Neck Surg 1998;118:545–50.

26. Lambros V. Volumizing the brow with hyaluronic acid fillers. Aesthet Surg J 2009;29:177–9.

Upper Lid Blepharoplasty
A Current Perspective

David M. Lieberman, MD[a], Vito C. Quatela, MD[b],*

KEYWORDS

- Upper eyelid blepharoplasty • Upper lid blepharoplasty • Brow position • Periorbital anatomy

KEY POINTS

- Upper eyelid blepharoplasty is one of the most common facial plastic surgeries performed in the United States.
- Understanding how brow position contributes to the upper eyelid appearance is essential.
- Consistent and desirable surgical outcomes are best achieved with a detailed knowledge of periorbital anatomy.
- The surgeon must take time to understand each patient's expectations and ensure that the surgical goals are realistic.
- Although complications are rare, a frank discussion of operative risks is necessary. The potential complications and their management are discussed.
- The goal of upper eyelid blepharoplasty is to create a sculpted upper lid with a visible pretarsal strip and subtle fullness along the lateral upper lid–brow complex. The trend toward volume preservation is discussed.

INTRODUCTION

People relate to each other through the eyes. In social interactions, we notice the eyes before any other facial feature. Over time, the eyelids and periorbital complex go through changes that convey the impression of fatigue, even if a person is well rested. These changes are often the first signs of aging noted by a patient, explaining why blepharoplasty is one of the most common facial plastic surgeries performed in the United States.[1]

The eyes are framed in a complex and dynamic bony and soft tissue landscape. This includes the upper and lower lids, brow and forehead, and the midface. Although this article focuses on the upper eyelids, aging and rejuvenation of each of these facial units must be evaluated in the proper context. As will be discussed, in evaluating candidacy for upper eyelid blepharoplasty, the surgeon and patient must critically assess the contribution of the eyebrow to the periorbital appearance.

The importance of upper eyelid rejuvenation is highlighted by its history. The original writings on eyelid surgery are from the Sushruta, a document created by an Indian surgeon 2000 years ago.[2] Over the ensuing centuries, surgeons continued to document their experience with eyelid surgery, with the focus on reduction of excess eyelid skin through either cauterization or resection. Although periorbital fat removal was previously described, it was Costanares in 1951 who described the anatomy of the orbital fat compartments.[3] In the following 3 decades, the predominant surgical wisdom was that removal of fat, orbicularis oculi, and skin was the key to restoring a youthful-appearing upper eyelid. It was not until the 1990s that conservation of volume in the upper eyelid became an essential part of surgical rejuvenation.

No Disclosures.
[a] Facial Plastic and Reconstructive Surgery, The Redwood Center for Facial Plastic Surgery, Palo Alto, CA, USA;
[b] Facial Plastic and Reconstructive Surgery, Lindsay House Center for Cosmetic and Reconstructive Surgery, 973 East Avenue, Rochester, NY 14607, USA
* Corresponding author.
E-mail address: vquatela@quatela.com

Clin Plastic Surg 40 (2013) 157–165
http://dx.doi.org/10.1016/j.cps.2012.07.005
0094-1298/13/$ – see front matter © 2013 Published by Elsevier Inc.

The youthful upper eyelid maintains a sharp upper lid crease with visible pretarsal skin. The subcutaneous layers contain sufficient elasticity and volume such that excess eyelid skin is minimized and the preseptal and pretarsal skin remains smooth and fluid as the lid moves. Redundant eyelid skin, upper lid fat protrusion, and lateral orbital hooding are all signs of aging. Similarly, a hollow upper lid can convey an aged appearance or the skeletal look characteristic of an aggressive upper blepharoplasty. The task of the esthetic surgeon is to strike the balance between excess soft tissue and volume depletion. This remains a debated facet of upper eyelid surgery and facial plastic surgery in general. The second ongoing controversy in upper eyelid surgery is incision design, as is discussed.

ANATOMY
Brow and Eyelid Topography

When assessing upper eyelid appearance, the brow position and shape must be evaluated. Brow ptosis can be the primary reason for an aged appearance of the upper lid complex. In women, a youthful brow starts at the orbital rim in the same axis as the alar-facial crease. The brow arches superiorly with the highest point over the lateral canthus, approximately 1 cm from the bony rim (**Fig. 1**).[4] Laterally, the brow descends but remains above the orbital rim. In men, the brow maintains a straight course along the bony orbital rim.

The upper lid crease is formed by the condensation of the levator aponeurosis with the orbital septum and orbicularis fascia and its insertion into the skin. In white women, the crease is typically 10 to 12 mm above the lash line. In men, it ranges from 7 to 8 mm.[5] The Asian upper lid crease is lower or absent because of a more inferior insertion of the distal aponeurosis into the orbital septum and variation in the aponeurosis insertion into the skin.[6]

The palpebral fissure is typically 28 to 30 mm wide and 9 to 10 mm high. The visible portion of the globe is almond shaped with the lateral canthal angle set on average 2 mm higher than the medial canthal angle. Although the inferior lid runs across the inferior limbus, the superior lid sits 2 mm inferior to the superior limbus. The most superior point of the upper eyelid is just nasal to the vertical mid-pupillary line (see **Fig. 1**).

Surgical Anatomy

The upper eyelid is divided into anterior and posterior lamellae (**Fig. 2**).[7] The anterior lamella consists of the thin lid skin, a subcutaneous layer, absent in the pretarsal area, and the orbicularis oculi muscle. The orbicularis is divided into 3 regions: the orbital portion, which interdigitates with the corrugators superiorly, the preseptal portion, and the pretarsal portion.

The posterior lamella consists of the conjunctiva, the tarsal plate, Muller muscle, and the levator aponeurosis. The conjunctiva is the epithelial mucous membrane lining the lid. The tarsal plate of the upper lid is a dense fibrous structure ranging from 10 to 12 mm in vertical height. Muller muscle

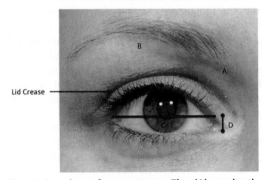

Fig. 1. Female surface anatomy. The (A) marks the medial brow along the orbital rim. The (B) shows the highest point of the brow at approximately the lateral canthus. The typical palpebral width, marked with a (C), ranges from 28 to 30 mm. The medial canthus, marked with a (D), is approximately 2 mm inferior to the lateral canthus. The natural supratarsal lid crease separates the taught pretarsal skin from the youthful fullness of the preseptal area.

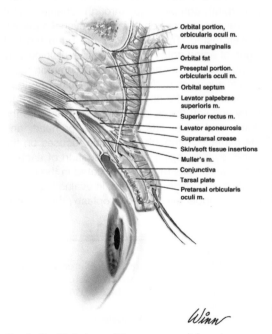

Orbital portion, orbicularis oculi m.
Arcus marginalis
Orbital fat
Preseptal portion, orbicularis oculi m.
Orbital septum
Levator palpebrae superioris m.
Superior rectus m.
Levator aponeurosis
Supratarsal crease
Skin/soft tissue insertions
Muller's m.
Conjunctiva
Tarsal plate
Pretarsal orbicularis oculi m.

Fig. 2. Sagittal view of the upper eyelid anatomy.

is a smooth muscle innervated by the sympathetic nervous system that lies deep to the levator aponeurosis. It inserts on the superior border of the tarsal plate. The levator aponeurosis is the fibrous extension of the levator palpebrae superioris and is the main upper lid retractor, controlled by the third cranial nerve. The aponeurosis inserts along the anterior aspect of the superior tarsus and fuses with the orbital septum, orbicularis, and skin at a variable point superior to the tarsus, forming the supratarsal crease.

The orbital septum, sometimes referred to as the middle lamella, begins along the arcus marginalis. It serves as a fibrous barrier between the anterior and posterior lamellae. Posterior to the septum, above the tarsal plate, is the orbital fat. Weakening of the septum causes bulging of the fat, a stigmata of the aging upper eyelid.

The orbital fat lies posterior to the septum and anterior to the levator aponeurosis, superior to the tarsal plate. There are 2 fat compartments: the central and medial fat pads (**Fig. 3**). These are separated by the trochlea of the superior oblique muscle. The central, or preaponeurotic, fat pad is larger and less vascular, with a more yellow appearance. The medial, or nasal fat pad is more dense and white in color. The lateral compartment consists of the lacrimal gland and a variable amount of associated fat.

EVALUATION FOR UPPER EYELID BLEPHAROPLASTY

Proper evaluation of surgical candidacy for upper eyelid blepharoplasty requires a thorough understanding of the correctable changes of the aged eyelid as well as the patient's medical, ophthalmologic, and psychological history. Perhaps most important is for the surgeon to pay close attention to the expectations of the patient.

Aging of the upper eyelid begins as early as the late 20s (**Fig. 4**). The skin thins farther from its already delicate baseline. Dynamic folds develop over the lateral orbicularis, known as crow's feet. As the elasticity of the subcutaneous tissue decreases, the dermatochalasis, or eyelid skin laxity, progresses, leading to hooding over the fixed pretarsal skin and muscle. Along with skin laxity, the orbicularis oris hypertrophies and relaxes, adding volume to the hooded preseptal tissue. Over time, the orbital septum weakens, allowing pseudoherniation of the medial and central fat pads and visible irregular fullness in these areas, known as steatoblepharon. Fullness in the lateral compartment can be caused by either a ptotic lacrimal gland or occasionally fat pseudoherniation.[8] If a ptotic lacrimal gland is present, a firm nodule can frequently be palpated just deep to the bony margin. If present, the gland can be suspended just under the orbital rim intraoperatively. As the brow descends, the thicker brow skin and soft tissue crowds the upper eyelid and contributes to the bulk of lateral hooding. It is crucial to determine the contribution of the brow to the upper eyelid appearance. For example, in cases of severe brow ptosis, excision of skin inferior to the brow during a blepharoplasty can cause worsening of brow drooping.[8] In these cases, a successful outcome requires a procedure to lift the brow.

Preoperative Photographs

To properly manage a patient's expectations, standardized preoperative photography must be performed. In addition, close-up pictures of the eyes from front and profile views in primary and up gaze must be obtained. Photographs should be reviewed with the patient to allow a discussion about preoperative asymmetry. Unless prompted,

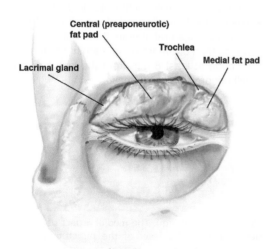

Fig. 3. Upper eyelid fat compartments and lacrimal gland.

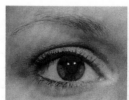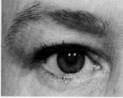

Fig. 4. Aging process of the upper eyelid. The image on the right highlights typical aging changes of the upper lid when compared with the youthful right eye on the left. Specifically dermatochalasis and steatoblepharon are apparent.

patients will frequently not recognize baseline facial, eyelid, and brow asymmetry until they are analyzing their appearance critically in the postoperative period. This is especially true of asymmetric palpebral fissures, which frequently are noticed by the patient only after eyelid surgery. A frank preoperative discussion will guide a patient's postoperative analysis of results. Reviewing photographs also facilitates the patient's understanding of how the brow is contributing to the upper eyelid appearance.

Ophthalmologic History

A detailed ophthalmologic history is essential before proceeding with upper eyelid blepharoplasty. A patient's history of dry-eye symptoms, ocular infections, visual disturbances, blink function, and prior surgical history is elicited. A standard vision test and extraocular muscle examination should be performed as part of the preoperative physical. Additionally, the senior author (VCQ) refers all blepharoplasty patients to an ophthalmologist for baseline visual acuity testing, Schirmer tear testing, and visual field testing for patients with possible compromise.

Baseline Ptosis

Recognizing baseline unilateral or bilateral ptosis is paramount. Ptosis should be documented to the nearest 0.5 mm and is best described using the margin-to-reflex distance-1 (MRD1), or distance from the pupillary light reflex to the upper lid margin.[9] Additionally, levator excursion should be noted. This is the lid mobility in millimeters from extreme upgaze to downgaze with the brow immobilized. Good excursion is 10 mm or greater, whereas moderate mobility is 5 to 9 mm and poor function is less than 4 mm. Patients with impaired levator excursion and documented ptosis should be counseled and provided a workup for ptosis correction, which is beyond the scope of this article.

Medical Comorbidities

Medical comorbidities must be assessed preoperatively to achieve safe and reliable results. A history of bleeding dyscrasias or conditions requiring anticoagulation, hypertension, and diabetes are elicited. Anticoagulation, including dietary supplements that disrupt the clotting cascade, must be stopped 2 weeks preoperatively. Patients with known thyroid disease may have ophthalmologic issues caused by their condition. Any condition that could contribute to dry-eye symptoms, including autoimmune and global inflammatory disease processes, should

be explored. If there is a predisposing factor for dry-eye pathology, the Schirmer test is performed. This is done via the standard ophthalmology referral in this center.

Patient Psychological Status

Finally, an assessment of the patient's psychological status is a key component of the preoperative evaluation. The surgeon must determine whether a patient's motivations for surgery are realistic and are aligned with a healthy psychological profile. Communicating honestly about a patient's preoperative expectations, about what is achievable, and about baseline asymmetries that may be accentuated postoperatively help to establish an honest dialogue. If there is concern on the surgeon's side regarding a patient's desires and expectations, or even the patient's psychological well-being, it is prudent to delay or cancel the surgical procedure and assist the patient in finding appropriate support.

SURGICAL PROCEDURE

- Surgical marking is performed in the preoperative area with the patient in the upright position and the eyes in neutral gaze (**Fig. 5**). The upper eyelids are cleaned with an alcohol swab to remove any grease and keep the marker line thin. The brows are elevated manually to allow full visualization of the upper lid skin and natural supratarsal crease. The brows are released periodically during the marking to fully appreciate the degree of skin laxity. Using a fine pen, the supratarsal crease is marked from the level of the puncta medially to the lateral canthus.
- The crease typically lies between 8 and 10 mm from the palpebral margin. If the natural crease is less than 8 mm from the margin, the marking is made at least 8 mm from the lash line. This will become the new crease.

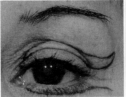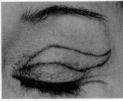

Fig. 5. Incision design. The medial aspect of the incision comes to the level of the punctum to avoid webbing. The lateral aspect of the incision extends past the lateral canthus along relaxed skin tension lines to treat lateral hooding. The most skin excised is at the level of the midpupillary line.

- The incision should not extend medial to the puncta to prevent webbing. Other investigators advocate using an M-plasty if more tissue requires excision medially.[8,10]
- As the incision approaches the lateral canthus, the vector becomes more horizontal and then rises toward a point between the lateral canthus and the lateral end of the brow. The lateral extent depends on a number of factors discussed as follows.
- The midpupillary line is marked. This is the point of maximal skin excision. The extent of excised upper lid skin depends on the degree of skin laxity. This can be estimated by grasping the redundant skin with a forceps. The medial aspect of the upper incision takes off from the inferior limb at a 30-degree angle. The lateral aspect of the upper incision contacts the lateral aspect of the inferior limb again at approximately a 30-degree angle (see **Fig. 5**). On closure, the lateral aspect of the upper lid excision should parallel the relaxed skin tension lines.
- The amount of excised skin lateral to the lateral canthus is primarily dictated by the severity of lateral hooding. For thin-skinned patients with significant hooding, the lateral aspect of the excision can extend 10 to 15 mm past the canthus. For thicker-skinned patients, men, and young women with minimal lateral orbital creasing, a conservative lateral excision is performed to minimize postoperative visibility of the incision. There is variation in the preferred incision pattern among surgeons. Several investigators do not extend the incisions beyond the lateral canthus and instead use a crescenteric shape. The senior author prefers the described pattern, as it allows simultaneous treatment of upper lid skin redundancy as well as lateral hooding, which is frequently a primary complaint of the patient.[8] If closed properly, this incision pattern heals exceptionally well with high patient satisfaction.
- Upper blepharoplasty can be performed under local anesthesia alone, with sedation, or under general anesthesia. In this center, local anesthesia with sedation is used. The local anesthesia is a combination of 2% lidocaine with 1:200,000 epinephrine and 0.25% bupivacaine with 1:200,000 epinephrine.
- Injections are performed with a 27-gauge needle deep to the skin and superficial to the orbicularis muscle (**Fig. 6**). Injections are performed precisely to avoid injury to the muscle and subsequent hematoma formation. No more than 1.5 mL is used for each lid. The lid is compressed against the supraorbital rim after

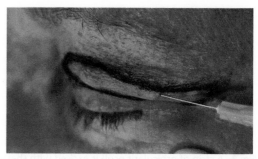

Fig. 6. Local anesthesia injection between the skin and orbicularis muscle. Injection proceeds from lateral to medial.

injection to restore the naturally thin appearance of the upper eyelid complex.

- After prepping and draping the patient, a no. 15 blade is used to make the inferior and then superior incisions, moving medially to laterally along each limb (**Fig. 7**A).
- A Q-tip is used to maintain tension on the lid during the incision.
- The skin is removed from laterally to medially using the scalpel blade to release any attachments between the skin and underlying muscle (see **Fig. 7**B).
- In this center, the senior author preserves the excised upper lid skin in a refrigerator, keeping it in saline-soaked gauze for 3 weeks. During this timeframe, the patient is monitored closely to ensure that the remaining upper lid skin is adequate for proper eye closure.
- In most cases, a strip of orbicularis muscle is then excised with sharp scissors from lateral to medial (**Fig. 8**). The depth increases as the excision progresses medially so as to protect the levator aponeurosis, which is located more superficially in the lateral lid. The excised edge of muscle is always under tension, again to prevent injury to the levator. The amount of muscle resected varies from person to person

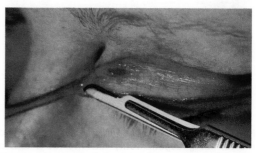

Fig. 7. Skin excision. The orbicularis oculi muscle is left intact.

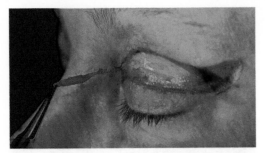

Fig. 8. A strip of orbicularis oculi is excised with sharp scissors, uncovering the orbital septum.

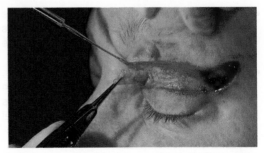

Fig. 10. The medial fat is treated in a similar manner.

and there is no consensus regarding the optimal treatment of the orbicularis.[11] The goal is to achieve optimal definition of the upper eyelid without creating a cadaveric appearance in a woman or a feminized look in a man. Additionally, removing a rim of muscle allows access to the orbital septum and the underlying fat compartments.

- The orbital septum over the central fat compartment is incised with scissors and a conservative amount of fat is teased into view (**Fig. 9**). The fat is either sculpted with bipolar cautery or excised and then sculpted. If excised, bipolar cautery is used to treat the excision line to prevent retraction of an open vessel into the postseptal space.
- Attention is turned to the medial fat pocket (**Fig. 10**). The medial brow is retracted upward and a small incision is made through the orbital septum. This fat is consistently paler than the central fat, helping confirm that the appropriate space has been entered. The fat is again teased gently into view. The volume of fat to be excised is determined by palpating the globe with the lid closed and assessing the bulge of the medial fat. The fat is treated in a similar fashion as described previously. The trochlea of the superior oblique muscle resides in-between the medial and central fat compartments. The

surgeon must be sure that cautery is applied to fat only and that muscle fibers or the trochlea itself are not receiving heat. The excised fat from each compartment is saved to allow comparison between eyes and minimize asymmetry postoperatively (**Fig. 11**). Meticulous hemostasis is kept at each stage of the surgery with bipolar cautery.

- The incision is closed from lateral to medial. A number of different closure techniques are described, such as subcuticular, running, interrupted, and skin glue.[8,9,12] Studies have looked at healing differences among closure techniques. Recently, no difference was found in cosmetic outcome or patient satisfaction when either absorbable or nonabsorbable suture was used.[13] In this center, the incision lateral to the lateral canthus is closed with vertical mattress 6-0 nylons. The rest of the incision is closed with a running locking 7-0 silk (**Fig. 12**). Care is taken to maximize eversion of the skin edges along the entire incision.

POSTOPERATIVE CARE FOR UPPER LID BLEPHAROPLASTY

At the conclusion of surgery, before leaving the operating room, antibiotic ointment is applied to the suture lines and the cornea. Ice packs are placed over the eyes in the recovery room. Patients continue icing for the first 48 hours and

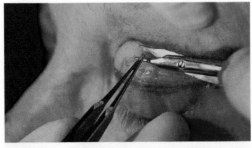

Fig. 9. The orbital septum is incised to allow access to the central (preaponeurotic) fat. The fat is teased through the orbital septum incision before being treated with cautery and excision.

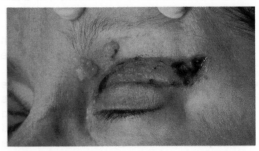

Fig. 11. Excised fat shown adjacent to the respective compartments.

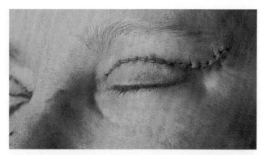

Fig. 12. The incision is closed in 2 segments. The lateral aspect is closed with 6-0 nylon sutures in a vertical mattress fashion. The thin skin of the lid is closed with a running locking 7-0 silk suture.

apply the ointment twice a day. Sutures are removed on postoperative day 3. Steri-strips are applied to the lateral aspect of the incisions. Full activity can resume 3 weeks after surgery. Patients are advised to avoid heavy lifting, bending over, and heavy exercise until that time. If medically appropriate, patients are kept on a short steroid taper to mitigate swelling. Immediate postoperative visits are on days 1, 3, 7, and 14 (**Figs. 13–16**).

COMPLICATIONS OF UPPER LID BLEPHAROPLASTY

Upper eyelid blepharoplasty can reliably be performed in a safe manner with consistent outcomes. When complications arise, they are typically minor. More serious complications can occur, however, and must be recognized immediately so that appropriate management can be implemented:

- Vision loss
- Dry eye or corneal irritation
- Diplopia
- Eyelid malposition and lagophthalmos

Vision Loss

The most severe complication after blepharoplasty is vision loss. This is most commonly a result of retrobulbar hemorrhage but has also been reported as a result of ischemic optic neuropathy, and globe perforation.[14–16] A recent retrospective study documented the incidence of retrobulbar hemorrhage at 0.05% and related permanent visual loss at 0.0045%, or 1 in 10,000.[14] Typical presentation can include severe orbital pain, proptosis, tense globe, opthalmoplegia, chemosis, and decreased visual acuity. Attention to hemostasis during the procedure is essential to avoid this rare but severe complication. If it is diagnosed in the postoperative setting, rising intraocular pressure must be treated within 2 hours of symptom onset to avoid vision compromise. The initial management is with topical and systemic medications to reduce intraocular pressure. Mannitol and systemic corticosteroids are often used. If vision is threatened, surgical decompression is indicated. The first step is to release the sutures and reopen the orbital septum widely. The postseptal space is explored and any active bleeding sites are cauterized. If the pressure remains high or concern regarding vision loss persists, a lateral canthotomy and cantholysis are performed. In refractory cases, bony decompression of the anterior orbit and orbital apex is performed.[15]

Dry Eye or Corneal Irritation

A much more common early postoperative issue is dry eye or corneal irritation. The complex mechanism of tear production and corneal lubrication

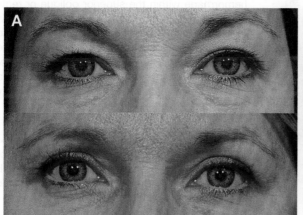

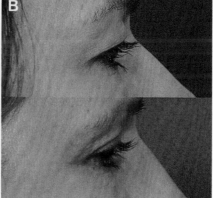

Fig. 13. (*A*) Before (*top*) and 6 months after (*bottom*) upper eyelid blepharoplasty in a 47-year-old female patient. (*B*) The same patient in profile view.

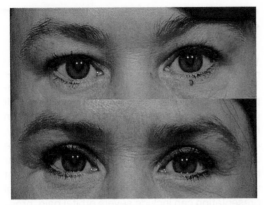

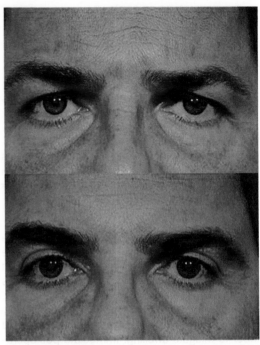

Fig. 14. Before (*top*) and 1.5 years after (*bottom*) upper eyelid blepharoplasty in a 52-year-old female patient.

can be disrupted temporarily after surgery, typically as a result of postoperative edema. Patients are maintained on ophthalmic antibiotic ointment for the first week postoperatively regardless of symptoms. When dry-eye symptoms occur, longer-term ocular lubrication with ointment and drops is implemented. In this center, moderate to severe chemosis, which can contribute to dry-eye symptoms, is treated with topical steroid and hypertonic saline drops. The drops are administered every 4 hours in an alternating fashion until the edema improves. If any signs of conjunctivitis arise, the patient is evaluated and started on appropriate topical antibiotic therapy.

Fig. 16. Before (*top*) and 1 year after (*bottom*) upper eyelid blepharoplasty in a 52-year-old male patient.

Immediate irritation following surgery can be a result of a corneal abrasion from either drying of the cornea intraoperatively or trauma to the corneal epithelium. Although an abrasion can cause significant discomfort, symptoms typically resolve within 24 hours. Management consists of more aggressive antibiotic ointment application over that period. If symptoms persist beyond 24 hours, ophthalmologic consultation is sought.

Diplopia

Diplopia following upper eyelid blepharoplasty is rare. It is thought to be caused by edema or hemorrhage within the superior oblique or rectus muscle. Injury to the trochlea with resultant brown syndrome, or restricted superior oblique function with limitations in upward gaze, has been reported after blepharoplasty.[17] Conservative management with reassurance is typically sufficient. Ophthalmologic consultation is requested if symptoms show no signs of improvement within 1 week.

Eyelid Malposition

Eyelid malposition can occur following upper eyelid surgery. Postoperative ptosis can be caused by either lid edema or ecchymosis, which should resolve with conservative treatment, or caused by levator dysfunction from injury or attenuation.[15] As mentioned, preoperative ptosis should be recognized and discussed with the

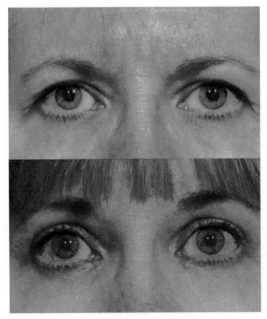

Fig. 15. Before (*top*) and 1 year after (*bottom*) upper eyelid blepharoplasty in a 56-year-old female patient.

patient to avoid dissatisfaction after surgery. Lagophthalmos, or incomplete lid closure, is not uncommon in the immediate postoperative period. An opening of 4 mm at the end of the procedure will allow for normal closure once the edema resolves.[8] An opening of 6 mm or greater risks persistent long-term lagophthalmos. This is typically a result of excessive skin excision or abnormal scarring between the septum and the anterior lamella. Incomplete closure frequently responds to conservative measures, including massage, taping, and aggressive ocular lubrication. If there is concern regarding the amount of lid skin resection and postoperative lagophthalmos, the strip of the excised skin is used as a full-thickness skin graft to prevent this. If this is noted in the postoperative period, options include raising the lower eyelid, skin grafting, or orbital-septal adhesion release.[15]

Patients are followed for a full year after surgery. If suture tunnels or milia occur, they are treated during an office visit. If the lateral scar widens during the healing process, scar excision is performed in the office. Rarely, persistence of fat herniation from the medial compartment is noted. The precise volume of fat to be removed is most difficult to predict in the medial compartment because of its posterior displacement when the patient is supine on the table. If this occurs, it also can typically be treated in the office setting through an approximately 5-mm opening at the medial aspect of the original incision.

SUMMARY

Upper eyelid blepharoplasty remains one of the most sought after procedures in facial plastic surgery. Over the past 2 decades, the ideal esthetic has evolved with a stronger emphasis on volume preservation and even replacement, specifically at the lateral lid and brow. Volume conservation should not, however, come at the expense of a heavy, ptotic-appearing lateral lid-brow complex. Consistent and desirable surgical outcomes are achieved only with a detailed knowledge of upper eyelid and brow anatomy and a thorough understanding of each patient's expectations. The eyelid cannot be evaluated in isolation but in the context of the brow, the lower lid, the globe position, and the bony skeleton. The senior author's goal is to create a sculpted upper lid with a visible pretarsal strip and subtle fullness along the lateral upper lid–brow complex. With conservative skin, muscle, and fat resection, the upper lid can be rejuvenated without leaving an overskeletonized result.

Although different surgeons advocate different incision techniques, the steps described in this article reliably result in a youthful and natural upper lid and lateral brow complex.

REFERENCES

1. American Academy of Facial Plastic and Reconstructive Surgery 2010 Membership Study. Available at: http://www.aafprs.org/media/stats_polls/aafprs Media2010.pdf. Accessed January 19, 2012.
2. Dupuis C, Rees TD. Historical notes on blepharoplasty. Plast Reconstr Surg 1971;47:246–51.
3. Castanares S. Blepharoplasty for herniated intraorbial fat; anatomical basis for a new approach. Plast Reconstr Surg 1951;8(1):46–58.
4. Cook TA, Brownrigg PJ, Wang TD, et al. The versatile midforehead browlift. Arch Otolaryngol Head Neck Surg 1989;115(2):163–8.
5. Most SP, Mobley SR, Larrabee WF Jr. Anatomy of the eyelids. Facial Plast Surg Clin North Am 2005;13(4): 487–92.
6. Doxanas MT, Anderson RL. Oriental eyelids. An anatomic study. Arch Ophthalmol 1984;102(8):1232–5.
7. Love LP, Farrior EH. Periocular anatomy and aging. Facial Plast Surg Clin North AM 2010;18(3):411–7.
8. Pastorek N. Upper-lid blepharoplasty. Facial Plast Surg 1996;12(2):157–69.
9. Gentile RD. Upper lid blepharoplasty. Facial Plast Surg Clin North Am 2005;13(4):511–24.
10. Rohrich RJ, Coberly DM, Fagien S, et al. Current concepts in aesthetic upper blepharoplasty. Plast Reconstr Surg 2004;113(3):32e–42e.
11. Hoorntje LE, van der Lei B, Stollenwerck GA, et al. Resecting orbicularis oculi muscle in upper eyelid blepharoplasty—a review of the literature. J Plast Reconstr Aesthet Surg 2010;63(5):787–92.
12. Parikh S, Most SP. Rejuvenation of the upper eyelid. Facial Plast Surg Clin North Am 2010;18(3):427–33.
13. Jaggi R, Hart R, Taylor SM. Absorbable suture compared with nonabsorbable suture in upper eyelid blepharoplasty closure. Arch Facial Plast Surg 2009;11(5):349–52.
14. Hass AN, Penne RB, Stefanyszyn MA, et al. Incidence of postblepharoplasty orbital hemorrhage and associated visual loss. Ophthal Plast Reconstr Surg 2004;20(6):426–32.
15. Lelli GJ Jr, Lisman RD. Blepharoplasty complications. Plast Reconstr Surg 2010;125(3):1007–17.
16. Morax S, Touitou V. Complications of blepharoplasty. Orbit 2006;25(4):303–18.
17. Neely KA, Ernest JT, Mottier M. Combined superior oblique paresis and Brown's syndrome after blepharoplasty. Am J Ophthalmol 1990;109(3):347–9.

Asian Upper Lid Blepharoplasty Surgery

Charles K. Lee, MD[a,b,*], Sang Tae Ahn, MD[c],
Nakyung Kim, MD[d]

KEYWORDS

- Asian eye • Asian blepharoplasty • Supratarsal crease • Eyelid surgery • Surgical technique

KEY POINTS

- Asian upper lid blepharoplasty is a common procedure that requires precise technique and understanding of key anatomic differences.
- The goal is to create a natural upper lid crease with manipulation of the tarso-levator junction and skin tension around the medial epicanthus.

INTRODUCTION

Upper lid blepharoplasty is the most common plastic surgery procedure in Asia and has consistently maintained its position over the past three decades as cultural acceptance and techniques have evolved. Eyelid aesthetics cannot be underestimated because they can exert significant social and economic influence in an extremely homogenous Asian society. A highly competitive culture mixed with modern values for beauty has created a constant demand for this procedure.

Surgical creation of the supratarsal crease has become synonymous with the term "double eyelid" surgery. The premise of the operation is to create a supratarsal crease that creates an eyelid that is more aesthetically pleasing. The term "double eyelid" is a bit of a misnomer, because creation of a supratarsal crease does not actually create another eyelid; it is simply a translation of the Korean term "ssang-cupul" (쌍꺼풀 双眼皮), which has come about from the Chinese character "ssang 双," which means "double" and the Korean character "cupul 꺼풀," which means "cover." It has been estimated that 30% to 50% of East Asians (China, Korea, and Japan) have a natural supratarsal crease.[1] The earliest procedures began in Japan in the early1900s, and have been more recently modified by Korean and Chinese plastic surgeons.[2]

The Asian blepharoplasty procedure has often been called a "westernizing" procedure. This description is a gross oversimplification of its role in function and form. Functionally, patients may request this procedure to address corneal irritation from eyelash inversion, ptosis, or pseudoptosis.[3] In form, patients may request this procedure for purely aesthetic reasons, but the most important principle to remember in Asian blepharoplasty is that is it not a "westernizing" procedure. Patients universally want a natural look that respects their Asian identity. They want a look that naturally "opens the eye" and brings out its inherent shape and beauty (**Fig. 1**). The tell-tale signs of a poor Asian blepharoplasty are an excessively high and thick supratarsal crease that is overly stylized and contrived. Correction of this disfigurement is fraught with complexities and unpredictable results.[4–6]

The key elements in Asian blepharoplasty require finesse, precision, and a clear understanding of anatomy. The patient's goals and priorities must be clearly defined. Despite satisfaction rates that vary widely (50%–90%), Asian upper lid blepharoplasty can be extremely rewarding and can provide a unique opportunity to create an expert

[a] St. Mary's Medical Center, San Francisco, CA, USA; [b] University of California, San Francisco, San Francisco, CA, USA; [c] Seoul St. Mary's Hospital, The Catholic University of Korea, 222 Banpo-daero, Seocho-gu, Seoul 137-701, Korea; [d] L Plastic Surgery – Form & Function, 2250 Hayes Street, Suite 508, San Francisco, CA 94117, USA
* Corresponding author. 2250 Hayes Street, Suite 508, San Francisco, CA 94117.
E-mail address: Lplasticsurgery@gmail.com

Clin Plastic Surg 40 (2013) 167–178
http://dx.doi.org/10.1016/j.cps.2012.07.004

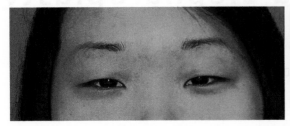
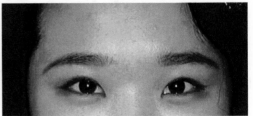

Fig. 1. Asian upper eyelid blepharoplasty. Natural result (preoperative and postoperative).

niche within an aesthetic eyelid practice (W.S. Yum, personal communication, GAAM Plastic Surgery, Gang Nam Gu, Seoul, Korea, 2008).[7]

ANATOMY OF THE ASIAN EYELID

The anatomy of the Asian eyelid has been studied in great detail over the past decades.[8–10] Despite some controversy, key anatomic differences remain: (1) an absent or short supratarsal crease, (2) a shorter tarsus, (3) descending preaponeurotic fat, and (4) minimal to absent connections between the levator aponeurosis to the upper lid dermis.

These internal anatomic differences combined with classic outer characteristics create the classic Asian eyelid (**Fig. 2**). Outer characteristics include an almond-shaped fissure with varying degrees of slant, lash ptosis, and medial epicanthal fold.

With these differences in mind, it is important to recognize functionally that the inferior extension of the orbital septum acts as a barrier between the dermis and the levator that leads to a poorly defined or absent crease. This "inferior extension," interchangeably known as the "preaponeurotic fat," descends close to the eyelid margin. This key anatomic difference allows the surgeon to perform the appropriate maneuvers to create or manipulate the supratarsal crease.[10–12] It also explains why certain techniques have advantages in creation, control, and longevity of the supratarsal crease.

The other anatomically important zone is the medial epicanthal fold, which may have a variable shape, presence, and severity. The epicanthal fold is the skin flap at the medial portion of the upper eyelid that descends along the side of nose and can obscure the medial globe and inner punctum making the pupils seem closer to the midline. In

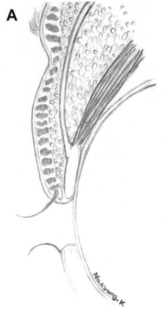
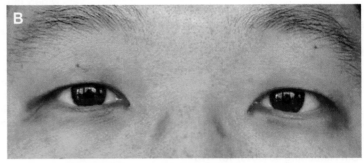

Fig. 2. (A) Asian upper eyelid anatomy. (B) Classic Asian eyelid: absent supratarsal crease, almond-shaped fissure, lash ptosis, medial epicanthal fold.

Table 1
Epicanthal fold classification

Fold Type	Fold Description	Types 1, 2, 3, 4: Top to Bottom
Type 1	No fold	
Type 2	Epicanthus tarsalis: upper eyelid skin covers the tarsal border as it nears the medial canthus	
Type 3	Epicanthus palpebralis: upper eyelid skin obscures the lacrimal lake, covering the medial angle of the palpebral fissure	
Type 4	Epicanthus inversus: lower eyelid skin crosses over the lacrimal lake, creating a reverse epicanthal fold	

severe cases, the eyes may appear "cross eyed," with the medial portion of the eye blunted by the web of the eipcanthal fold. Several types of medical epicanthal folds have been described (**Table 1**).[13] The most common in Asians is types 2 and 3, with either being amenable to epicanthoplasty. Identifying its severity and functional significance is critical in performing a successful Asian upper lid blepharoplasty, which now combines treatment of both areas simultaneously.

These anatomic points can be contrasted to the Caucasian upper eyelid (**Fig. 3**), where the septum fuses with the levator 5 to 10 mm above the tarsal border. This higher point of fusion allows interdigitations of the levator to the subdermal surface creating the higher supratarsal crease that is characteristic of the white eyelid. The supratarsal crease is typically a semilunar shape with a parallel crease.

EVALUATION

A thorough evaluation of the eyelid is performed at the initial consultation. In addition to the standard evaluation, it is critical to understand the patient's sense of aesthetics regarding the eye and their goals. It is easy to simply "create a fold"; it is much more difficult to create one that is functional and aesthetically pleasing. When a patient brings in photographs demanding that their eyelid look like a specific "movie star," it is important to caution and emphasize that the fold shape is not necessarily a function of the surgery and technique, but just as much their inherent anatomy and "crease tendency." The "crease tendency" is a term the authors have used with patients to demonstrate where their supratarsal crease "wants to go" when choosing different fold heights. Showing patients crease

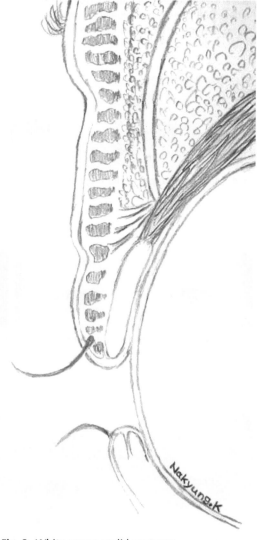

Fig. 3. White upper eyelid anatomy.

shape and height immediately in the mirror during the consultation can address patient expectation dramatically.

Fold Height

In the initial evaluation phase, the first point to address is the patient's sense of fold height. Most patients already come with some idea of fold height, in the range of low, moderate, and high. The moderate height, the most commonly requested, indicates that the patient is looking for a natural-appearing supratarsal crease. The high fold height is typically requested to attract greater attention to the fold, particularly for ease of makeup application. The low fold height is typically reserved for the male patient who desires a subtle fold (**Fig. 4**). Measuring the tarsal height by flipping the lid open on the conjuctival side can determine if a high fold is even technically achievable. At this time, it is good to note the degree of lash ptosis,

the angle at which eyelashes are pointing from the globe.

Selection of fold height naturally follows to create a crease shape. The shape can be a parallel crease (**Fig. 5**) or a nasally tapered crease (**Fig. 6**). In general, a high fold yields a parallel crease, whereas a moderate to low fold yields a nasally tapered crease. Crease heights are measured with key millimeter measurements in mind: 5 to 6 mm is a low crease, 7 to 8 mm is a moderate crease, and 9 to 10 mm is a high crease. These are guidelines and have to be adjusted when skin excision is involved. Measurements are best done with a surgical caliper.

Medial Epicanthus

Next, the medial epicanthus is addressed. The medial epicanthal fold must first be recognized, and then should be addressed based on patient expectation. In general, the stronger the medial epicanthal fold, the more tendency there is to

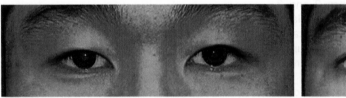

Fig. 4. Male Asian upper eyelid blepharoplasty, low fold height (preoperative and postoperative).

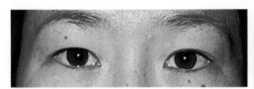
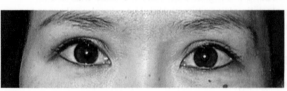

Fig. 5. Parallel crease, moderate fold height (preoperative and postoperative).

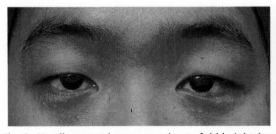
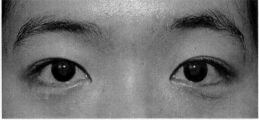

Fig. 6. Nasally tapered crease, moderate fold height (preoperative and postoperative).

create a nasally tapered crease. If the patient desires a parallel crease or specifically wants the epicanthal fold diminished, the medial epicanthoplasty procedure must be discussed in detail.[14]

Symmetry

Patients may also present with asymmetric or multiple folds (**Fig. 7**).[15,16] These elements must be pointed out explaining the greater variability and potential higher degree of difficulty in obtaining exact symmetry. Adding to the complexity is identifying degrees of subclinical ptosis and pseudoptosis. Subclinical ptosis should be suspected when a patient shows significant frontalis strain (**Fig. 8**, left). With the frontalis muscle overcompensating before surgery, the frontalis relaxes

after the blepharoplasty (see **Fig. 8**, right), which makes the ptosis even more apparent.

Skin and Fat Excision

Pseudoptosis and degrees of preaponeurotic fat must also be addressed. Both elements may be addressed with skin and fat excision. Skin removal is a function of age, skin quality, and dermatochalasis. In Asian blepharoplasty, conservative skin removal is the norm; younger patients may have 1 to 2 mm of skin removed, and older patients may have 3 to 5 mm removed.[17] Preaponeurotic fat excess should be estimated. The puffier the upper lid appears, the more fat that needs to be excised (**Fig. 9**).

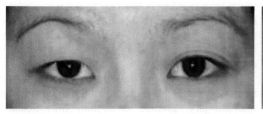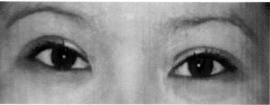

Fig. 7. Asymmetric crease, high fold (preoperative and postoperative).

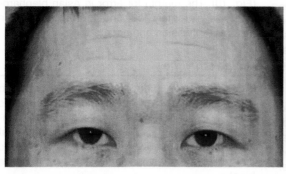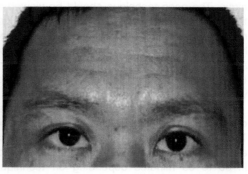

Fig. 8. Subclinical ptosis with levator advancement. Note relaxed frontalis postprocedure (left is preprocedure, right is postprocedure).

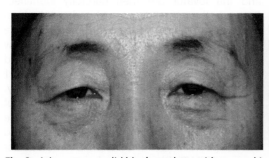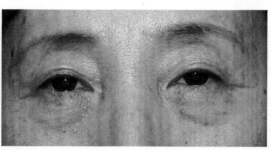

Fig. 9. Asian upper eyelid blepharoplasty with excess skin excision, natural supratarsal crease result (before and after).

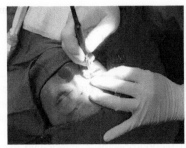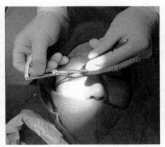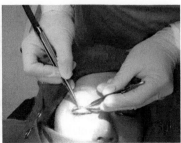

Fig. 10. Using fine instruments, surgical caliper, 7–0 monofilament suture.

Preoperative Photography

Photographic documentation for planning and record keeping is vital for any elective surgery procedure. Besides the anteroposterior, lateral, and oblique views, it is helpful to take an anteroposterior photograph with the eyes closed. This can assist in the planning and marking phase.

PATIENT PERSPECTIVE

After a thorough evaluation, it is time to discuss technical details with the patient; this converges onto an open or closed technique. In general, the more anatomic elements that need to be addressed, the greater the need for an open technique. The open technique should be viewed as the gold standard and the closed technique reserved for eyelids that require minimal change, have minimal fat, or may already have a crease. A detailed discussion with the patient regarding the advantages and disadvantages of an open versus closed technique is critical.

After the technical details have been mapped out, options regarding anesthetic are discussed. The procedure can be performed under local anesthesia with or without intravenous sedation in 30 to 90 minutes depending on technique. Patients need to take a week away from work or before making any social appearances; it is important to reemphasize the possibility for swelling and asymmetry, particularly in the early period, up to 3 months.

SURGICAL PROCEDURE

The procedure begins with the eyelid markings performed in the upright position. A fine-tipped surgical marking pen, a smooth wire, and a caliper can assist greatly in creating sharp, definitive markings. A symmetric midline mark at the high point of the limbus is a useful reference point on each side. The new supratarsal crease is drawn extending from the medial to the lateral canthus. The crease

heights are checked in the upright and supine position; after the patient is in the supine position, the marks are completed, including the medial epicanthoplasty marks if needed. There can never be too much time spent with attention to detail in confirming the skin markings. Local anesthetic (1% lidocaine plus epinephrine) is placed symmetrically into the upper lids, being careful to avoid skin distortion.

The authors' technical approach to eyelid surgery is similar in principle to their approach in microsurgery: precise dissection with delicate instruments aided by ×3 or greater loupe magnification; minimal cautery (bipolar preferred); and the use of fine sutures (7–0 monofilament suture) (**Fig. 10**). The margin for error in Asian blepharoplasty is extremely low and this approach can maximize precision and accuracy.

Open Technique

The skin incision is made with dissection carried down through the orbicularis; excess muscle is carefully excised. Next, the orbital septum is identified and orbital septal fat/preaponeurotic fat conservatively removed if needed. Hemostatic control of the fat vasculature is done with the bipolar.

The glistening levator aponeurosis is then identified down toward the superior border of the tarsus. The lid over the tarsus, the tarsal plate, and the levator are then carefully identified. Suture is then carefully placed horizontally from the tarsus or levator to the subdermis or muscle of the lower flap margin depending on how much of a distinct fold is desired (**Figs. 11** and **12**). Eyelash eversion can be controlled with 1 to 2 mm of lower skin advancement cranially. Fine sutures minimize the possibility of knot prominence. Three points of fixation that are spaced evenly over the lid are performed and the lid position is checked on both sides for symmetry (M.S. Lee, personal communications,

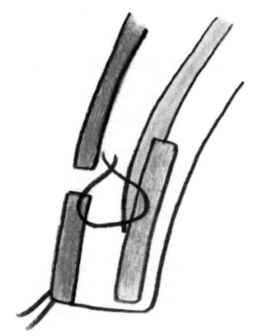

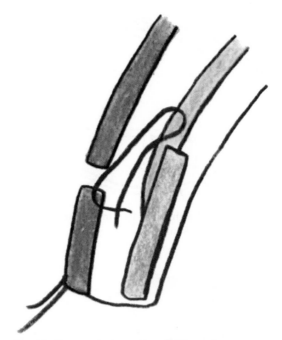

Fig. 11. Open technique: levator, tarsus to dermis. (*Courtesy of* S.T. Ahn.)

Fig. 12. Open technique. Levator above the tarsus, to the dermis; tendency toward a deep or high fold. (*Courtesy of* S.T. Ahn.)

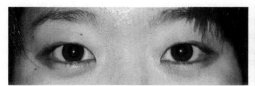

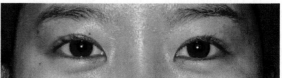

Fig. 13. Closed technique with interrupted suture (preoperative and postoperative).

M Plastic Surgery, Daegu, Korea, 2008). The crease heights are checked throughout with the surgical caliper.

In between each eyelid procedure, the exposed wound can be covered with an iced wet gauze, which is soaked with a mixed solution of 20 mL saline, 40 mg triamcinolone, 1% xylocaine, and 1:100,000 epinephrine, to reduce intraoperative and postoperative bleeding and swelling. The skin is closed temporarily with 4–5 sutures. Before full closure of both eyelids, the patient is asked to sit up and the shape and symmetry of the folds are checked. A minor touch up, if needed, is done and the skin is closed with interrupted sutures (**Fig. 13**).[2]

Closed Technique

Suture placement can be done sequentially (**Fig. 14**) or continuously (**Fig. 15**).[18–21] Dr Ahn's suture method uses two nonabsorbable sutures with anchoring of the tarsus to the deep dermis. Three small 1-mm incisions (medial, central, lateral) are made along the marked crease line, spaced evenly apart. A 6–0 monofilament suture with straightened needle is passed through the medial incision, tarsal plate, and conjunctiva. Coming back through the conjuctival puncture site, the needle is advanced toward the center incision subconjunctivally. Coming out and back to the conjunctiva, the needle is passed through the tarsal plate and central incision. Coming back to the central incision, the needle is advanced toward the medial incision subdermally. The suture is placed through the tarsus and then a segment of overlying dermis with the knot buried. Another suture is done from the lateral, through the center, to the lateral. Skin closure is not necessary.

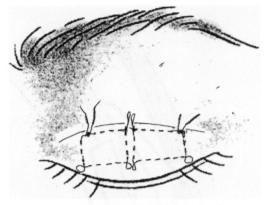

Fig. 14. Closed technique. Two interrupted sutures. (*Courtesy of* S.T. Ahn.)

Table 2 Open versus closed technique		
	Advantages	**Disadvantages**
Open technique	Optimal control of skin, fat, and levator More durable fold	Longer scar Longer recovery
Closed technique	Faster recovery Less scarring	Less control of fat, levator, and skin Less durable fold

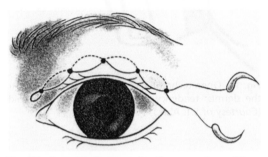

Fig. 15. Closed technique. Continuous suture. (*Courtesy of* S.T. Ahn.)

Open Versus Closed Technique

There are advantages and disadvantages to the open technique versus the closed technique (**Table 2**). The key advantages of the open technique lie in its versatility and ability to control the elements of the blepharoplasty: skin and fat excision, precise placement of suture from the tarsus to levator to dermis, ultimately leading to more durable supratarsal crease. The disadvantages lie in the longer recovery from the greater dissection and the possibility of a longer scar. The closed technique or nonincision technique has a faster recovery and less chance of scar. The disadvantages are its inability to completely address the preaponeurotic fat and orbital septum, which leads to its variable longevity. A detailed discussion about the benefits and risks should be part of the preoperative evaluation.

Medial Epicanthoplasty

The medial epicanthoplasty can be performed in conjunction with the blepharoplasty or separately (**Fig. 16**). Multiple variations exist on the tension-relieving techniques using Z- or W-plasty techniques.[15,22] More recently, minimal scar techniques have come to the forefront.[13,20,23–28] The authors prefer the skin redraping method (**Fig. 17**), which has been described by Oh and colleagues.[6] In this method a horizontal line is drawn from the new medial epicanthus by way of the edge of the epicanthal fold to 2 mm medial to the lacrimal lake. The line is continued to the subciliary line of the lower lid. The length of the subciliary incision is just enough to treat the skin excess and dog-ear. After the skin flap is raised, the dense connective tissue and hypertrophic orbicularis oculi muscle are exposed and resected. By redraping the skin flap, the epicanthal fold and skin tension are dissipated. The excess skin is trimmed, the dog-ear is removed, and the skin is closed.

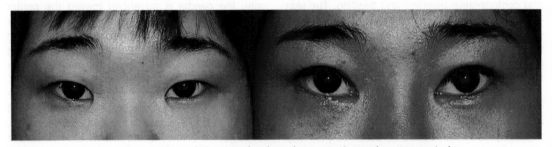

Fig. 16. Asian blepharoplasty with medial epicanthoplasty (preoperative and postoperative).

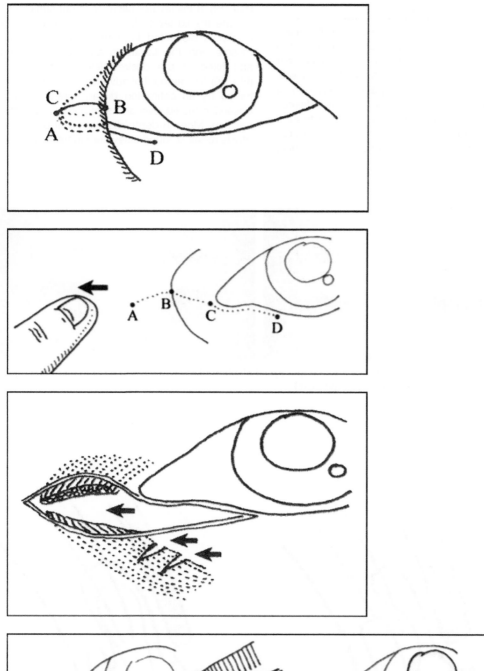

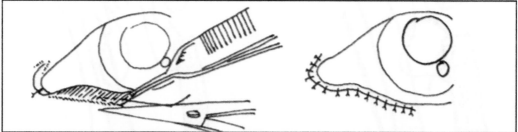

Fig. 17. Skin redraping method for medial epicanthoplasty. (*Modified from* Oh YW, Seul CH, Yoo WM. Medial epicanthoplasty using the skin redraping method. Plast Reconstr Surg 2007;119(2):703–10.)

Levator Advancement

Performing a levator advancement can be direct because the levator has already been dissected free during the blepharoplasty. An advancement of 2 to 4 mm can address the issue of "subclinical ptosis" (**Fig. 18**). When a patient with normal levator function without pathologic ptosis desires a larger eye with an increased palpebral fissure, the distal 2 to 4 mm of levator can be plicated simply without further dissection or shortening

(**Fig. 19**). If the levator plication is not sufficient to elevate the lid level, the posterior surface of the levator is dissected from the tarsus and Müller muscle and the tarsus is advanced superiorly and fixed at the desired level of the levator (**Fig. 20**). The amount of advancement is not determined by an estimated distance but rather by observing the lid level and symmetry in the sitting position. More in-depth discussion of ptosis and ptosis repair is found elsewhere in this issue.

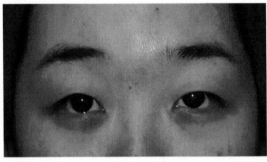
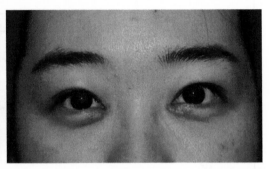

Fig. 18. Patient with subclinical ptosis. Asian upper eyelid blepharoplasty with levator advancement and medial epicanthoplasty (preoperative and postoperative).

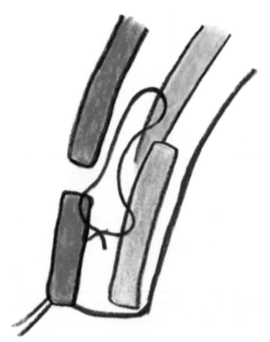

Fig. 19. Levator plication. (*Courtesy of* S.T. Ahn.)

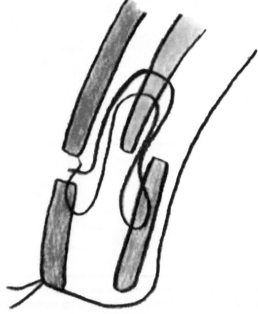

Fig. 20. Tarsal-levator advancement. (*Courtesy of* S.T. Ahn.)

AFTER CARE

Postoperative care is similar to standard blepharoplasty procedures. The patient is instructed to keep the head of the bed elevated for 1 week to reduce edema and sutures are typically removed within 1 week. Eye makeup may be used after the sutures are removed and contact lenses can be resumed after 3 weeks. The definitive fold height and shape can be reasonably determined at 3 weeks, and by 6 weeks the patient is allowed to return to full activities without restrictions.

COMPLICATIONS

The most common complication after Asian blepharoplasty is asymmetry. It is the first, second, and third most common complaint and up to one-third of patients may have some form of asymmetry. Disciplined management of asymmetry is crucial for a satisfactory outcome, preoperatively and postoperatively. If a subtle asymmetry is noted, patience is the best course of action until 4 to 6 months. Confidence in one's markings and technique give the patient and surgeon the perseverance to wait the appropriate time. Photographic documentation during each of the visits can help reassure the patient that the asymmetry is resolving over time.

Other complications include a fading fold where the newly created supratarsal crease begins to lose its crisp line. This condition most commonly follows a limited/nonincision technique because the suture may be holding too many layers between the dermis and levator. As a result, the fold begins to fade. More serious complications of blepharoplasty are covered elsewhere in this issue. Hematoma can best be avoided with meticulous dissection and compulsive attention to hemostasis, especially during orbital fat removal.

A number of techniques address these complications. Diagnosing the correct anatomic reasons that are causing the issues determines the technique used to address the problem. Typically, an open technique is used to perform a needed adhyesiolysis between the levator and orbicularis, levator advancement, or fat grafting as necessary. Results after revisional surgery are much more variable.[14,29–33]

SUMMARY

Asian upper lid blepharoplasty is a complex procedure that requires comprehensive understanding of the anatomy and precise surgical technique.[11] The creation of the supratarsal crease has gone through many evolutions in technique but the principles and goals remain the same: a functional, natural-appearing eyelid crease that brings out the beauty of the Asian eye. Recent advances in the treatment of the medial canthus and subclinical ptosis have improved functional and aesthetic outcomes of Asian upper lid blepharoplasty. The lateral canthus, subbrow orbital aesthetics, and revisional techniques are newer areas where one can expect advances in Asian upper lid blepharoplasty.[34,35]

REFERENCES

1. Cho M, Glavas IP. Anatomic properties of the upper eyelid in Asian Americans. Dermatol Surg 2009; 35(11):1736–40.
2. Kim HN, Kim JH. Various clinical application of the bead stitch method. J Korean Soc Aesthetic Plast Surg 2006;12(2):125–9.
3. Lee TE, Lee JM, Lee H, et al. Lash ptosis and associated factors in Asians. Ann Plast Surg 2010;65(4): 407–10.
4. Nagasao T, Shimizu Y, Ding W, et al. Morphological analysis of the upper eyelid tarsus in Asians. Ann Plast Surg 2011;66(2):196–201.
5. Nguyen MQ, Hsu PW, Dinh TA. Asian blepharoplasty. Semin Plast Surg 2009;23(3):185–97.
6. Oh YW, Seul CH, Yoo WM. Medial epicanthoplasty using the skin redraping method. Plast Reconstr Surg 2007;119(2):703–10.
7. Park DH, Choi WS, Song CH. Anatomy of upper eyelid in Koreans. J Korean Soc Aesthetic Plast Surg 2006;12(1):1–6.
8. Hwang K, Kim DJ, Hwang SH. Thickness of Korean upper eyelid skin at different levels. J Craniofac Surg 2006;17(1):54–6.
9. Ichinose A, Tahara S. Extended preseptal fat resection in Asian blepharoplasty. Ann Plast Surg 2008; 60(2):121–6.
10. Kakizaki H, Leibovitch I, Selva D, et al. Orbital septum attachment on the levator aponeurosis in Asians: in vivo and cadaver study. Ophthalmology 2009;116(10):2031–5.
11. Kikkawa DO, Kim JW. Asian blepharoplasty. Int Ophthalmol Clin 1997;37(3):193–204 [review].
12. Wong JK. Aesthetic surgery in Asians. Curr Opin Otolaryngol Head Neck Surg 2009;17(4):279–86 [review].
13. Park JI. Modified Z-epicanthoplasty in the Asian eyelid. Arch Facial Plast Surg 2000;2(1):43–7.
14. Park SG, Jung KI, Choi JY. The preferred shape of supratarsal fold in 979 double eyelid operation candidates. J Korean Soc Aesthetic Plast Surg 2005;11(2):195–200.
15. Kim DH, Yoon SW, Kim CH. Epicanthoplasty using the Y-M plasty. Archives of Aesthetic Plastic Surgery 2011;17(2):112–8.

16. Lew DH, Kang JH, Cho IC. Surgical correction of multiple upper eyelid folds in East Asians. Plast Reconstr Surg 2011;127(3):1323–31.

17. Chang HJ, Ko DH. The measurement method of skin amount to be excised in the upper blepharoplasty. J Korean Soc Aesthetic Plast Surg 2001;7(2):87–91.

18. Lam SM, Kim YK. Partial-incision technique for creation of the double eyelid. Aesthet Surg J 2003;23(3): 170–6.

19. Park SG, Lee SK, Baek RM. A new interpretation of ptosis-like eyes through the results of small-incision double eyelid operation. J Korean Soc Plast Reconstr Surg 2006;33(4):449–53.

20. Park SG, Song IG, Choi JH, et al. Epicanthoplasty using modified Uchicda method to shift a superomedial direction. J Korean Soc Plast Reconstr Surg 2007;34(6):807–12.

21. Yoon IM, Hong JK, Yoo G. Double eyelid operation using partial incision and continuous buried suture. J Korean Soc Plast Reconstr Surg 2003; 30(5):674–6.

22. Chen W, Li S, Li Y, et al. Medial epicanthoplasty using the palpebral margin incision method. J Plast Reconstr Aesthet Surg 2009;62(12):1621–6.

23. Lee MA, Yoon ES, Shin YW, et al. Epicanthoplasty with simple excision technique. J Korean Soc Aesthetic Plast Surg 2006;12(2):108–11.

24. Lee YH, Lee SW, Baek RM. Correction of the epicanthal fold with invisible scar. J Korean Soc Plast Reconstr Surg 2005;32(3):299–303.

25. Lu JJ, Yang K, Jin XL, et al. Epicanthoplasty with double eyelidplasty incorporating modified Z-plasty for Chinese patients. J Plast Reconstr Aesthet Surg 2011;64(4):462–6.

26. Tianyi L, Haiyan S, Fei L, et al. Blepharoptosis correction by excision of levator muscle and tarsus in Asians. J Craniofac Surg 2010;21(3):652–5.

27. Yoo WM, Park SH, Kwag DR. Root z-epicanthoplasty in Asian eyelids. Plast Reconstr Surg 2002;109(6): 2067–71 [discussion: 2072–3].

28. Zhang H, Zhuang H, Yu H, et al. A new Z-epicanthoplasty and a concomitant double eyelidplasty in Chinese eyelids. Plast Reconstr Surg 2006;118(4): 900–7.

29. Chan HC, Yoon DJ, Kang CU, et al. Correction of high fold without skin excision. J Korean Soc Plast Reconstr Surg 2009;36(5):649–53.

30. Kim BG, Youn DY. Revision of high fold with pretarsal fibromuscular flap. J Korean Soc Aesthetic Plast Surg 2006;12(1):19–22.

31. Kruavit A. Asian blepharoplasty: an 18-year experience in 6215 patients. Aesthet Surg J 2009;29(4):272–83.

32. Kwon YS, Heo J. Secondary blepharoplasty using various methods. J Korean Soc Aesthetic Plast Surg 2006;12(2):130–4.

33. Takayanagi S. Case studies in Asian blepharoplasty. Aesthet Surg J 2011;31(2):171–9.

34. Cha JH, Woo SM, Kim JW, et al. Sub-brow resection via relocation of retro-orbicularis oculi fat and preseptal fat unit. J Korean Soc Plast Reconstr Surg 2011;38(4):477–84.

35. Han BK, Jung HS. Lateral canthoplasty using lateral canthotomy and YV advancement. J Korean Soc Plast Reconstr Surg 2007;34(5):641–6.

Revision Blepharoplasty

Natalie A. Stanciu, MD, Tanuj Nakra, MD*

KEYWORDS

- Blepharoplasty • Plastic surgery • Surgical procedures

KEY POINTS

- Functional and/or cosmetic complications can arise from upper blepharoplasty surgery.
- A detailed understanding of anatomy is an essential component of successful revision.
- Revision options include surgical and nonsurgical interventions.
- A successful outcome to revision surgery depends on a clear understanding of the patient's complaint, clinically identifying the problem, and clearly delineating realistic expectations for revision.
- One of the most common complications of blepharoplasty is dry eye syndrome, for which there are a variety of nonsurgical options.
- The most common cosmetic complications are crease and/or fold, under- and overcorrection, asymmetry, and volume loss.
- Maintenance of racial and gender characteristics is critical to patient satisfaction.
- Maintaining a nonjudgmental attitude toward other physicians is vital to creating a healthy relationship with the patient.

INTRODUCTION

Blepharoplasty surgery is typically a routine and rewarding procedure. However, on occasion, it can lead to adverse outcomes. Proper preoperative evaluation, patient selection, and appropriate procedure customization will prevent most complications. However, even in the best of hands, patient dissatisfaction may result from unrealistic expectations, inappropriate surgical plan, over- or undercorrection, asymmetry, or an unexpected surgical event. The patient who is dissatisfied may present from the physicians' own practice or as a referral. This article characterizes upper blepharoplasty complications and elaborates on available treatment options for revision blepharoplasty.

One of the first hurdles in managing a patient who requires revision surgery is to understand the emotional needs of a dissatisfied patient and how to delicately navigate the revision process. The psychological status of a dissatisfied patient is often complex and requires time and attention to properly navigate. The ultimate success of revision

blepharoplasty depends on listening carefully to the patient's concerns and outlining a realistic plan developed to meet her or his goals.

Whether the patient's primary blepharoplasty was performed for cosmetic or functional reasons, the ensuing complication can be cosmetic, functional, or both. Therefore, a common tactic in addressing blepharoplasty revisions is to divide the complications into two categories: functional or cosmetic. This article presents techniques to recognize the categories of blepharoplasty complications and ultimately identify options for managing these problems. It is important to understand that even the finest surgeons will have some patients who suffer unexpected outcomes and that, fortunately, most complications can be managed appropriately.

EVALUATION
Subjective Complaints

The most important part of the patient interview is understanding the patient's primary complaint. What are the patient concerns? Is there a problem

Texas Oculoplastic Consultants, 3705 Medical Parkway, Suite 120, Austin, TX 78705, USA
* Corresponding author.
E-mail address: TNakra@tocaustin.com

Clin Plastic Surg 40 (2013) 179–189
http://dx.doi.org/10.1016/j.cps.2012.06.006

with dryness, irritation, difficulty blinking, or closing the eye? Or is the patient more concerned about the cosmetic appearance with respect to symmetry, scarring, and volume? The patient's own words often help make the distinction as to whether the issue is functional or cosmetic. Identification of the patient's concerns is the basis for the process of identifying options available for addressing the problem.

Physical Examination

We will review specific components of the physical examination that are relevant to a patient who presents for revision upper eyelid surgery. See the article by Lam and colleagues elsewhere in this issue for the pertinent anatomy when examining a patient undergoing primary upper eyelid blepharoplasty.

Standard measurements
The margin reflex distance (MRD1), along with the levator-muscle function (LF), is important to record when documenting uncorrected ptosis after blepharoplasty. The MRD1 is the distance from a light reflex centered on the pupil to the upper lid margin when the patient is staring at a light source in primary gaze. A normal measurement is roughly 3 to 4 mm. A lesser value indicates upper eyelid ptosis. The LF is the upper lid excursion from down to up gaze (with the brow immobilized), with a normal value of approximately 15. A patient who has undergone standalone upper blepharoplasty may have had preexisting ptosis that was overlooked. Excising redundant eyelid skin should not cause ptosis (low MRD1). If a patient underwent only blepharoplasty and the MRD1 is low after the procedure, it is likely that there was preoperative ptosis that not addressed in the primary procedure.[1]

Another important anatomic measurement is the height of the anterior lamella present from lid margin to brow. A measurement of less than 20 mm is a significant indicator of excessive skin excision. It is important to document whether there is subtle eversion of the lid or inability to close the eyelid due to anterior lamellar shortage.

Orbicularis function
Lagophthalmos (poor lid closure) may result not only from aggressive skin excision but also from damage to the orbicularis muscle itself. It is not uncommon for skin and muscle to be excised together during upper blepharoplasty so recording the function of the muscle following such surgery is critical.[2,3] This is especially important for patients who may have had preoperative underlying weakness such as facial nerve palsy or Parkinson's disease. In such cases, removing muscle

at the time of surgery will lead to further impairment in orbicularis function with poor eyelid closure. Eversion of the eyelid margin on forced closure is suggestive of orbicularis damage.

Lacrimal function and basal secretion test
One of the most common complaints after blepharoplasty surgery is immediate postoperative dry eye symptoms. These complaints typically resolve within a few weeks. When the problem persists, there may be underlying of dry eye pathology that was unmasked by the procedure. Alternatively, aggressive skin excision or orbicularis damage may have caused de novo ocular exposure and dry eye symptoms. Lacrimal gland function can be assessed with a Schirmer test, which documents basal tear secretion and identifies if there is a quantitative problem with tear production.[4] The slit lamp examination should include evaluation of meibomian gland function through tear film breakup time (TBUT; the time it takes for tears to evaporate), which will indicate if a qualitative disturbance in tear quality is present. This involves placing fluorescein drops in the eyes, asking the patient to blink, and assessing the time it takes for the dyed tears to evaporate. It is relevant to document the presence of tear instability and dysfunction in the setting of aggressive skin removal and/or diminished orbicularis function because diminished tear quality may further exacerbate the symptoms of dry eye.

Crease and upper eyelid position and contour
A significant factor affecting the satisfaction of a patient after upper blepharoplasty is the symmetry in the eyelid position, crease, fold, and contour. Typical racial and gender variations should be taken into account. Typical female eyelid anatomy features a higher lid crease in contrast to male eyelid anatomy. Asian patients may prefer to maintain their lid with the crease in its anatomically low normal position. These individualized patient preferences are much better discussed before the surgery instead of after.

Brow position
In the previous section, the MRD1 was discussed as it relates to uncorrected ptosis. Equally important is evaluating the height and contour of the brow. Patients may complain of "droopiness" of the eyelid temporally, alleging that not enough eyelid skin was removed at the time of blepharoplasty surgery, when, in fact, the low position of the brow causes the temporal eyelid hooding. Additionally a persistent "heavy" feeling after blepharoplasty surgery may relate to untreated brow ptosis.

Lash anatomy

Oftentimes overlooked preoperatively, the postoperative eyelash position may be a source of dissatisfaction for the patient. Eyelash ptosis (an inferiorly directed lash position) may lead to discomfort and visual compromise for the patient. Recognizing and addressing this subtle issue can lead to a functional, as well as cosmetic, benefit for the patient.

Medial and lateral canthus

Generally, canthal appearance and function is unaffected by upper blepharoplasty procedures. However the canthal anatomy itself may affect the outcome of the surgery. Patients who have canthal or upper eyelid laxity may experience suboptimal ptosis correction when added to primary blepharoplasty. Patients with frank floppy eyelid syndrome require lid tightening at the time of primary surgery to address their upper eyelid functional compromise. Untreated laxity may lead to exacerbation of symptoms after blepharoplasty due to weakening of the orbicularis muscle as a consequence of surgery.

Also, particularly in Asian patients, the medial canthus may be altered after surgery when an epicanthal fold is present. Scarring and webbing of the medial canthus in Asian patient can occur with manipulation of the epicanthal fold. Reviewing preoperative photographs can be helpful in understanding the natural genetic phenotype.

COMPLICATIONS

After identifying the anatomic changes in a patient with a blepharoplasty complication, the revision surgeon can turn his or her attention to analysis and categorization of the problem and correction of the deficit. There are two general categories of upper blepharoplasty complications: functional and cosmetic. Some deficits fall into both categories and some patients have a combination of the two. Nevertheless, it is useful to analyze each

Functional Complications	Cosmetic Complications
Lagophthalmos	Hollowing
Orbicularis damage	Scarring
Dry eyes	Crease, contour, and eyelash irregularity
Untreated ptosis	Medial canthal/ epicanthal irregularity
Undercorrection	

component of the problem to customize the most effective management plan.

FUNCTIONAL COMPLICATIONS
Lagophthalmos

Skin overresection

Excess skin excision in upper blepharoplasty is one of the most common complications of surgery (**Fig. 1**). Blepharoplasty surgeons often focus on maximizing the surgical outcome by aggressively debulking the eyelid. This excision-based approach to surgery can lead to potentially significant problems with eyelid closure. A rule of thumb to avoid skin-shortage–related lagophthalmos is to ensure that at least 20 mm of skin remains from inferior brow to lid margin. This assumes normal brow position and the measurement can be altered based on brow location if brow lifting is not added. Using the "skin pinch" test during marking for skin excision will also help prevent skin shortage issues. In this technique, the proposed excess skin is captured with a forceps while observing the position of the lid margin.[1] If the lid margin everts and/or there is more than mild degrees of lagophthalmos, less skin is engaged for safe excision.[1]

When a patient presents with lagophthalmos (related to skin shortage) after blepharoplasty there are surgical and nonsurgical management options.

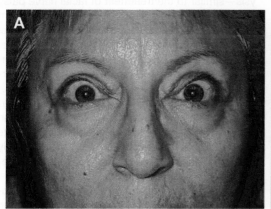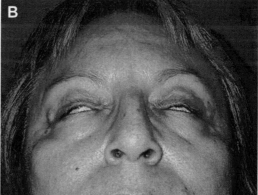

Fig. 1. (A) Postoperative blepharoplasty excessive skin excision with scleral show and (B) lagophthalmos.

Surgical options for lagophthalmos correction

In cases in which limitation of eyelid closure is severe, the definitive treatment is skin grafting.

- The eyelid skin is among the thinnest on the body. As such, appropriate harvest sites should best match the skin of the eyelid and include, in descending order, skin from the:
  - Opposite upper lid
  - Postauricular area
  - Supraclavicular area.

If donor skin in these harvest sites is inadequate, the inner upper arm, inner thigh, or, rarely, foreskin can be considered.

The recipient bed on the eyelid is typically fashioned through an eyelid crease incision. Secondarily, a supralash incision can be used. A marginal traction suture is used to place the upper lid on downward stretch. Dissection can be performed in the subcutaneous plane as needed to fully expand the defect with care to avoid damage to the orbicularis muscle (which can further limit eyelid closure). Hemostasis is assured but overzealous cautery must be avoided to maintain blood supply to the grafted skin.

Once fully created, the recipient bed is measured horizontally and vertically. The dimensions are noted and an appropriately sized full-thickness graft is harvested. The graft is thinned of subcutaneous tissue as needed, its size is adjusted as appropriate, and the graft is secured to the recipient bed with fibrin tissue glue and/or circumferential sutures. Focal 1 mm full-thickness skin ports can be created throughout the graft to allow egress of blood. The upper eyelid can be placed on stretch with a reverse Frost suture to optimize healing and the eye firmly patched for up to 7 days. In the most severe cases, a permanent lateral tarsorrhaphy and/or lid recession (levator or Mueller's muscle) can be added.

Nonsurgical options for lagophthalmos correction

In more subtle cases of lagophthalmos related to skin shortage, or when the patients does not desire further surgical intervention, less invasive maneuvers are used to help address patient symptoms.

One elegant option is the use of chemodenervation to induce brow depression. The brow and upper eyelid are intimately related. As brow position changes the eyelid is secondarily effected. Changing the brow position with neurotoxin (Botox, Dysport) can induce brow depression and mechanical pressure on the upper eyelid, with resultant improved eyelid closure and reduction of exposure symptoms. It is important to counsel the patient on the potential consequences of this procedure, including brow immobility and ptosis.

Another nonsurgical option to reduce lagophthalmos is the addition of hyaluronic acid gel fillers to the upper lid. In this instance the filler is not added solely for volume augmentation but also to create a lamellar and/or scar expansion and, potentially, as a load (weight) to aid in closure.

Using tape to aid in closing the eyelids during sleep can be helpful in reducing nocturnal lagophthalmos.

Orbicularis Damage

The strength and tone of the orbicularis muscle may be impaired after blepharoplasty surgery with or without postoperative skin deficiency. Orbicularis weakness is more commonly seen when transcutaneous lower lid surgery and/or canthal suspension is added; however, it is also seen with stand-alone upper blepharoplasty. The orbicularis muscle is innervated by the zygomatic branch of the facial nerve, which enters the muscle lateral to the lateral canthus. Extended lateral incisions and the addition of canthal suspensions (when lower lid surgery is added) can contribute to orbicularis weakness.

In upper blepharoplasty, the preseptal orbicularis is often resected with the skin in the course of tissue excision, which can affect the involuntary lid closure. Involuntary blink is critical for the tear pump mechanics, reflex tear production, and maintaining tear film stability. Testing for orbicularis weakness is performed by asking the patient to maximally squeeze their eyelids shut while the examiner simultaneously opposes this action with digital counterpressure on the eyelids. Orbicularis weakness is confirmed with ease of lid opening or, in less severe cases, eversion of the eyelid margin.

Surgical treatment of orbicularis damage

Unfortunately there is no definitive surgical treatment to improve orbicularis muscle function.

Insertion of an upper eyelid gold weight is the ultimate solution for advanced orbicularis paralysis—similar to the treatment of facial nerve palsy patients. An appropriately sized gold or platinum weight can be surgically implanted in the pretarsal space via an upper eyelid incision. A nonsurgical equivalent of the eyelid gold weight can be accomplished by injecting hyaluronic acid into the pretarsal space to act as an upper eyelid load.

Canthal suspension procedures with associated muscle tightening may improve the length-tension dynamics of the orbicularis, thereby maximizing its contractility. Canthoplasty is a low-risk, minimally invasive maneuver that may be worthwhile—especially in the setting of upper eyelid laxity.

Other surgical options for improving the problems related to orbicularis weakness include skin grafting and partial lateral tarsorrhaphy.

Nonsurgical options for treating orbicularis damage

Nonsurgical supportive therapy for orbicularis function deficit–related lagophthalmos include therapies to improve ocular lubrication (see later discussion on nonsurgical management of dry eye).

Dry Eye

Perhaps the most common problem a patient faces after upper blepharoplasty is new or worsening dry eye symptoms. Patients may complain of grittiness, foreign-body sensation, blurring, discharge, and red eyes. The problem is often multifactorial, related to skin deficiency, poor lid closure, and reduced tear production. The patient may have had an unrecognized preexisting dry eye condition that was exacerbated by surgery. Preoperatively, patients manifesting even subtle degrees of dry eye should have the condition detailed in depth and maximally managed before proceeding with blepharoplasty. If it is deemed safe for patients with dry eye syndrome to proceed with surgery, they will be better equipped to handle side effects should they occur after surgery.

When treating postoperative dry eye, it is important to determine whether the problem is a qualitative (tear quality) or quantitative (tear production) in nature, or a combination. The Schirmer and TBUT measurements previously described will help differentiate the nature of the problem. Dry eye symptoms can be very troublesome to patients. Fortunately there are a variety of treatment options to minimize dry eye symptoms.

Surgical options for treating dry eye

Conservative management is the best initial option.

If symptoms persist, or are severe enough to warrant a procedure, then lacrimal punctual occlusion by cautery or open intracanalicular suturing is a useful step toward improving ocular surface lubrication.

Last resort options include (as previously mentioned) skin grafting, upper eyelid gold weight placement, and permanent lateral tarsorrhaphy.

Nonsurgical options for treating dry eye

The frequent use of preservative-free artificial tears and ointment is the initial step in treating dry eyes.

If symptoms persist, punctual occlusion (with plugs) should be considered. Punctal and canalicular plugs come in a variety of shapes and sizes, but they are all designed to obstruct lacrimal outflow and maximize ocular surface lubrication. Ideally, intracanalicular plugs, along with small punctual plugs, should be avoided because these tend to migrate and are difficult to retrieve if necessary.

Once the quantitative component of tears has been maximized, efforts to improve the qualitative component (quality of tears), if needed, is useful. Lid hygiene maneuvers (baby shampoo, lid scrubs) and warm compresses may increase the lipophilic component of the tear film and prevent tear evaporation. The use of oral fish oil 1000 mg by mouth twice per day has also been known to improve ocular lubrication.

It is helpful to spend time with patients discussing specific environmental factors that might worsen dry symptoms, such as overhead and tabletop fans, and factors that can reduce ambient humidity (local climate, season, and home thermoregulation.) Using a humidifier in the bedroom at night can be a useful adjuvant therapy.

Finally, taping the eyelids closed at night and tissue expansion or lid load with hyaluronic acid filler can be considered when eyelid closure is a significant causative factor.

Untreated Ptosis

Management of ptosis begins with identifying the problem. The MRD1 is recorded and used as reference for the severity of ptosis. The LF should be documented to plan the appropriate procedure for correction. Unrecognized preoperative ptosis masked by dermatochalasis at the time of initial evaluation is, as previously mentioned, a common cause of ptosis after blepharoplasty (**Fig. 2**). Excess skin does not lead to true eyelid ptosis and lid position should always be determined preoperatively.

It is important to recognize that overcompensation for a contralateral ptosis (Hering's law) may give the appearance of upper eyelid retraction in the nonptotic eyelid. The surgeon must distinguish this condition from true eyelid retraction by observing the position of the supposedly retracted eyelid while the contralateral, presumably ptotic eyelid, is either manually elevated or occluded.

Surgical correction of untreated ptosis

The surgical procedure selected for the correction of ptosis depends on the severity of the problem.

For patients with mild ptosis (less than 2 mm) a phenylephrine test (instillation of a phenylephrine 2.5% drop to the affected eye, twice, spaced 5 minutes apart) may be used to assess whether a posterior approach procedure is appropriate (see article by Martin elsewhere in this issue). If lid position corrects to the desired height, posterior approach surgery is favored with the benefit of being less invasive and having a better likelihood of achieving a more natural contour (see **Fig. 2**C).

For cases in which ptosis is more severe (>3 mm) and/or there is a poor phenylephrine response, an anterior approach levator advancement (see article by Martin elsewhere in this issue) or a full-thickness resection are more appropriate choices. The anterior

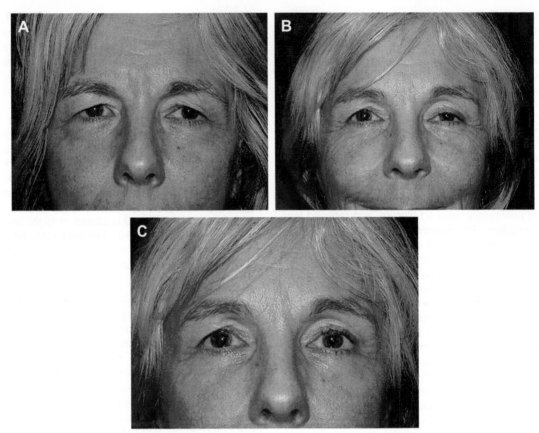

Fig. 2. (*A*) Preoperative dermatochalasis and masked ptosis on the left side. (*B*) Postoperative dermatochalasis ptosis on the left side. (*C*) Postoperative ptosis repair via posterior approach conjunctival mullerectomy.

approach offers the added benefit of intraoperative adjustments in lid height contour and/or adjustments in lid crease position.

See later discussion concerning crease adjustments Cosmetic Complications.

Nonsurgical correction options for untreated ptosis

Neurotoxins can be useful in cases in which patients are opposed to having any additional surgery. Chemodenervation is used to weaken the eyelid protractor, the orbicularis, which can produce mild lid elevation. Ideal patients have very mild ptosis (1–2 mm), and may be treated with 5 to15 units of botulinum toxin to the lateral canthal and pretarsal locations of the orbicularis muscle. The potential exacerbation of dry eyes should be weighed before considering this treatment option.

Undercorrection of Blepharoplasty

When assessing a patient with an undercorrected upper blepharoplasty, it is far better to have taken too little skin than too much skin. In the setting of a true undercorrection, additional skin excision can easily be performed under local anesthesia

in the office. The important question is whether there was a true surgical undercorrection versus unrecognized brow ptosis, simulating the appearance of redundant upper eyelid skin.

Patients with significant dermatochalasis often compensate by raising their forehead in an effort to maintain a clear axis of vision. After blepharoplasty, the drive to raise the forehead is removed, and the brow reverts back to its natural position. In this instance, latent brow ptosis becomes unmasked by the blepharoplasty procedure. This is especially common in the temporal brow region where native brow ptosis is most pronounced. It is critical to recognize this problem preoperatively, so the possibility of lateral eyelid fullness persisting after surgery can be discussed with the patient. When patients understand the anatomic problem, they can make informed decisions as to whether to add a brow lift or accept the limitations of blepharoplasty alone.

Surgical options for blepharoplasty undercorrection

If there is true undercorrection evidenced by excess skin folds without brow ptosis, and in the setting of adequate eyelid closure, then touch-up blepharoplasty revision is warranted.

Care must be taken to ensure that excessive skin removal is conservative to maintain optimal lid function.

These procedures can be safely performed in the office under local anesthesia only.

If the problem is brow ptosis, some form of brow lifting (chemical vs surgical) is indicated (see articles by Nahai and colleagues, Terella and Wang, Walrath and McCord, and Langsdon and Velargo elsewhere in this issue).

COSMETIC COMPLICATIONS

The functional blepharoplasty patient is often more forgiving of postoperative complications than the patient seeking aesthetic rejuvenation. Aesthetic patients have typically paid a substantial sum of money for their elective surgery, have high expectations for an optimal aesthetic outcome, and are often less tolerant of deviations from their expectations. It is important to recognize that patient satisfaction in cosmetic blepharoplasty (like all cosmetic procedures) is personalized and that that the dictum "beauty is in the eye of the beholder" often overrides reality. This section focuses on recognizing cosmetic blepharoplasty complications from an objective viewpoint, as well as understanding those surgical problems that may render patients dissatisfied with their surgical outcome.

Hollowing

Traditional blepharoplasty surgery techniques involve aggressive excision of various amounts of skin, muscle, and fat. This often leads to gaunt postoperative results that exacerbate the aged eyelid instead of restoring youth (**Fig. 3**A).[5,6] Contemporary surgery has shifted toward a more conservative approach of tissue excision to prevent postoperative

eyelid hollowing. When sulcus depression does develop after surgery, there are several treatment options to address the issue.

Surgical correction of hollowing

Autologous fat transfer can be employed for treating periorbital hollowing, whether age-related or iatrogenic in nature.[7]

Fat can be harvested from numerous sites, including the abdomen, flanks, inner thighs, and inner knees using a microliposuction technique. Low-pressure hand aspiration is preferred to suction-assisted fat cell harvesting to reduce pressure gradient related cell lysis.

Transcutaneous injections of harvested fat that have been prepared with gravitational decanting or centrifugation can be delivered to the periorbital area (see **Fig. 3**B). The increased vascularity of the orbicularis muscle provides an ideal environment for injected fat. Care is taken to inject small aliquots of fat, typically 0.05 to 0.1 cc per pass of the cannula, to avoid lumpiness and irregularity. Placing the patient at a 45° supine position aids intraoperative analysis of contour and symmetry.

Additional periorbital injection sites include the temple, the brow, the perinasal midfacial soft tissue, and the malar region.

A surgical alternative for soft tissue volume augmentation is using free pearl fat grafts.[8] Open periumbilical or submental incisions can be used to harvest free fat pearls. A preseptal dissection performed to the arcus marginalis via an upper eyelid crease incision allows access to the supraorbital rim soft. Here, the placement of free pearl fat grafts to the subbrow fat pad can help adding volume to the superior sulcus.

Nonsurgical options for hollowing

Often the first choice for the treatment of iatrogenic volume loss is nonsurgical filler injections.

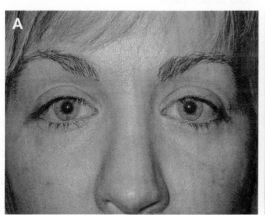 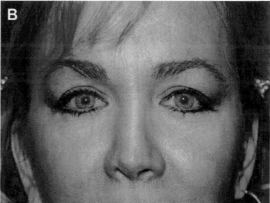

Fig. 3. (*A*) Postoperative lash ptosis and hollowed sulcus after blepharoplasty. (*B*) After repair using lash rotation sutures and autologous fat transfer to the subbrow region.

Hyaluronic acid gel filler is an ideal periorbital soft tissue volumizer for multiple reasons, including ease of injection, relative low risk, reversibility, and performance as an excellent soft tissue proxy. An initial injection of a single syringe allows the patient to "dip a toe in" and experience the benefits of revolumization.

Filler volume injections for upper eyelid hollowing ideally are performed with attention to the brow fat pad and the postseptal superior orbit. Any irregularity or desire for reversal can be accomplished via hyaluronidase enzyme if necessary.

Other fillers, such as hydroxyapatite and poly-L-lactic acid are less desirable in the periorbital region owing to increased risk of nodules and irregularity.

Scarring

Postoperative scarring is a troublesome complication of upper blepharoplasty. A variety of causes lead to scarring, including:

- Infection
- Wound dehiscence
- Impaired healing from cautery-related thermal injury
- Peculiarities of individual patient skin anatomy
- Predisposition to scarring.

Scarring can occur even with flawless surgical technique. It is important to resist the temptation to rush to revision because it is wise to allow scar maturation before proceeding with further surgery. Ideally, revision should wait up to 6 to 12 months. During healing, the patient is instructed to massage the scarred tissue and avoid sun exposure. A variety of over-the-counter preparations (eg, creams) may be of benefit in reducing scar formation. The OTC creams which are silicone based available for reducing scar formation include Prosil, Scarfade and Xeragel. When planning revision, it is important to discuss with the patient the reality that scar revision will only result in an incremental improvement. An expectation for a perfect result is not realistic.

Surgical correction for scars

Successful scar revision often requires adequate residual skin because resection of the eyelid scar is often the first step in revision. Correcting a scar with excision that will lead to poor lid closure would just trade one problem for a new and, maybe, worse problem.

Scar revision is often combined with crease reformation procedures to allow for ideal symmetric placement of the eyelid crease and redraping of the anterior lamella.

Careful measurement with a caliper and precise incision with either a number 15 scalpel blade or carbon dioxide laser is the ideal approach to these revision procedures.

Meticulous closure with tension-reducing suturing techniques completes the procedure.

Nonsurgical correction for scars

Nonsurgical solutions for improving eyelid scarring are indicated for early treatment during scar maturation and for superficial textural cicatricial skin irregularities. In addition, for those patients who would benefit from incision revision procedures but do not wish to have further surgery, these nonsurgical treatments may be of benefit.

Injections with antimetabolites, such as 5-fluorouracil, (5-FU) can be useful in reducing scar thickness and cicatrization[9–11] and are ideal biologic scar modulators in the early healing after blepharoplasty. Ideally, these injections are most helpful from as early as 3 to 4 weeks postoperatively with less utility after 6 months. In contrast to the hyperpigmentation, skin thinning, and telangiectasia-inducing side effects of depot steroid injections, 5-FU does not typically lead to these unwanted side-effects.

Fractionated laser resurfacing may also improve eyelid scarring. These lasers, both fractionated carbon dioxide and erbium modalities, can provide deep (subepithelial) and superficial (epithelial) treatments that may be efficacious with scarring. Fractionated treatments may require several sessions to achieve the desired goal. The physician must take caution to pretreat and posttreat pigmented patients (Type III–V on the Fitzpatrick scale) with hydroquinone because they are prone to postinflammatory hyperpigmentation with laser applications.

Another option for superficial epithelial remodeling to improve scar appearance is 25% to 30% trichloroacetic acid peeling. The risks for postinflammatory hyperpigmentation are applicable to skin peels.

A simple nonsurgical alternative is instructing the patient on cosmetic make-up tips to further camouflage the scar.

Crease, Contour, and Eyelash Irregularity

One of the complexities of blepharoplasty surgery is that it is not only essential to understand the internal functional anatomy but also to be aware of the delicate external framework. The eyelid crease and contour are formed by a complicated relationship of the levator muscle, tarsus, and skin, and are exquisitely sensitive to surgical eyelid manipulation. Patients may be most unhappy after surgery because it alters the most obvious and visible aspects of their eyelid appearance—the eyelid crease and contour.

Eyelid crease

A normal appearance is a fairly symmetric upper eyelid crease with an upper eyelid margin forming a smooth arch with the highest point positioned between the medial limbus and the pupil.[12]

The distance of the lid crease from the eyelid margin is additionally pertinent because it relates to gender and demographic variations. Preserving a patient's gender and racially defining characteristics is critical to the external satisfaction with blepharoplasty surgery (**Fig. 4**).

Generally, white males have a lower crease (roughly 6 mm from the lid margin).

White females generally have a crease (typically 8 mm) above the margin.

Male eyelids tend to be slightly more ptotic and full compared with female eyelids.

Asian eyelid creases in both men and women range from no crease to 8 mm.

Patients of Central American and Mexican descent often have the features of the Asian eyelid.

Having discussed these "ideal" measurements, it is important to identify preoperative inherent eyelid asymmetries and to discuss this with the patient because perfect symmetry may is not a realistic goal of surgery. In addition, despite assumed gender and racial preferences, each patient may have different expectations for their appearance and, again, it is important that the surgeon have an understanding of the patients' specific goals before surgery.

Eyelid contour

Blepharoplasty surgery can also affect eyelid contour. If there has been an over-resection of skin and/or muscle medially or laterally, the contour peak may shift in that direction. This is also true of the eyelid crease, related to disruption of the levator attachments to the pretarsal skin, overexcision of preaponeurotic fat with superior cicatrization of the crease, and irregular skin healing.

Eyelash contour

Changes to the eyelash contour can occur following blepharoplasty. Specifically, disruption of the levator slips to the pretarsal skin can lead to eyelash ptosis following blepharoplasty.

Independent specific analysis of each upper eyelid for contour, crease location, and eyelash position allows for appropriate revision surgery design.

Surgical correction of crease, contour, and eyelash irregularity

Surgical correction of the crease, contour, and eyelash position are among the most unpredictable eyelid revision procedures. Therefore, lengthy and detailed preoperative patient counseling regarding the limit of realistic surgical outcomes are necessary before proceeding with any interventional plan. If the crease height is imperfect or asymmetric, careful planning with caliper measurements and analysis of globe position brow position are helpful tools.

Crease height can be adjusted by the full-thickness suture techniques (especially in Asian lids) if the intent is to raise the height.[13] This has the advantage of being minimally invasive; however, is less predictable though, perhaps, less permanent.

The traditional crease formation surgery involves open exposure via an incision at the desired crease location with fixation of the inferior incision edge orbicularis to the levator-tarsus complex using multiple interrupted sutures.

If there is lash ptosis, additional cephalad traction on the orbicularis can rotate the lash trajectory upwards (see **Fig. 3**).

Uneven contour of the eyelid margin can be corrected using single sutures placed in an interrupted horizontal mattress fashion positioned from

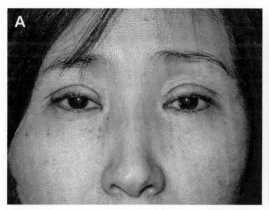
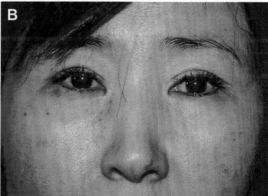

Fig. 4. (A) Postoperative blepharoplasty of Asian patient with inappropriately placed "high" eyelid crease as well as uncorrected ptosis. (B) Postoperative reformation of crease using "pang" sutures and posterior ptosis repair.

the superior tarsus to the levator aponeurosis edge in the desired location. The patient can be brought into an upright position during the surgical procedure to check the contour by requesting dynamic interaction from the patient in opening the eyes.

Nonsurgical correction of crease, contour, and eyelash irregularity

Hyaluronic acid gel fillers can be a dramatic nonsurgical tool in the treatment of contour and crease irregularities. These fillers, injected below or above the crease, can expand or mechanically compress the crease to manipulate its position.

Further options include manipulating the brow position to camouflage eyelid crease irregularity. Elevation of the brow via botulinum toxin injection to the brow depressors will highlight hollowness above the crease, whereas depressing the brow by injecting into the brow elevators will camouflage an irregular crease.

Clever makeup can further help provide nonsurgical improvements to irregular eyelid deficits after blepharoplasty.

Medial Canthal and/or Epicanthal Irregularity

The most unforgiving area of the upper eyelid leading to cicatricial changes is the medial canthus and epicanthal fold (if present). Asian, Eastern European, and Hispanic eyelids have a genetic predisposition toward the epicanthal fold. Because the fold is exquisitely sensitive to microvector changes in skin tension, it is critical to avoid incisions approaching or on the epicanthal fold. Once the fold is violated, it is difficult to predict the effect on epicanthal-fold healing.

Surgical correction of medial canthal and/or epicanthal irregularities

Surgical repair of canthal webs and/or irregularities[10] include a variety of Z-plasty, local tissue rearrangements, consideration of the regional vectors of force, and dorsal nasal augmentation to provide anterior traction on the fold.

Nonsurgical correction of medial canthal and/or epicanthal irregularities

As noted previously, biomodulation early in the healing process with 5-FU can be of benefit. Unlike corticosteroids, 5-FU does not affect the melanocytes and does not cause soft tissue depression and/or contraction. Additional options include hyaluronic acid fillers to shape and/or camouflage the epicanthal anatomy.

Dorsal nasal filler augmentation can be a tool in providing an anterior vector of pull on the scarred canthal tissues.

SUMMARY

Upper blepharoplasty is one of the most commonly performed functional and cosmetic facial surgeries. Although generally a straightforward procedure, as with all surgery, complications can occur. Some of these problems are minor and easy to address and some are troublesome and can be challenging to overcome. As upper blepharoplasty is such a staple in the facial surgeon's practice, it is important to be familiar with the range of potential adverse outcomes that may occur after surgery.

Equally important to understanding and managing complications is the manner in which the dissatisfied patient is dealt with. A nonjudgmental approach, which details the problem in depth, reviews treatment options, stresses realistic expectations to revision, and emphasizes that the goal is "better" but not "perfect," is essential to a successful outcome. When this approach is taken, patients are more comfortable, understanding, and better educated about their problem. In the end, they are more apt to be happy with the revision therapy or procedure that is undertaken.

REFERENCES

1. Nerad JA. Oculoplastic surgery. 1st edition. St Louis (MO): Mosby Inc; 2001.
2. Nahai F. Clinical decision-making in aesthetic eyelid surgery. In: Foad Nahai, editor. The art of aesthetic surgery. 1st edition. St Louis (MO): Quality Medical Publishing Inc; 2005.
3. Nakra T, Shorr N. Ophthalmic plastic surgery. In: Kraushar MF, editor. Risk prevention in ophthalmology. New York: Springer; 2008.
4. Codner MA, Hanna MK. Upper and lower blepharoplasty. In: Foad Nahai, editor. The art of aesthetic surgery. 1st edition. St Louis (MO): Quality Medical Publishing Inc; 2005.
5. Massry GG, Hartstein MA. The lift and fill lower blepharoplasty. Ophthal Plast Reconstr Surg 2012; 28:213–8.
6. Massry GG. Nasal fat preservation in upper eyelid blepharoplasty. Ophthal Plast Reconstr Surg 2011; 27:352–5.
7. Cook T, Nakra T, Shorr N, et al. Facial recontouring with autologous fat. Facial Plast Surg 2004;20(2):145–7.
8. Shorr N, Christenbury JD, Goldberg RA. Free autogenous "pearl fat" grafts to the eyelids. Ophthal Plast Reconstr Surg 1988;4(1):37–40.
9. Taban M, Lee S, Hoenig JA, et al. Postoperative wound modulation in aesthetic and eyelid periorbital surgery. In: Massry GG, Murphy M, Azizzadeh B, editors. Master techniques in blepharoplasty and periorbital rejuvenation. New York: Springer; 2012. p. 307–12.

10. Massry GG. Cicarricial canthal webs. Ophthal Plast Reconstr Surg 2011;27(6):426–30.
11. Massry GG. The external browpexy. Ophthal Plast Reconstr Surg 2012;28:90–5.
12. Buchanon AG, Hilds JB. The beautiful eye: perception of beauty in the periocular area. In: Massry GG, Murphy M, Azizzadeh B, editors. Master techniques in blepharoplasty and periorbital rejuvenation. New York: Springer; 2012. p. 25–9.
13. Pang HG. Surgical formation of the upper lid fold. Arch Ophthalmol 1961;65:783–4.

FURTHER READINGS

Codner MA, Day CR, Hester TR, et al. Management of mundane to complex blepharoplasty problems. Perspect Plast Surg 2001;15:15.

Codner MA, Kikkawa DO, Korn BS, et al. Blepharoplasty and brow lift. Plast Reconstr Surg 2010; 126(1):1e–17e.

Codner MA, Pacella JS. Minor complications after blepharoplasty: dry eyes, chemosis, granulomas, ptosis, and scleral show. Plast Reconstr Surg 2010;125:2.

Culbertson WW, Ostler HB. The floppy eyelid syndrome. Am J Ophthalmol 1981;92:568.

Dailey RA. Upper eyelid blepharoplasty. Focal points: clinical modules for ophthalmologists. San Francisco (CA): American Academy of Ophthalmology; 1995. module 8.

Demartelaere SL, Blaydon SM, Tovilla-Canales JC, et al. A permanent and reversible procedure to block tear drainage for treatment of dry eye. Ophthal Plast Reconstr Surg 2006;5:352–5.

Demere M, Wood T, Austin W. Eye complications with blepharoplasty or other eyelid surgery. Plast Reconstr Surg 1974;53:634–7.

Frueh BR, Musch DC. Evaluation of levator muscle integrity on ptosis with levator force measurement. Ophthalmology 1996;103:244–55.

Lelli GR Jr, Lisman RD. Blepharoplasty complications. Plast Reconstr Surg 2010;125(3):1007–17.

Lisman RD, Hyde K, Smith B. Complications of blepharoplasty. Clin Plast Surg 1988;15:309–35.

Lowry JC, Bartley GB. Complications of blepharoplasty [review]. Surv Ophthalmol 1994;38:327–50.

McCord CD, Fort DT, Hanna K, et al. Lateral canthal anchoring: special situations. Plast Reconstr Surg 2005;15:116.

Morax S, Touitou V. Complications of blepharoplasty. Orbit 2006;25(4).

Neuhaus RW. Complications of blepharoplasty. Focal points: clinical modules for ophthalmologists. San Francisco (CA): American Academy of Ophthalmology; 1990. module 3.

Rees TD, Latrenta GS. The role of Schirmer's test and orbital morphology in predicting dry-eye syndrome after blepharoplasty. Plast Reconstr Surg 1988;82:619.

Shorr N, Goldberg RA, MacCann JD, et al. Upper eyelid skin grafting: an effective treatment for Lagophthalmos following blepharoplasty. Plast Reconstr Surg 2003;112:1444–8.

Tenzel RR. Surgical treatment of complications of cosmetic blepharoplasty. Clin Plast Surg 1978;5:517–23.

Adjunctive Fat Grafting to the Upper Lid and Brow

Ryan M. Collar, MD*, Kofi D. Boahene, MD,
Patrick J. Byrne, MD

KEYWORDS

- Fat grafting • Aging face • Cosmetic surgery • Facial rejuvenation

KEY POINTS

- Lipoatrophy and volume loss are significant components of upper lid and brow aging.
- The aging process of the upper eyelid may lead to deep hollowing of the upper lid with increased upper eyelid show and a skeletonized supraorbital rim appearance without significant dermatochalasis.
- Traditional blepharoplasty, even with fat preservation, does little to rejuvenate patients with severe lipoatrophy and skeletonization. This population requires volume restoration instead of soft tissue removal.
- Fat transposition techniques, autologous fat grafting, and hyaluronic acid fillers are reliable choices for volume augmentation of the upper eyelid.
- Autologous fat is biocompatible, naturally integrates into the host tissues without producing an inflammatory reaction, and is potentially permanent.
- Fat grafting may be used alone or in conjunction with other procedures such as blepharoplasty and browlift techniques as part of the treatment of periorbital aging.

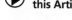

Video of Fat Transfer Showing Technique of Suborbicularis Injection with Micro Cannula Accompanies this Article at http://www.plasticsurgery.theclinics.com/

INTRODUCTION

Lipoatrophy and volume loss are now recognized as significant components of upper lid and brow aging[1–4] Traditional upper lid blepharoplasty techniques that focus on soft tissue excision of skin and fat do not treat volume loss.[5] Therefore, recent technical advances aim to provide volume restoration for upper periorbital rejuvenation in select patients. These advances include autologous fat transfer techniques[6–10] and other novel maneuvers of local fat transposition.[11–13]

PATTERNS OF UPPER LID AND BROW AGING

The youthful brow–upper lid complex is full and convex. The upper lid crease is sharp, and pretarsal show, the amount of exposed upper lid skin visible when the eye is open, is minimal. The lateral upper lid and brow are particularly full and round and transition smoothly without orbital rim skeletonization into the adjacent temple esthetic unit (**Fig. 1**).[14]

Solar damage, gravitational forces, and lipoatrophy together cause upper lid and brow aging. Solar damage leads to skin degeneration with fine rhytids and increased elastosis. Gravitational forces initiate slow downward descent of soft tissue with resultant laxity and ptotic appearance. Lipoatrophy leads to volume loss and an overall deflated form. These 3 components–skin degeneration, laxity, and deflation–each manifest in varying degrees across patients. This variability leads to distinct presentations of upper periorbital aging.

Division of Facial Plastic and Reconstructive Surgery, Johns Hopkins School of Medicine, 601 N, Caroline St 6th Floor, Baltimore, MD 21287, USA
* Corresponding author.
E-mail address: ryanmcollar@gmail.com

Clin Plastic Surg 40 (2013) 191–199
http://dx.doi.org/10.1016/j.cps.2012.07.006
0094-1298/13/$ – see front matter © 2013 Elsevier Inc. All rights reserved.

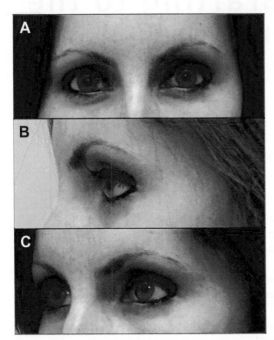

Fig. 1. Frontal (*A*), side (*B*), and oblique (*C*) views of the youthful upper lid and brow demonstrating sharp supratarsal crease, minimal pretarsal show, and ample soft tissue coverage of the bony orbital rim with smooth transition into the temple esthetic unit.

The present discussion focuses primarily on lipoatrophy and periorbital deflation. Several recent studies have described patterns of upper lid fat pad changes during the aging process.[8] It seems that the nasal fat pad volume resists atrophy, whereas the central pad atrophies extensively.[5] Clinical experience suggests the rate and degree of this atrophy vary considerably, with some patients presenting in their fifth and sixth decades with severe changes of atrophy and others maintaining upper lid volume indefinitely.

With this in mind, a simplified methodology may place patients in 2 distinct categories—those with dermatochalasis and those with hollowing.[15]

Those in the "dermatochalasis category" present with pronounced upper lid skin degeneration and laxity but no clinically significant lipoatrophy. This category contains most patients who seek upper lid rejuvenation. Findings include a blunted and obscured upper lid crease, with loss of pretarsal show as a result of upper lid skin redundancy and accumulation of orbital fat (**Fig. 2**C–D).

Conversely, those in the "hollowing category" have pronounced, perhaps premature, upper lid lipoatrophy and deflation that are severe compared with the impact of elastosis and laxity. In such cases, there is deep hollowing of the upper lid,

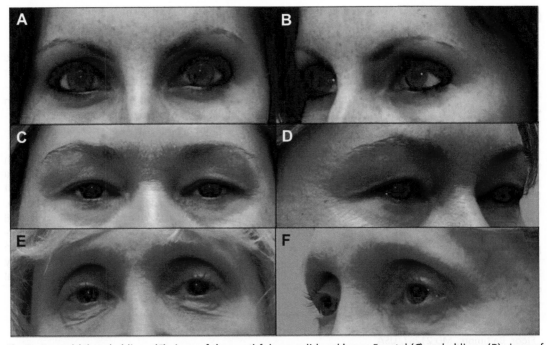

Fig. 2. Frontal (*A*) and oblique (*B*) views of the youthful upper lid and brow. Frontal (*C*) and oblique (*D*) views of the aging upper lid and brow marked by dermatochalasis and accumulation of orbital fat. Frontal (*E*) and oblique (*F*) views of the aging upper lid and brow as a result of lipoatrophy with excessive upper eyelid show, hollowing, and skeletonization of the bony orbit.

particularly at the central fat pad, with increased upper eyelid show and a skeletonized supraorbital rim appearance without significant dermatochalasis (see **Fig. 2**E–F). On initial inspection, one often suspects such patients have previously undergone an overly aggressive upper lid blepharoplasty with fat excision.

Although upper periorbital aging represents more of a spectrum than a dichotomy, this delineation may be useful in considering treatment regimens for a given patient's presentation.

VOLUME RESTORATION FOR UPPER LID AND BROW REJUVENATION

Traditional blepharoplasty aims to rejuvenate the upper periorbita by excising excess skin and postseptal fat.[9] This approach may be valuable for patients in the dermatochalasis category as described. For these patients, the removal of excess skin, and sometimes a degree of fat, may lead to a more youthful pretarsal show and defined supratarsal crease (**Fig. 3**).

However, blepharoplasty, even with fat preservation, does little to rejuvenate patients in the hollowing category, with little dermatochalasis but severe lipoatrophy and skeletonization. This population requires volume restoration instead of soft tissue removal. Techniques include pedicled fat transposition procedures, akin to those developed by Loeb and Hamra,[16] within the lower lid to smooth the lid–cheek junction,[16] and autologous fat grafting.

Pedicled Fat Transposition

Shorr and colleagues[15] describe transposing pedicled fat from the central compartment of the upper lid into the lateral lid and brow deep to the orbicularis muscle to create youthful lateral fullness with

subjective success without complications in 31 patients at a 2-year follow-up. However, because the central fat pad undergoes most age-related atrophy, there may be risk in further depleting it surgically. Such endeavors could accelerate the deepening of the central sulcus over time.

Orbital Fat Relocation

Park and colleagues[16] describes an "orbital fat relocation" procedure in which both fat pads are dissected to the Whitnall ligament and relocated anteroinferiorly between the conjoined tendon of the levator aponeurosis, the orbicularis muscle, and the skin flap. Although the follow-up was only 4 months, the group reported good esthetic results in 50 Korean and Chinese patients without complications.

Medial Fat Pad Transposition

Massry[17] has described a technique in which the medial fat pad, which is resistant to atrophy, is transposed laterally in a pedicled fashion into the medial compartment and affixed to the arcus marginalis to slow or prevent postoperative hollowing after routine upper lid blepharoplasty. In 65 patients, he reports no new formation of the superior sulcus deformity during an 11-month follow-up. He reports 2 cases of temporary mechanical ptosis early in the series that is attributed to incomplete freeing of the nasal fat pad causing undue tension on the levator aponeurosis at the time of fat transfer.

Hyaluronic Acid Filler

Instead of using fat grafting, Morley and colleagues[17] and others[18] describe the use of hyaluronic acid filler to treat upper lid hollowing or

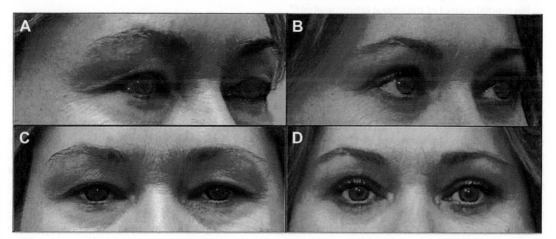

Fig. 3. Traditional upper lid blepharoplasty for a patient with dermatochalasis and upper lid fat accumulation. Oblique (*A*) and frontal (*C*) preoperative views. Oblique (*B*) and frontal (*D*) postoperative views.

excessive postblepharoplasty eyelid show with an 85% success rate. Hyaluronic acid treatment may have a niche for less severe cases with modest medial "A"-shaped hollowing and in those patients open to serially repeated treatments.

Autologous Fat Transfer

After falling out of favor because of unreliable results and the introduction of safe commercial facial fillers, the general use of autologous fat transplantation has again gained interest among plastic surgeons. The efforts of Coleman and others have refined the procurement process, in part stimulating this revival because clinical and animal data now support fat inosculation and long-term survival.[19–21] Many believe fat to be the ideal filler: it is autologous and biocompatible, it naturally integrates into the host tissues without producing an inflammatory reaction, and it is potentially permanent.[22]

Several groups have reported on fat transfer for upper lid and brow rejuvenation with promising results.[10–14] The remainder of this article reviews the relevant anatomy, perioperative considerations, and complications of upper lid and brow autologous fat transfer.

ANATOMY OF EYELID

The extremely thin skin of the eyelid is firmly connected to the underlying orbicularis oculi (OO) muscle through fine connective tissue attachments. The OO is divided into pretarsal, preseptal, and orbital components. The medial canthal tendon is a continuation of superficial and deep heads of the pretarsal OO inserting onto the anterior and posterior lacrimal crest, respectively. Similarly, the lateral canthal tendon is a coalescence of OO laterally inserting onto the tubercle of Whitnall on the medial aspect of the lateral orbital wall.[23,24]

Deep to the thin OO is the orbital septum (OS). The OS is a thin fibrous sheet extending from the arcus marginalis of the orbital rim to its fusion with the levator aponeurosis (LA) just cephalad to the superior tarsal border. The LA is an extension of the levator palpebra superioris that arises at the undersurface of the lesser wing of the sphenoid at the orbital apex. After 40 mm of anterior intraconal extension, the levator palpebra superioris transitions into the LA approximately10 mm behind the OS. After the LA fuses with the OS, some LA fibers descend to insert into the lower third of the anterior surface of the tarsal plate, the pretarsal OO, and the overlying skin. The latter attachment, which is approximately 10 mm from the lid margin, forms the upper lid crease in the Western eyelid.[25,26]

Between the OS and the LA, there are 2 preaponeurotic fat collections, the nasal and central fat pads, that are separated by the superior oblique muscle tendon. The nasal fat is white, akin to intraconal fat, and postulated to be of neural crest lineage, perhaps underpinning its resistance to atrophy. This fat pad is an extraconal extension of intraconal fat and is not separated from orbital fat by the LA. Central fat is yellow, similar to adipose tissue throughout the body, and of mesodermal origin. It is subject to significant volume loss with aging and is separated from intraconal orbital fat by the LA. The lacrimal gland occupies the lateral aspect of the orbit and is divided into orbital and palpebral lobes by a lateral extension of the LA.[25,26]

PATIENT EVALUATION

For all patients, it is critical to elucidate one's motivation for esthetic surgery, a history of any previous periorbital pathologic conditions or procedures, and the precise physical aspects for which modification is desired. Photography is crucial and is performed with each consultation to guide conversation. Often, youthful photographs of the patient play a role in effectively identifying and communicating the patient's specific periorbital aging pattern.

Global Treatment Strategy

Typically, patients present for a consultation to discuss facial aging in general, and the upper lid–brow complex is only a small focus of their overall attention. In these cases, it is important to clarify and prioritize a patient's concerns to effectively create a global treatment strategy with intelligent timing of the various procedures and operations she or he may desire.

Eye and Brow Aging Assessment

The key to the upper eyelid and brow examination is identifying the relative impact of skin degeneration, soft tissue laxity, and lipoatrophy on the patient's presentation of periorbital aging. This assessment will guide the surgeon to selecting the optimal maneuver for rejuvenation.

This examination therefore includes an assessment of the patient's pretarsal show, presence of dermatochalasis, position of the superior sulcus, solar damage and rhytid formation, the degree of lipoatrophy and skeletonization, and postseptal fat compartments that are most affected. Further, the degree of volume loss overlying the lateral and lid brow region, and the affect this has on a smooth transition into the temple region, is appraised. The overall location of the brow is noted in relation to the supraorbital rim so as to determine to the potential complementary role of brow-lifting procedures.

For those patients with a significant lipoatrophy and resultant periorbital hollowing, particularly with volume depletion of lateral lid–brow complex, fat augmentation may be considered. In patients with little dermatochalasis and acceptable brow position, this may be performed independently. Fat transfer may also be considered in conjunction with other procedures, such as fat transfer to the temple, blepharoplasty, or brow lift, based on the clinical findings and desires of the patient. Fat transfer to the temple is of particular importance in patients with concomitant temple lipoatrophy, which is typically the case, because adding volume to the lateral lid and brow without also treating the temple will only exaggerate the appearance of temporal hollowing.

PATIENT PERSPECTIVE AND EXPECTATIONS

The key aspects in managing patient expectations in upper lid and brow fat transfer include accurate projection of downtime, expected degree of improvement, and longevity of the transplant.

Upper lid fat transfer incites fairly significant bruising, inflammation, and edema. Edema tends to subside during approximately 1 week, but complete resolution of bruising requires up to a month to completely disappear, a reality that should be clearly communicated to patients. Animal models have revealed an early inflammatory response histologically after fat transfer followed by sequestration of nonviable tissue but with viable vascularized fat present at least 1 year after transplant.[27] Such studies coincide with clinical experience insofar as initial results immediately after the procedure are often better than the ultimate final result. This should be effectively conveyed to the patient to avoid disappointment as edema resolves with time.

The long-term viability of transplanted fat and the longevity of the result are the focuses of significant debate.[10,22] Most reported clinical data are subjective and based on review of photography. Kaminer and colleagues[25] reported more than 250 autologous fat transplants, stating that correction of many soft tissue defects lasted 5 years or longer. They did note the occasional use of touch-up procedures to optimize outcomes. Rubin and Hoefflin[26] reported more than 100 injections with a 60% rate of viable fat at 1 year.[27] Another group reported that 83% of patients have persistent volume improvement after fat transfer to the lower lid after 3 years.[26] More recent reports have introduced objective measures. Meier and colleagues[28] attempted to clinically quantify the proportion of implanted fat that survives in midface rejuvenation using 3-dimensional imaging. They found that approximately 32% of the volume initially injected is present at 16 months.[28]

Long-term viability results specific to upper periorbital autologous fat transfer are not currently available. Based on available data and clinical experience, the authors counsel patients that results are somewhat unpredictable and that multiple procedures may be required to achieve a desired result.

SURGICAL PROCEDURE
Fat Harvest

The senior author uses a modification of Coleman's method for fat harvest and preparation as previously described.[20,24,27] Data suggest that Coleman's cannula-based technique leads to superior adipocyte structural integrity and functional viability compared with traditional liposuction methods.[29]

- The harvest procedure is typically performed under local anesthesia and oral sedation when being performed alone.
- The ideal donor site is selected preoperatively. Many sites are possible, but the most commonly used sites are the abdomen and the upper lateral thigh.
- The region from which the fat is to be harvested is injected with tumescence (0.1% lidocaine and 1/1,000,000 epinephrine) using a Tulip multihole anesthetic tumescent infiltrator (1.6 mm × 15 cm, Tulip Medical Products, San Diego, CA, USA). Typically, 40 mL of tumescence is evenly infiltrated into the subcutaneous plane. Fifteen minutes is allowed for vasoconstriction to occur before beginning the harvest.
- The harvest site is then prepared and draped in sterile fashion.
- A Triport Harvester (2.4 mm × 15 cm, Tulip Medical Products) is attached to a 10 mL luer-lok syringe. A stab incision is made and harvest is performed using a fanning motion of the cannula with plunger withdrawn within the subcutaneous plane while placing the nondominant hand over the skin to gauge cannula depth.

SURGICAL NOTE: Ports are best directed away from the dermis to avoid damage. Any dimpling of the skin suggests the cannula is too superficial and may lead to untoward contour irregularity at the donor site.

- After sufficient fat has been removed, the stab incision is closed with 5-0 fast-absorbing gut suture.

Fat Preparation

Coleman emphasizes the necessity to remove nonviable components of the fat aspirate such as oil, red blood cells, and tumescence through either centrifugation or sedimentation.[22,24,27]

The process of centrifugation has been challenged by Rohrich and colleagues,[30] who found no quantitative difference in adipocyte viability between centrifuged and noncentrifuged cells. Ramon and colleagues[31] found no difference in fat graft weight or volume between aspirates that were centrifuged and those that were simply wiped with a sponge to remove debris. In fact, the centrifuged fat was found to have a greater degree of fibrosis on histologic evaluation relative to the latter group.

Washing the aspirate has also been suggested to improve survival. Marques and colleagues[32] performed media washings with lactated Ringer's solution and reported increased graft survival at 1 year relative to nonwashed media.

In the authors' center, fat aspirates are not centrifuged. Harvested fat is washed with lactated Ringer's solution using a strainer to remove oil, red blood cells, and tumescence. Once washed, the fat is transferred to 1-mL syringes for transfer into the upper lid and brow area (**Fig. 4**).

Fat Transfer

Because of the delicate nature of upper lid tissue, Tulip micro injector cannulas (0.7 mm × 4 cm or 0.9 mm × 5 cm, Tulip Medical Products) are used to transfer fat to minimize postprocedural edema and bruising (see **Fig. 4**).

- The upper lids and brows are first anesthetized with a small volume of 1% lidocaine with 1:100,000 epinephrine.
- Under sterile conditions, a small stab incision is made in the lateral brow.

SURGICAL NOTE: Although some authors[11] support subcutaneous injection in the upper lid area, we use a suborbicularis injection plane. Subcutaneous injection may increase the risk of contour irregularity given the thin nature of upper lid skin.

- The micro injector cannula is used in a fanning motion to lay 0.1 to 0.2 mL of fat per pass along the trajectory of the upper lid superior to the tarsal crease, extending superiorly toward the upper lid sulcus below the skeletonized orbital rim (**Fig. 5**, Video 1).
- Injections are then transitioned into the lateral brow region, this time delivering fat into a supraperiosteal plane to develop youthful lateral fullness.
- For medial "A-frame" deformities, a small volume, 0.5 mL, may be delivered medially. In sum, typically 1 to 3 mL is injected per upper periorbita.
- The desired result is one of modest overcorrection,[29,33] with minimal pretarsal show, obliteration of the hallowing below the orbital rim, and an emphasis on filling the lateral brow (see **Fig. 5**).

Fat grafting may be used alone or in conjunction with other procedures as part of a treatment plan for patients with periorbital aging. In patients with brow ptosis and significant lipoatrophy and upper lid hallowing, brow lift and upper lid volume

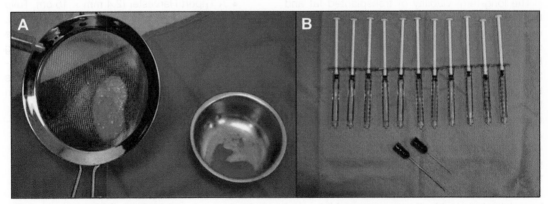

Fig. 4. Harvested fat in strainer before washing (*A*) fat prepared for injection after washing with 0.9-mm and 1.2-mm Tulip micro cannulas (*B*).

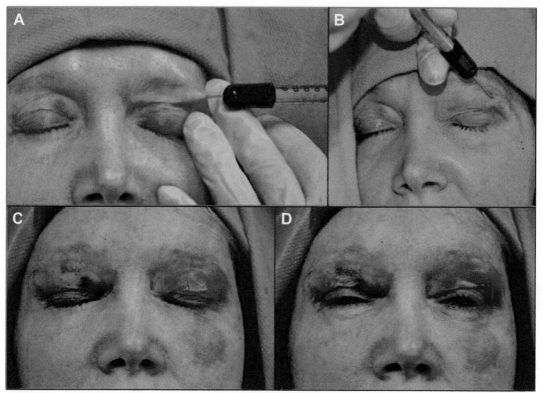

Fig. 5. Fat injection into sub-OO tissue plane of the upper lid (*A*) and supraperiosteal plane of the lateral brow (*B*) with 0.9-mm micro injector cannula. (*C, D*) Immediate postoperative appearance.

augmentation may be performed at the same operation. Generally, fat grafting and blepharoplasty are not performed together. For patients undergoing blepharoplasty for dermatochalasis, fat grafting may be considered as an adjunctive procedure if the patient seems volume depleted and/or skeletoninzed after blepharoplasty.

AFTERCARE OF FAT GRAFTING

Aftercare includes standard wound care and avoidance of strenuous activity. Routine antibiotics are not required. Pain is typically modest. Bruising may be concealed with makeup after 1 week. Some groups advocate postoperative botulinum toxin treatment to the temporal brow as a means to increase graft survival.[34]

COMPLICATIONS

Fat transfer is a relatively safe procedure. Complications include[11,35]:

- Contour irregularity
- Fat embolism with stroke or blindness
- Asymmetry
- Infection and fat migration

Patients should be counseled that asymmetry is expected to some degree with fat transfer. Contour irregularity can be minimized through suborbicularis injection in the lid and supraperiosteal injection in the brow. Infection is rare but can be devastating if severe. This can be avoided with strict adherence to sterile technique during fat preparation and transfer. Obagi and colleagues[7] reported only a single clinically relevant infection in 250 lipotransfer cases.

The most feared complication of fat transfer is fat embolism and stroke or blindness, with several case reports in the literature.[36–40] This can be prevented by avoiding sharp needles and using a smaller syringe to minimize delivery pressure.

SUMMARY

Lipoatrophy is one element that underlies the aging process in the upper lid and brow. In patients with severe lid and brow lipoatrophy marked by deflation, hollowing, increased upper eyelid show, and skeletonization of the bony orbital rim, traditional blepharoplasty techniques will not effectively rejuvenate the periorbita. Several adjunctive fat grafting techniques have recently been described to treat this patient

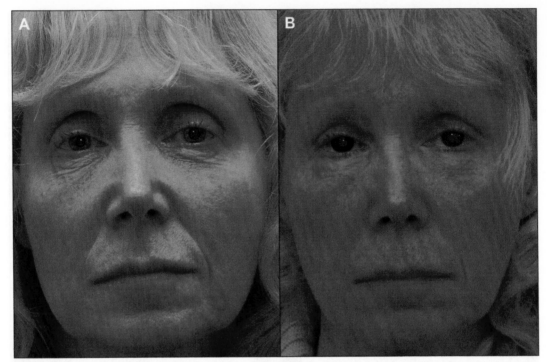

Fig. 6. Upper lid and brow autologous fat transfer. Pre-operative frontal view (*A*) and postoperative frontal view (*B*) at 6 months.

population. Pedicled fat transposition procedures are intriguing but limited data are present and long-term follow-up data are pending. Autologous fat transfer, which has been described in detail here, seems to be advantageous for this patient population, although data on longevity of results are largely subjective, photography based, and not specific to the upper lid and brow (**Fig. 6**). Extended follow-up data and further objective measure of the degree of volume enhancement are needed.

VIDEO

Video related to this article can be found online at http://dx.doi.org/10.1016/j.cps.2012.07.006.

REFERENCES

1. Oh SR, Chokthaweesak W, Annunziata CC, Priel A, Korn BS, Kikkawa DO. Analysis of eyelid fat pad changes with aging. Ophthal Plast Reconstr Surg. 2011;27:348–51.
2. Zimbler MS, Kokoska MS, Thomas JR. Anatomy and pathophysiology of facial aging. Facial Plast Surg Clin North Am. 2001;9:179–87.
3. Coleman S, Saboeiro A, Sengelmann R. A comparison of lipoatrophy and aging: volume deficits in the face. Aesthetic Plast Surg. 2009;33:14–21.
4. Donath AS, Glasgold RA, Glasgold MJ. Volume loss versus gravity: new concepts in facial aging. Curr Opin Otolaryngol Head Neck Surg. 2007 Aug;15:238–43.
5. McCord CD Jr. Techniques in blepharoplasty. Ophthalmic Surg 1979;10:40–55.
6. Minton TJ, Williams EF. Lipotransfer in the upper third of the face. Facial Plast Surg 2010;26:362–8.
7. Kranendonk S, Obagi S. Autologous fat transfer for periorbital rejuvenation: indications, technique, and complications. Dermatol Surg 2007;33:572–8.
8. Trepsat F. Periorbital rejuvenation combining fat grafting and blepharoplasties. Aesthetic Plast Surg 2003;27:243–53.
9. Chen HH, Williams EF. Lipotransfer in the upper third of the face. Curr Opin Otolaryngol Head Neck Surg 2011;19:289–94.
10. Ciuci PM, Obagi S. Rejuvenation of the periorbital complex with autologous fat transfer: current therapy. J Oral Maxillofac Surg 2008;66:1686–93.
11. Sozer SO, Agullo FJ, Palladino H, et al. Pedicle fat flap to increase lateral fullness in upper blepharoplasty. Aesthet Surg J 2010;30:161–5.
12. Park SK, Kim BG, Shin YH. Correction of superior sulcus deformity with orbital fat anatomic repositioning and fat graft applied to retroorbicularis oculi fat for Asian eyelids. Aesthetic Plast Surg 2011;35:162–70.
13. Massry GG. Nasal fat preservation in upper eyelid blepharoplasty. Ophthal Plast Reconstr Surg 2011;27:352–5.

14. Fagien S. Advanced rejuvenative upper blepharoplasty: enhancing aesthetics of the upper periorbita. Plast Reconstr Surg 2002;110:278–91.

15. Shorr N, Hoenig JA, Goldberg RA, et al. Fat preservation to rejuvenate the lower eyelid. Arch Facial Plast Surg 1999;1:38–9.

16. Hamra ST. Arcus marginalis release and orbital fat preservation in midface rejuvenation. Plast Reconstr Surg 1995;96:354–62.

17. Morley AM, Taban M, Malhotra R, et al. Use of hyaluronic acid gel for upper eyelid filling and contouring. Ophthal Plast Reconstr Surg 2009;25:440–4.

18. Liew S, Nguyen DQ. Nonsurgical volumetric upper periorbital rejuvenation: a plastic surgeon's perspective. Aesthetic Plast Surg 2011;35:319–25.

19. Coleman SR. Long-term survival of fat transplants: controlled demonstrations. Aesthetic Plast Surg 1995;19:421–5.

20. Coleman SR. Structural fat grafting. St Louis (MO): Quality Medical Publishing; 2004.

21. Coleman SR. Structural fat grafting: more than a permanent filler. Plast Reconstr Surg 2006;118:108S.

22. Bucky LP, Percec I. The science of autologous fat grafting: views on current and future approaches to neoadipogenesis. Aesthet Surg J 2008;28:313–21.

23. Kakizaki H, Malhotra R, Selva D. Upper eyelid anatomy: an update. Ann Plast Surg 2009;63:336–43.

24. Persichetti P, Di Lella F, Delfino S, et al. Adipose compartments of the upper eyelid: anatomy applied to blepharoplasty. Plast Reconstr Surg 2004;113: 373–8.

25. Kaminer MS, Omura NE. Autologous fat transplantation. Arch Dermatol 2001;137:812.

26. Rubin A, Hoefflin SM. Fat purification: survival of the fittest. Plast Reconstr Surg 2002;109:1463.

27. Brucker M, Sati S, Spangenberger A, et al. Long-term fate of transplanted autologous fat in a novel rabbit facial model. Plast Reconstr Surg 2008;122:749–54.

28. Meier JD, Glasgold RA, Glasgold MJ. Autologous fat grafting: long-term evidence of its efficacy in midfacial rejuvenation. Arch Facial Plast Surg 2009;11:24–8.

29. Pu LL, Coleman SR, Cui X, et al. Autologous fat grafts harvested and refined by the Coleman technique: a comparative study. Plast Reconstr Surg 2008;122:932–7.

30. Rohrich RJ, Sorokin ES, Brown SA. In search of improved fat transfer viability: a quantitative analysis of the role of centrifugation and harvest site. Plast Reconstr Surg 2004;113:391.

31. Ramon Y, Shoshani O, Peled IJ, et al. Enhancing the take of injected adipose tissue by a simple method for concentrating fat cells. Plast Reconstr Surg 2005;115:197.

32. Marques A, Brenda E, Saldiva PH. Autologous fat grafts: a quantitative and morphometric study in rabbits. Scand J Plast Reconstr Surg Hand Surg 1994;28:241.

33. Xie Y, Zheng DN, Li QF, et al. An integrated fat grafting technique for cosmetic facial contouring. J Plast Reconstr Aesthet Surg 2010;63:270–6.

34. Holck DE, Lopez MA. Periocular autologous fat transfer. Facial Plast Surg Clin North Am 2008;16:417–27.

35. Kaufman MR, Miller TA, Huang C. Autologous fat transfer for facial recontouring: is there science behind the art? Plast Reconstr Surg 2007;119:2287–96.

36. Feinendegen DL, Baumgartner RW, Vuadens P. Autologous fat injection for soft tissue augmentation in the face: a safe procedure? Aesthetic Plast Surg 1998;22:163.

37. Dreizen NG, Framm L. Sudden unilateral visual loss after autologous fat injection into the glabellar area. Am J Ophthalmol 1989;107:85.

38. Egido JA, Arroyo R, Marcos A. Middle cerebral artery embolism and unilateral visual loss after autologous fat injection into the glabellar area. Stroke 1993;24:615.

39. Thaunat O, Thaler F, Loirat P. Cerebral fat embolism induced by facial fat injection. Plast Reconstr Surg 2004;113:2235.

40. Yoon SS, Chang DI, Chung KC. Acute fatal stroke immediately following autologous fat injection into the face. Neurology 2003;61:1151.

Ptosis Repair in Aesthetic Blepharoplasty

John J. Martin Jr, MD

KEYWORDS

- Ptosis • Blepharoplasty • Aging face • Eyelids • Surgical technique • Plastic surgery
- Cosmetic surgery

KEY POINTS

- Upper eyelid ptosis is not an uncommon finding during evaluation for blepharoplasty surgery.
- A detailed examination of eyelid position is critical in recognizing ptosis before performing blepharoplasty surgery.
- Missing a preexisting ptosis can lead to an unhappy patient even if blepharoplasty surgery is performed successfully.
- The surgeon must be aware of the multiple causes of ptosis and how to rule out potential pathologic processes that can be associated with ptosis.
- The most common etiology of ptosis is involutional, related to attenuation of the levator aponeurosis tendon.
- A clear understanding of eyelid anatomy is essential to successful ptosis repair.
- There are 2 standard techniques for the repair eyelid ptosis: an external levator resection and a posterior-approach Müller muscle–conjunctival resection.
- The surgeon should be prepared to manage dry-eye–related symptoms, as these can easily occur after ptosis repair.
- Revisional ptosis repair is far more common and complex than revision blepharoplasty surgery.

 Three surgical technique videos accompany this article, showing the author's approach to: External levator resection, Pretarsal aponeurosis resection, and Müller's muscle–conjunctival resection. Available at: http://www.plasticsurgery.theclinics.com/

INTRODUCTION

Upper blepharoplasty is one of the most common cosmetic procedures performed today. Eyelid changes associated with age include dermatochalasis, fat herniation, and lax/redundant orbicularis muscle. Blepharoplasty can be performed to selectively remove excessive skin, muscle, and fat from the eyelid. Often, patients with dermatochalasis also have upper eyelid ptosis, which is a lowered position of the eyelid margin when the eye is in primary position. A normal eyelid rests in a position where the eyelid margin is approximately 3.5 to 4.5 mm above the central pupil. An upper eyelid is considered to have functional ptosis when the upper lid margin rests 2.5 mm or less from the center of the pupil.[1] Ptosis should be repaired at the time of blepharoplasty surgery. If not, ptosis is often more apparent after surgery because it is unmasked by the lid debulking inherent to blepharoplasty. In addition, the patient does not know that their lid droop is due to ptosis. If ptosis is undiagnosed and apparent after blepharoplasty, the patient will be unhappy and feel surgery was not successful.[1–5]

There are 2 muscles responsible for elevating the upper lid, the levator palpebrae superioris and the Müller muscle. Their location in the eyelid is

2912 South Douglas Road, Coral Gables, FL 33134, USA
E-mail address: jjmjrmd@comcast.net

Clin Plastic Surg 40 (2013) 201–212
http://dx.doi.org/10.1016/j.cps.2012.06.007

posterior to the orbital septum and deep to the eyelid fat pads, which is important because the fat pads act as an anatomic landmark or barrier to the surgeon as to where these vital eyelid-elevating muscles are. In turn, this allows a level of protection from inducing ptosis during upper blepharoplasty surgery by avoiding surgical manipulations deep to the fat pads. When performing stand-alone upper-lid blepharoplasty these muscles should be left undisturbed. Because they are deeper structures of the eyelid, correcting concurrent ptosis while performing blepharoplasty surgery requires a more detailed knowledge and familiarity with upper eyelid anatomy. In addition, ptosis correction is more challenging, complex, and time consuming than blepharoplasty alone, and can result in additional postoperative complications such as abnormalities in eyelid height and contour.

There are 2 standard surgical options to address ptosis in conjunction with blepharoplasty.

1. An anterior approach is performed by resection and advancement of the levator aponeurosis through the same incision that is used for the blepharoplasty procedure.
2. Conversely, a Müller muscle–conjunctival resection is performed from the posterior aspect of the eyelid.

Levator surgery is more complex and time consuming, and requires the cooperation of the patient. The posterior approach is easier and more appropriate to the less experienced ptosis surgeon if the patient is a good candidate. Both procedures are reviewed here in detail.

EYELID ANATOMY

A detailed description of eyelid anatomy is found in the article by Lam and colleagues elsewhere in this publication. Reviewed here is the relevant anatomy specific to ptosis repair. A general concept is that the various tissue layers of the eyelid are different if a cross section were to be taken beneath the eyelid crease as opposed to above the eyelid crease.

Starting anteriorly, one finds the following layers:

Below the Crease	Above the Crease
Skin	Skin
Orbicularis muscle	Orbicularis muscle
Tarsus	Orbital septum
Conjunctiva	Orbital fat
	Levator aponeurosis tendon
	Müller muscle
	Conjunctiva

As the eyelid-elevating muscles exist primarily above the crease, the balance of ptosis surgery occurs at this level, and understanding eyelid anatomy in this area is the foundation of attaining good surgical results.

Levator Palpebrae Superioris Muscle

The levator palpebrae superioris muscle provides the majority of muscle elevation of the upper eyelid. It is a striated muscle that arises from the lesser wing of the sphenoid at the orbital apex, and is approximately 40 mm in length. It passes anteriorly in a common muscle sheath with the superior rectus muscle. It is innervated by the superior division of cranial nerve (CN) III. The levator transitions from muscle to aponeurosis tendon about 15 to 17 mm above the superior tarsal border. The aponeurosis inserts into the anterior and superior aspects of the tarsal plate. It also sends attachments through the pretarsal orbicularis to the skin to form the upper eyelid crease.[6–9]

Müller Muscle

The Müller muscle is a smooth, autonomically innervated muscle that originates from the levator muscle, approximately 15 mm above the superior tarsal border. It is found just posterior to the levator aponeurosis, and is intimately associated with the conjunctiva on its posterior surface. The peripheral vascular arcade lies on the anterior surface of the Müller muscle and acts as an anatomic landmark to the location of the muscle, which attaches to the superior tarsal border.[10–12]

Orbicularis Oculi Muscle

While the 2 retractors of the eyelids (eyelid-opening muscles) already described are the basis of ptosis surgery, the protractor of the eyelids, the orbicularis oculi muscle, is also important in ptosis and blepharoplasty surgery, as maintaining its function is critical to lid closure, blink, and corneal integrity. The orbicularis oculi is a sphincter-like muscle that overlies the orbital rim and eyelids, and functions to close the upper and lower lids. It is separated into an orbital and palpebral segment. The palpebral segment is further subdivided into a preseptal and pretarsal component. The muscle is innervated by CN VII, and postoperative weakness results in a paretic/paralytic lagophthalmos. The muscle lies just beneath the skin, with its terminal portion visible as the gray line on the eyelid margins.

Orbital Septum

Posterior to the preseptal orbicularis is the orbital septum, a fibrous connective-tissue structure that lies just anterior to the orbital/eyelid fat pads. It arises at the superior arcus marginalis and extends to insert on the levator aponeurosis in Caucasians. The orbital septum inserts lower (on to tarsus) in Asian eyelids, thus allowing the eyelid fat to sit lower than in Caucasian lids. In part this leads to the fuller appearance of Asian lids and lower or indistinct eyelid crease. The orbital septum is a critical structure in eyelid surgery, as it defines the division of the eyelid proper from the orbit. Violation of the orbital septum (a necessary step in levator advancement ptosis surgery) exposes orbital fat and the underlying levator aponeurosis.

There are 2 fat pads in the upper eyelid. The nasal fat is lighter, denser, and in continuity with deeper orbital fat, because the levator aponeurosis does not separate the nasal fat from the extraconal and intraconal orbital fat, which is also why nasal fat can be approached transconjunctivally. The central fat is also called preaponeurotic fat, as it lies anterior to the levator aponeurosis. It is more yellow, less dense, and separated from deeper orbital fat by the levator aponeurosis. In the lateral upper lid there is no fat pad (as opposed to the lower lid). In the upper eyelid this space is occupied by the lacrimal gland.

Tarsus

The tarsus is a dense fibrous connective tissue that provides the structured framework and form of the eyelids. It averages 10 mm in height in the upper lid and 4 to 5 mm in the lower lid. It tends to be taller in females and shorter in Asians (7–8 mm). The tarsus is the attachment point for the levator aponeurosis (on its anterior surface) and Müller muscle (at its superior edge). When performing levator ptosis repair, the tarsus is exposed and the levator aponeurosis reattached to its anterior surface. In posterior-approach ptosis surgery the tarsus is seen through the conjunctiva, but left undisturbed. Rather, the conjunctiva and Müller muscle are resutured to its superior extent. The tarsus contains numerous sebaceous adnexal structures called meibomian glands, which provide the outer layer of the tear film to prevent tear evaporation. Approximately one-third of the tarsus lies medial to an imaginary vertical line drawn through the pupil, and two-thirds lies lateral to this point.

Vascular System in Eyelids

The eyelids contain a rich vascular supply, formed from an anastomosis of the external and internal carotid arteries. The 2 branches of this system in the upper lid are the marginal and peripheral arcades. The marginal arcade lies just above the lid margin and the peripheral arcade just above the tarsus. Visualization of the peripheral arcade is very helpful in identifying the Müller muscle when approached through the skin, because it runs on its surface 1 to 3 mm above the superior border of the tarsus. Müller muscle can be infiltrated by fibrofatty tissue, making it difficult to identify. In these cases the peripheral arcade is a very helpful landmark. The marginal arcade runs 3 mm above the eyelid margin on the anterior tarsal surface. It is important to avoid disturbing the marginal arcade during surgery because this can lead to excessive bleeding, bruising, lash loss, trichiasis, lid notches, and other deficits of the eyelid margin.

ETIOLOGY OF PTOSIS

When evaluating a patient for upper eyelid surgery, it is important to both recognize the presence and etiology of ptosis. There are various causes of adult ptosis, typically divided into 4 categories:

1. Aponeurotic (involutional)
2. Myogenic
3. Neurogenic
4. Mechanical

Aponeurotic

The most common form of ptosis is aponeurotic or involutional, in which an attenuated and/or disinserted aponeurosis results in a drooping of the upper lid.[13] This ptosis is most commonly observed as an age-related process (hence the term involutional), but can also be seen after trauma, in chronic allergic eyelid disease, after surgery, as a familial trait, in floppy eyelid syndrome, during prolonged topical steroid use, and with long-term use of contact lenses. This type of ptosis is characterized by good levator function (at least 12 mm), a high lid crease (greater than 10 mm), and thinning of the eyelid tissue so that the iris color can occasionally be seen through the eyelid.[14,15]

Myogenic

Myogenic ptosis occurs in disorders that decrease levator muscle strength and contractility. Congenital ptosis is the most common form of myogenic ptosis. Acquired myogenic ptosis can result from myasthenia gravis (MG), myotonic dystrophy, and chronic progressive external ophthalmoplegia (CPEO). These conditions will result in a decreased levator function (less than 12 mm). MG is an autoimmune disease of the neuromuscular junction that can affect the levator muscle. This condition is characterized by variable degrees of ptosis that becomes more severe with fatigue. Patients should be questioned about diplopia and difficulty swallowing or breathing. A diagnosis can be made with a tensilon test or by testing levels of acetylcholine receptor antibodies in the patient's blood. In the office, applying an ice pack to the affected eyelid for 2 minutes may temporarily lift the eyelid and suggest the diagnosis. Also, there is an association of MG with Graves disease and thymoma. For these reasons, if MG is suspected a prompt referral to a neuro-ophthalmologist is recommended.

CPEO can present in the second decade of life. Ptosis is often severe. The condition also affects the extraocular muscles, thus patients turn their head instead of moving the eyes to put objects into view. CPEO limits the Bell phenomenon whereby the globe supraducts during eyelid closure to maximize corneal protection. Severe corneal exposure is a risk of ptosis repair in these patients. As with MG, prompt patient referral is mandated if this condition is suspected.

Neurogenic

Neurogenic ptosis occurs in any disease that affects the third cranial nerve, such as Horner syndrome and third nerve palsy.

Third nerve palsy can present with ptosis and a dilated pupil. In the acute setting it represents a potential medical emergency. Horner syndrome is characterized by ipsilateral ptosis, miosis (constricted pupil), and anhidrosis. It is caused by a denervation of the sympathetic pathway somewhere between the hypothalamus and the eyelid. It typically presents with 1 to 2 mm of ptosis caused by loss of tone in Müller muscle. Any patient presenting with ptosis and pupillary changes should be referred to the appropriate setting.

Mechanical

Mechanical ptosis can occur when there is increased weight on the upper lid. A mass (such as a chalazion), significant excess skin, chronic edema, and other conditions can lead to this form of ptosis. The primary condition requires evaluation and treatment before proceeding to ptosis repair.

EXAMINATION

Patients presenting for blepharoplasty evaluation do not know the cause of their lid droop. It is incumbent on the surgeon to identify whether ptosis is present. No matter how successful the blepharoplasty surgery, patients will be unhappy if their lids still droop after surgery from unrecognized ptosis. If ptosis is noted on the preoperative evaluation, a detailed and directed history is essential. It is important to question the duration and severity of the ptosis, and whether there is associated diplopia or variability to the lid height during the day. If there is any suspicion of a neurologic process, prompt referral is suggested.

Pupil, Extraocular, Cornea

A brief evaluation of the pupillary response and extraocular movements is important to rule out the aforementioned potential neurologic processes. In the presence of a miotic or dilated pupil, or any suggestion of a motility disturbance, a referral to an ophthalmologist is mandated. A corneal evaluation with specific attention to ruling out a dry-eye condition is important when ptosis surgery is considered. It is more common to develop a dry eye after combined blepharoplasty and ptosis repair than after blepharoplasty alone. As the most common cause of ptosis seen is aponeurotic in nature, the remainder of the discussion elaborates this condition.

Ptosis Measurements

When assessing ptosis for surgical correction, there are a variety of measurements and clinical examination techniques that allows the selection of the best procedure to perform. The margin reflex distance 1 (MRD1) determines the degree of ptosis that is present, if any. With the patient in primary gaze, a light is shone on the eyes and a corneal light reflex is seen mid-pupil. The distance of the light reflex to the upper lid margin is the MRD1. This measurement of ptosis is better than the vertical palpebral fissure height, as lower lid position can affect the latter measurement. A normal MRD1 is between 3.5 and 4.5 mm. An MRD1 less than 2.5 mm should be considered as clinically significant ptosis.

Levator Function

The levator function (LF) measures the upper lid excursion. It is determined with the brow manually fixated. In this setting, excursion of the upper lid margin as the patient looks from extreme downgaze to full upgaze is measured. Normal LF should be between 14 and 16 mm. Patients with aponeurotic ptosis should have a normal or slightly reduced LF. If the LF is abnormal, a more detailed ptosis evaluation by a specialist (oculoplastic surgeon) is needed.

The upper eyelid crease height should also be evaluated. In the normal setting, in Caucasians the upper lid crease should measure approximately 10 mm from the central lid margin in women and 8 mm in men. In aponeurotic ptosis, the crease is usually higher or absent, and there is sometimes a deep superior sulcus.

Lid Fatigue

Finally, assessing lid fatigue is useful in ruling out MG. The patient is asked to stare at the examiner's finger that is placed in front of, and above, the patient's head; this forces the patient to elevate the upper lid for a sustained period. The patient should be able to maintain this lid position for 1 minute. If the lid fatigues (drops) with this maneuver, lid fatigue is present and referral to a neuro-ophthalmologist suggested.

Phenylephrine Test

Once these measurements have been assessed, a phenylephrine (PE) test should be performed to identify whether a posterior-approach ptosis repair can be performed. PE drops (2.5%) are instilled into the ptotic eye (eyes), and repeated in 3 to 5 minutes. PE will stimulate Müller muscle and should result in 2 to 3 mm of lid elevation. If this occurs a posterior approach can be considered.

PATIENT PERSPECTIVE

Many patients who present for upper eyelid surgery are unaware of what ptosis is and that it may be present and contributing to their upper lid fullness. Patients typically are concerned only with eyelid appearance and not with the cause of their heavy lids. When present, it is important to show patients that both dermatochalasis and ptosis exist, and to explain that the ptosis component should be addressed simultaneously. The addition of ptosis surgery will often result in a longer healing time and more swelling than if performing blepharoplasty alone. In addition, patients may also have more postoperative dryness as the eyelid height is elevated, leading to altered blink in the early healing phase. Contour abnormalities are also more common when adding ptosis repair to blepharoplasty, and this should be explained to the patient. Patients who undergo ptosis repair should also be counseled that the rate of revisional surgery is greater than for patients who undergo blepharoplasty alone.

OPTIONS FOR SURGICAL REPAIR OF THE EYELID

The author's most common method for repairing upper eyelid ptosis is an anterior-approach external levator resection (ELR), which can be performed in the same setting as for upper eyelid blepharoplasty. In a recent survey of oculoplastics specialists, surgeons preferred the ELR when performing ptosis repair concurrent with blepharoplasty.[16] Jones and colleagues[17] were the first to describe an external aponeurosis repair for ptosis in 1975. It has also been shown that in involutional (aponeurotic) ptosis, an attenuated aponeurosis is present, confirming this as a rational and anatomic approach for its repair.[14,18] Since that time there have been numerous reports describing this technique and demonstrating its success for ptosis repair.[19–21]

An internal approach for ptosis correction was initially described by Fasanella and Servat[22] in 1961, in which they everted the eyelid and resected a portion of the superior tarsus to advance the levator. In 1975 Putterman and Urist[11,12] described an alternative internal approach that preserves the tarsus: the Müller muscle–conjunctival resection. This procedure is an excellent alternative to ptosis repair when performing simultaneous blepharoplasty.

The author's technique for both ELR and Müller muscle–conjunctival resection are now described. Both procedures are usually preformed with either local or local-sedation anesthesia.

SURGICAL DESCRIPTION
External Levator Aponeurosis Resection

 See video: External levator resection.

When combining an external ptosis repair with blepharoplasty, the standard eyelid crease incision is used to access the levator muscle.

- A lid crease is marked between 8 and 10 mm above the lid margin centrally. If the patient's native crease is close to this level, it should be used. However, in involutional ptosis the crease is often elevated. The crease is then completed by tapering it in an arc nasally and temporally.
- Excess skin for excision can be determined using a Green forceps. One arm of the forceps is placed on the crease and the other above it, approximating the amount of skin to be excised. Gentle closure of the forceps will allow a determination of the amount of skin that can be safely removed. The end point is pinching skin with the forceps without creating eversion of the lid margin. This point is marked.
- The pinch maneuver is performed nasally, centrally, and temporally, and the marks are then made continuous and connected to the fabricated eyelid crease (**Fig. 1A, B**). Most surgeons use this as a guide and resect less than the maximum amount of skin possible to leave a slight fullness to

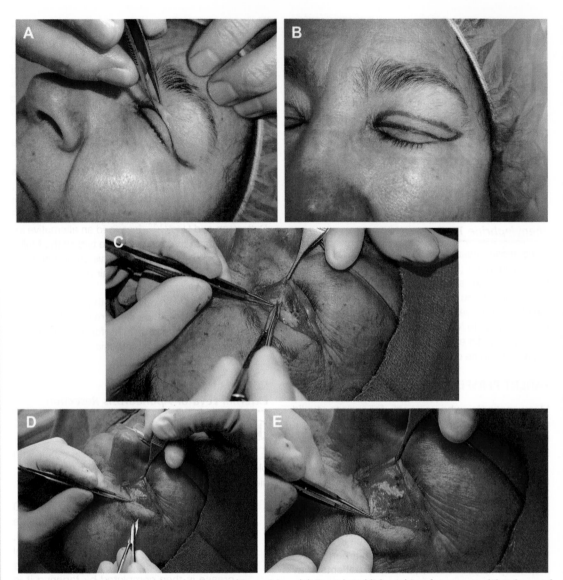

Fig. 1. (*A*) Green's forceps used to determine skin excision. (*B*) Completed lid marking for surgery. (*C*) Release of aponeurosis from tarsus. (*D*) Bare tarsus exposed. (*E*) Aponeurosis separated from Müller muscle.

the lid. There should always be at least 10 mm of skin remaining between the upper mark and the brow.

- A local anesthetic consisting of xylocaine 1% with 1:100,000 epinephrine is injected subcutaneously into the upper eyelid. The eyelid is then prepped with betadine, and the epinephrine allowed to take effect for 10 minutes before incision.
- An incision is made along the previously marked lines with at #15 Barde-Parker blade. Alternatively, a bovie with a Colorado needle microdissector or a CO_2 laser can be used.
- A skin or skin-muscle flap is excised with any of the aforementioned cutting devices,

and all bleeding controlled. Leaving adequate orbicularis will decrease the risk of lagophthalmos and altered blink after surgery.

- Orbital fat is identified as a prominence under the orbital septum. If there is difficulty in identifying the septum, the superior orbital rim is palpated. Just inferior to the rim will be the orbital fat pads.
- A small amount of local anesthetic is injected into this area to aid in elevating septal tissue.
- The septum is then opened along the length of the wound, and orbital fat is exposed. Excess nasal fat can be excised, but all central fat should be preserved to prevent

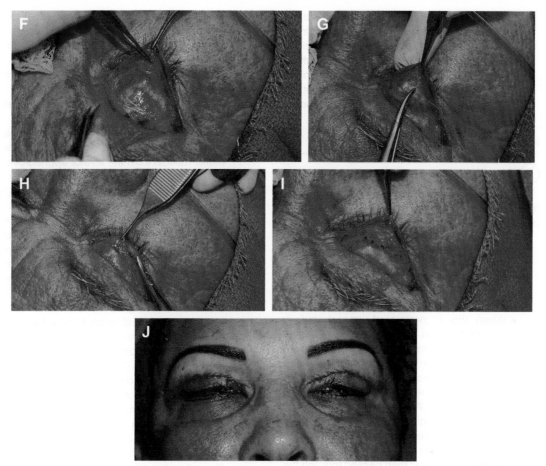

Fig. 1. (*F*) Levator free of any adhesions. (*G*) Partial thickness suture through tarsus. (*H*) Tarsal suture engaged to aponeurosis. (*I*) Three sutures placed along tarsus. (*J*) Lid gapping after closure.

a postoperative superior sulcus deformity. If the patient has a deep central sulcus, the nasal pad fat can be repositioned centrally.[23]

- After reflecting eyelid fat, the levator muscle and attenuated aponeurosis are evident. The anterior edge of the aponeurosis is isolated by cutting directly perpendicular to the tarsus, just below its superior border (**Fig. 1**C, D).

- The aponeurosis is then separated from the underlying Müller muscle with sharp dissection or light cutting cautery (**Fig. 1**E).

- Any remaining bands between the aponeurosis and the septum can be gently released so that the levator is easily advanced without undue tension (**Fig. 1**F).

- Once the aponeurosis is free, a 6-0 double-armed Vicryl suture is passed at partial thickness through the superior portion of the tarsus. Both arms of the suture are passed through the aponeurosis, and the suture is looped into a temporary knot (**Fig. 1**G, H).

- The lid should be everted to make sure that the suture has not gone full thickness through the tarsus.

- The patient is asked to open the eyes and the suture is adjusted until the desired lid height is achieved. A permanent knot is then tied. Two additional Vicryl sutures are placed medially and laterally for support and stability (see **Fig. 1**I). The sutures are adjusted until proper height and contour are obtained.

- After tying down the suture, it can be passed through the subcutaneous tissue of the inferior wound margin to help recreate the eyelid crease. The skin is then closed with a running 6-0 plain gut or Prolene suture.

- In bilateral cases surgeons typically perform all steps on both lids until the point where the central vicryl suture is placed. The patient can then open the eyes to check for lid height and contour symmetry; this is preferred in the seated position. If the patient is sedated and cannot adequately open the eyelids to evaluate the lid height, check the amount of "gapping" of the lid, which should be the same on both sides (**Fig. 1**J).[24]

Pretarsal Aponeurosis Resection

 See video: Pretarsal aponeurosis resection.

An alternative simplified technique is based on the attachment of the aponeurosis to the upper portion of the anterior face of the tarsus.

- Instead of releasing the entire aponeurosis from the tarsus, a rectangular segment of aponeurosis measuring 4 mm in width by 8 mm in length is resected from the superior anterior face of the tarsus (**Fig. 2**A, B).
- When this is performed, bare tarsus is exposed, which is important in obtaining a permanent correction (**Fig. 2**C).[19]
- The newly cut edge of aponeurosis is then advanced and hooked to the distal aponeurosis still attached to tarsus with two 6-0 Vicryl sutures (**Fig. 2**D, E). Because the aponeurosis is quite thin in this area, some of the orbicularis muscle will be included in the suture bite.
- The Vicryl suture is then passed through the subcutaneous tissue of the inferior wound margin to recreate the lid crease.
- As before, the patient is asked to open the eyes to check for contour and symmetry. The surgeon can also assess symmetry by the amount of aponeurosis advanced by measuring from the previously placed aponeurotic suture to the aponeurosis/ levator muscle junction (**Fig. 2**F). This distance should be the same on both sides, and is easily evaluated.
- The skin is then closed. The author prefers to initially place one suture centrally to line up the skin edges before complete closure (**Fig. 2**G).

Müller Muscle–Conjunctival Resection

 See video: Müller's muscle–conjunctival resection.

This surgical procedure excellent for patients who have a good response to the PE test.

- The lid crease and ellipse of skin to be excised are marked as with the ELR procedure.

- Using the same anesthetic as with ELR, a supraorbital nerve block is administered and a subcutaneous injection to the demarcated skin is given.
- The skin markings are scored and the lid is then everted over a Desmarres retractor.
- The superior border of the tarsus is outlined with a marking pen (**Fig. 3**A).
- The conjunctiva superior to the tarsus is gently pulled with a forceps to separate the Müller muscle from the levator aponeurosis.
- Calipers are used to mark the appropriate tissue excision above the superior tarsus (8 mm is typical for full correction) (**Fig. 3**B, C).
- The clamp is then placed to encompass the demarcated tissue (conjunctiva and Müller muscle) (**Fig. 3**D). Recent studies have demonstrated that some levator aponeurotic fibers are incorporated in the resected tissue. This aponeurotic resection may play an important role in eyelid elevation.[11] In lieu of a ptosis clamp, small hemostats can be used.
- A 6-0 double-armed plain suture is then run along the underside of the clamp starting at its temporal edge (**Fig. 3**E).
- Once the medial edge of the clamp has been reached, an incision along the undersurface of the clamp is made with a #15 Barde-Parker blade (**Fig. 3**F). The clamp is then removed. Careful cautery can be applied to assure hemostasis.
- The suture is run from the medial end temporally, hooking the conjunctiva and Müller muscle to the superior edge of the tarsus (**Fig. 3**G).
- At the temporal edge, the two ends of the suture are passed through the wound so that the knot will be buried when the suture is tied (**Fig. 3**H).
- The lid is then reinverted and a standard blepharoplasty is performed.

The amount of surgical resection should be based on the result of the preoperative PE test. The elevation seen with the test will be the amount of correction attained with an 8-mm resection of tissue. If the patient had more elevation than desired with the PE test, less than 8 mm of Müller muscle should be resected. If the elevation was not sufficient to correct the amount of ptosis, up to 9 to 10 mm of tissue can be resected. The amount of resection is refined with surgical experience.

Fig. 4 demonstrates 2 representative examples of aesthetic ptosis repair in association with upper blepharoplasty. Both patients underwent posterior-approach surgery, as this is the most

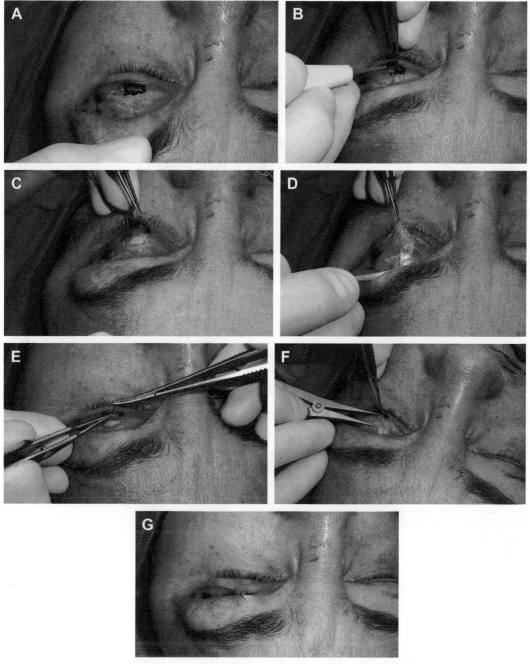

Fig. 2. (*A*) Rectangle of aponeurosis marked over tarsus. (*B*) Excision of aponeurosis. (*C*) Bare tarsus. (*D, E*) Edge of aponeurosis advanced and sutured to distal aponeurosis. (*F*) Measuring suture line to levator/aponeurosis junction. (*G*) Central suture for skin closure.

common procedure performed by the novice ptosis surgeon.

POSTOPERATIVE CARE

For both surgeries there will be swelling and bruising postoperatively. Ice or cold compresses

should be applied for the first 48 to 72 hours to help decrease edema, and then warm compresses 4 times a day for the next several days. An antibiotic/steroid ointment of choice can be used 3 times a day over the suture line and into the eye at bedtime. Most patients have some dryness after surgery, and artificial tears are recommended 4

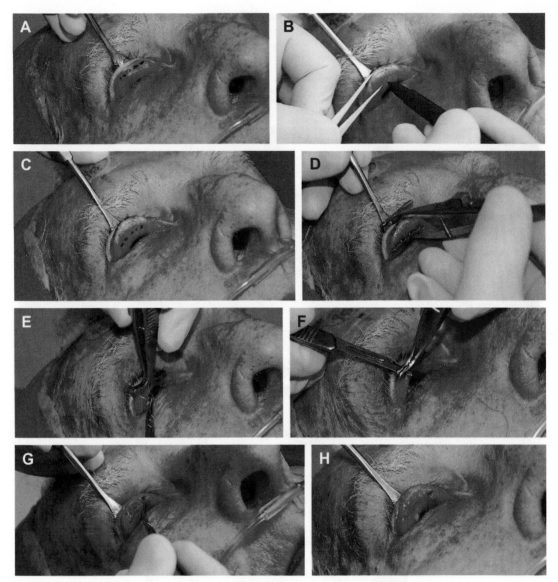

Fig. 3. (*A*) Superior border of tarsus marked. (*B*) Measuring 8 mm above tarsus. (*C*) Markings on conjunctiva. (*D*) Placement of clamp on markings. (*E*) Suture run on underside of clamp. (*F*) Clamp and tissue excised with #15 blade. (*G*) Conjunctiva sutured to edge of tarsus. (*H*) Suture tied and buried temporally.

times a day for at least the first week. Pain is minimal and acetaminophen should be all that is needed for any discomfort. If using nondissolvable sutures, they are removed 1 week postoperatively.

COMPLICATIONS IN PTOSIS REPAIR

By combining blepharoplasty and ptosis repair there is typically an increase in swelling and healing time. In addition, as the eyelid-elevating muscles are resected, there is an increased incidence of contour and lid height abnormalities compared with blepharoplasty performed alone.

Almost all patients will experience some dryness postoperatively. Patients are advised to use artificial tear drops throughout the day, and ointment at bedtime if there is significant irritation. For very symptomatic patients a punctal plug may be needed until the dryness resolves.

Over and undercorrection of lid height can occur. Early undercorrections should be followed until lid edema has resolved. Berlin and Vestal[18] reported that some ELR patients experience a drop in lid height at 2 to 4 months after surgery. These investigators believed that this recurrence of ptosis could be related to aponeurotic

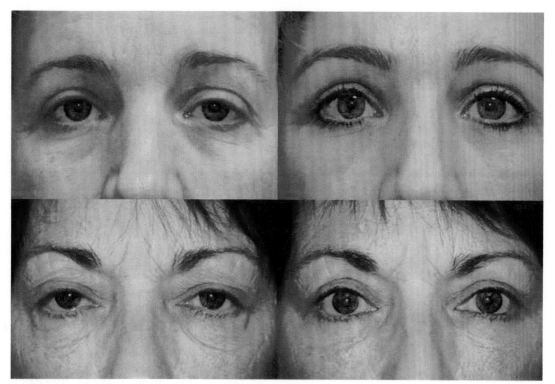

Fig. 4. (*Left*) Above and below are 2 women who presented for aesthetic eyelid rejuvenation. Both women manifested dermatochalasis and true eyelid ptosis, and both underwent upper blepharoplasty and ptosis repair via Müller muscle–conjunctival resection. (*Right*) Note improvement in upper lid position (corrected MRD1) as the ptosis was addressed, and in the contour and appearance of the upper lid in general. (*Courtesy of* Dr Guy Massry, MD.)

slippage from the tarsus if the internal sutures resorbed too quickly, or to a stretching of the aponeurosis postoperatively. Moreover, they found that patients with larger amounts of ptosis preoperatively had a higher incidence of undercorrection.

Early adjustments of lid height can be performed at 3 to 4 days after surgery if there is not significant edema. This procedure can be performed in the office with little or no anesthesia by adjusting suture tension in the ELR procedure.[25] If edema has not resolved, it is best to wait before further manipulation. With time the undercorrected lid may come up as the mechanical effect of the edema decreases. If the lid is still undercorrected at 6 months, a revision surgery can be performed. In posterior-approach surgery an undercorrection can be addressed with a repeat procedure, or an ELR if there is poor response to PE testing.

For overcorrections, warm compresses should be continued for several weeks and the lid massaged inferiorly. Lubricant drops and ointment should be used until the lid has dropped to an acceptable level. If this does not occur, the lid will have to be lowered surgically. In posterior-

approach surgery, the lid can often be everted in the office and the wound gaped in the early postoperative period to adjust an overcorrection.

Contour abnormalities such as peaking usually improve with time and massage. Alternatively, adjustments of the internal sutures or the placement of additional sutures may be necessary.

SUMMARY

Upper eyelid blepharoplasty is one of the most common cosmetic surgeries performed today. Many patients presenting with the complaint of upper eyelid fullness will have dermatochalasis with a concurrent ptosis of the upper lid. To achieve a good cosmetic result the ptosis correction should be performed at the same time as the blepharoplasty, and this can be accomplished by an ELR or Müller muscle–conjunctival resection. With experience, both procedures result in excellent results and a high level of patient satisfaction.

VIDEOS

Videos related to this article can be found online at http://dx.doi.org/10.1016/j.cps.2012.06.007.

REFERENCES

1. Massry G. Ptosis repair for the cosmetic surgeon. Facial Plast Surg Clin North Am 2005;13(4):533–9.
2. Older JJ. Upper lid blepharoplasty and ptosis repair using a transcutaneous approach. Ophthal Plast Reconstr Surg 1994;10(2):146–9.
3. Wilkins RB, Patipa M. The recognition of acquired ptosis in patients considered for upper eyelid blepharoplasty. Plast Reconstr Surg 1982;70(4):431–4.
4. Carraway JH, Tran P. Blepharoplasty with ptosis repair. Aesthet Surg J 2009;29(1):54–61.
5. Gausas RE. Technique for combined blepharoplasty and ptosis correction. Facial Plast Surg 1999;15(3):193–201.
6. Lemke BN, Stasior OG, Rosenberg PN. The surgical relations of the levator palpebrae superioris muscle. Ophthal Plast Reconstr Surg 1988;4(1):25–30.
7. Stasior GO, Lemke BN, Wallow IH, et al. Levator aponeurosis elastic fiber network. Ophthal Plast Reconstr Surg 1993;9(1):1–10.
8. Anderson RL, Beard C. The levator aponeurosis—attachments and their clinical significance. Arch Ophthalmol 1977;95:1437–41.
9. Collins JR, Beard C, Wood I. Experimental and clinical data on the insertion of the levator palpebrae superioris muscle. Am J Ophthalmol 1978;85:792–801.
10. Morris CL, Morris WR, Fleming JC. A histological analysis of the Müllerectomy: redefining its mechanism in ptosis repair. Plast Reconstr Surg 2011;127(6):2333–41.
11. Putterman AM, Urist MJ. Müller muscle-conjunctiva resection. Technique for treatment of blepharoptosis. Arch Ophthalmol 1975;93(8):619–23.
12. Putterman AM, Fett DR. Müller's muscle in the treatment of upper eyelid ptosis: a ten-year study. Ophthalmic Surg 1986;17(6):54–60.
13. Martin JJ, Tenzel RR. Acquired ptosis: dehiscences and disinsertions. Are they real or iatrogenic? Ophthal Plast Reconstr Surg 1998;8(2):130–2.
14. Finsterer J. Ptosis: causes, presentation, and management. Aesthetic Plast Surg 2003;27(3):193–204.
15. Cahill KV, Bradley EA, Meyer DR, et al. Functional indications for upper eyelid ptosis and blepharoplasty surgery a report by the American Academy of Ophthalmology. Ophthalmology 2011;118(12):2510–7.
16. Aakalu VK, Setabutr P. Current ptosis management: a national survey of ASOPRS members. Ophthal Plast Reconstr Surg 2011;27(4):270–6.
17. Jones LT, Quickert MH, Wobig JL. The cure of ptosis by aponeurotic repair. Arch Ophthalmol 1975;93(8):629–34.
18. Berlin AJ, Vestal KP. Levator aponeurosis surgery. A retrospective review. Ophthalmology 1989;96(7):1033–6.
19. Anderson RL, Dixon RS. Aponeurotic ptosis surgery. Arch Ophthalmol 1979;97(6):1123–8.
20. McCord CD, Tanenbaum M, Nunery WR. Oculoplastic surgery, Chapter 7. New York: Raven Press; 1995.
21. Tenzel RR. Orbit and oculoplastics, Chapter 2. Textbook of ophthalmology, vol. 4. New York: Gower Medical Publishing; 1993.
22. Fasanella RM, Servat J. Levator resection for minimal ptosis: another simplified operation. Arch Ophthalmol 1961;65:493–6.
23. Massry GG. Nasal fat preservation in upper eyelid blepharoplasty. Ophthal Plast Reconstr Surg 2011;27(5):352–5.
24. McCord CD, Seify H, Codner MA. Transblepharoplasty ptosis repair: three-step technique. Plast Reconstr Surg 2007;120(4):1037–44.
25. Dortzbach RK, Kronish JW. Early revision in the office for adults after unsatisfactory blepharoptosis correction. Am J Ophthalmol 1993;115:68–75.

Blepharoplasty Complications
Prevention and Management

Katherine M. Whipple, MD[a], Lee Hooi Lim, MBBS[a,b],
Bobby S. Korn, MD, PhD[a], Don O. Kikkawa, MD[a],*

KEYWORDS

- Blepharoplasty • Complications • Eyelid • Cosmetic surgery

KEY POINTS

- Preoperative assessment and counseling of expectations is essential to avoid complications and to maximize patient satisfaction after blepharoplasty surgery.
- Photograph the patient before surgery at multiple angles to help address patient concerns if questions arise after surgery.
- Upper eyelid blepharoplasty markings should take into account the patient's natural eyelid crease, desired crease placement, and ethnic background.
- Eyelid fullness is a sign of youth; avoid excessive resection of soft tissue.
- Become familiar with the management of all complications of surgery.
- Be cautious of the possibility of dry eye syndrome in the patient who has had previous laser in situ keratomileusis and is undergoing blepharoplasty.
- Avoid the temptation to intervene too early after surgery when unexpected results occur. Many imperfections resolve spontaneously.
- Blepharoplasty revisions are expected. It is important not to intervene until stability has been attained.

INTRODUCTION

Blepharoplasty is one of the most common cosmetic operations performed in the United States.[1] In addition to cosmetic improvement, patients may also benefit from functional improvement with increased field of vision and quality of life.[2,3] As the population continues to age, the demand for both cosmetic and functional blepharoplasty will increase.

With the growth of the information age, patient expectations and desires for precise results and minimal downtime after surgery are growing. Even patients undergoing functional blepharoplasty expect a rejuvenated appearance. In essence, every patient is a cosmetic patient. However, even in the most skilled hands, delayed healing, other complications, or unexpected results may occur. Unless properly counseled, patients may perceive normal healing (postoperative bruising and swelling) as an untoward effect; however, with the proper patient education, surgeon skill, and training, most adverse outcomes of blepharoplasty can be minimized and prevented.

It is important to recognize not only how but why complications from blepharoplasty occur. Most postoperative complications are in 1 of 4 categories:

1. Inaccurate preoperative assessment
2. Improper surgical technique
3. Miscalculations in judgment
4. Idiosyncratic outcome (unexplained complication)

[a] Division of Oculofacial Plastic and Reconstructive Surgery, Department of Ophthalmology, University of California-San Diego, Shiley Eye Center, 9415 Campus Point Drive, La Jolla, CA 92093, USA; [b] Oculoplastic Department, Singapore National Eye Center, Singapore
* Corresponding author.
E-mail address: dkikkawa@ucsd.edu

Clin Plastic Surg 40 (2013) 213–224
http://dx.doi.org/10.1016/j.cps.2012.07.002

Categorizing unexpected results into 1 of these 4 groups and recalling each of them before surgery is important and helps to continually improve surgeon skills and results.

PREOPERATIVE CONSIDERATIONS

The cornerstone of any successful operation is an adequate preoperative evaluation, consisting of a patient history, examination, and medical evaluation. Patient counseling should stress expected results, normal time frame and range of wound healing response, possible unexpected results, and potential need for revision. Preoperative evaluation for blepharoplasty and brow ptosis is discussed elsewhere in this issue by Czyz and colleagues. A detailed photodocumentation of the preoperative state is an essential step in the surgery. Preoperative photographs of the eyelids and periorbita at multiple angles serve as a basis for comparison after surgery, and may help dispel patient concerns about supposed changes that were present before surgery.

INTRAOPERATIVE CONSIDERATIONS
Anesthesia

Most blepharoplasty procedures are performed under local anesthesia with or without monitored anesthesia care. General anesthesia can be used if additional facial surgery is added. Even when performed under general anesthesia, local anesthetic with vasoconstrictors is administered to aid in hemostasis. The type of anesthetic used should be individualized to each patient and according to surgeon preference.

We use a 1:1 mixture of 2% Xylocaine with epinephrine 1:100,000 and 0.75% bupivacaine. For upper eyelid blepharoplasty, we typically inject 2–4 mL per lid. Potential risks of anesthetic injection are intravascular injection and damage to vital orbital structures (**Fig. 1**).[4] Our injection technique always directs the needle away from the globe. In addition, gentle traction is applied to the upper eyelid to separate it from the globe, minimizing the risk of globe penetration (**Fig. 2**). To completely anesthetize the deeper nasal fat pat, we inject additional anesthetic retroseptally in this quadrant (**Fig. 3**).

If lower eyelid surgery is added, we typically perform surgery with monitored anesthesia care. Additional sedation is often needed during local anesthetic injection for patient comfort. It may be helpful to have an assistant steady the head during injection for added support. To decrease the risk of sneezing during administration of local anesthetic, the addition of fentanyl or alfentanil to propofol infusion has been advocated.[5] Fifteen minutes should be allowed after injection to achieve the hemostatic effect of the epinephrine before incision.

Marking and Measuring

Marking eyelid crease
The skin marking for blepharoplasty is one of the most crucial portions of the operation. Although the technical aspect of blepharoplasty is straightforward, marking is an art. We typically mark within the patient's natural eyelid crease unless an altered lid crease is desired. If no crease or an ill-defined crease is present, our general guidelines are to mark the eyelid crease 7 to 8 mm above the lash line centrally in white men and 8 to 10 mm in white women (**Fig. 4**). The degree of lateral hooding, medial skin redundancy, and ethnicity also influence marking placement.[6,7] For example, in Asian patients, the eyelid crease should be marked lower, no higher than 5 to 6 mm above the lash line in men and 6 to 7 mm in women. The crease is completed across the length of the lid, tapering medially at the

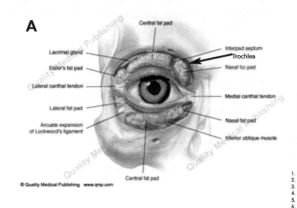

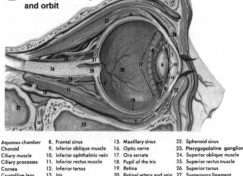

1. Aqueous chamber	8. Frontal sinus
2. Choroid	9. Inferior oblique muscle
3. Ciliary muscle	10. Inferior ophthalmic vein
4. Ciliary processes	11. Inferior rectus muscle
5. Cornea	12. Inferior tarsus
6. Crystalline lens	13. Iris
7. Frontal bone	14. Lateral rectus muscle

15. Maxillary sinus	22. Sphenoid sinus
16. Optic nerve	23. Pterygopalatine ganglion
17. Ora serrata	24. Superior oblique muscle
18. Pupil of the iris	25. Superior rectus muscle
19. Retina	26. Superior tarsus
20. Retinal artery and vein	27. Suspensory ligament
21. Sclera	28. Vitreous chamber

Fig. 1. Normal orbital anatomy showing location of globe and trochlea.

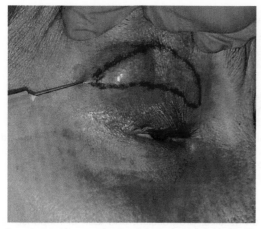

Fig. 2. Local anesthetic injected subcutaneously, creating a wave of anesthetic that proceeds from the needle tip. Note gentle elevation of lid away from globe.

upper punctum and laterally at the lateral canthus. When lateral hooding is significant, the marking should extend laterally past the canthus, angled superiorly for a length sufficient to reduce lateral skin excess. Medial skin redundancy, when present, is best managed by angling the skin marking superiorly 3 to 4 mm medial to the superior punctum. If the marking is angled inferiorly, aesthetically displeasing medial canthal webbing may occur and the incision is more noticeable.

Marking skin excision

The amount of skin to be removed is assessed with the pinch technique using a nontoothed forceps. The skin excess is pinched between the

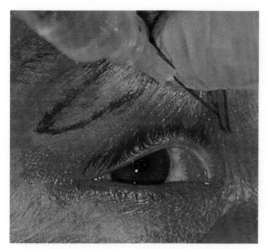

Fig. 3. The lid is retracted upwards from the globe to inject the deeper nasal fat pad.

arms of the forceps with the lower arm beginning at the demarcated crease. The intervening skin is incorporated between the arms of the forceps (**Fig. 5**). This technique is performed in the nasal, central, and temporal eyelid, with the excess skin marked at each point. The points are then connected in an arc and made continuous with the crease to form an ellipse for excision. Varying amounts of skin can be incorporated into the pinch depending on the desired result. The end point of redundant skin marking should not exceed mild eversion of the lashes.

Postoperative Complications

- Hemorrhage
- Infection
- Corneal abrasion
- Diplopia
- Lagophthalmos
- Ptosis
- Lacrimal gland injury
- Asymmetric eyelid crease
- Residual excess skin
- Sulcus deformity
- Canthal webbing
- Fire/skin burn/singed lashes

Hemorrhage prevention

No matter how meticulous the surgical technique, bleeding is inevitable with skin incisions, and bruising should be expected following surgery. Bleeding is especially inevitable in blepharoplasty because the eyelid has a rich vascular supply. Whether or not to stop anticoagulation for elective blepharoplasty is continually debated.[8] The preoperative evaluation should include a thorough history of anticoagulant use, including herbs and supplements.[9,10] When possible, these medications and supplements should be discontinued. Our practice is to discontinue medications 7 to 10 days before surgery if the medication or supplement is taken for preventative reasons. However, if the medication is to treat a disease, the prescribing physician should be consulted as to whether the medication can be discontinued in the perioperative period. Current recommendations suggest anticoagulation therapy be discontinued before blepharoplasty, lacrimal surgery, and orbital surgery; however, randomized controlled studies substantiating this have not been performed.[11] There is anecdotal evidence that *Arnica montana* reduces ecchymosis following blepharoplasty. However, in the only reported placebo-controlled, randomized, double-masked study, there was no evidence to suggest that *A montana* reduces or improves ecchymosis resolution following surgery.[12]

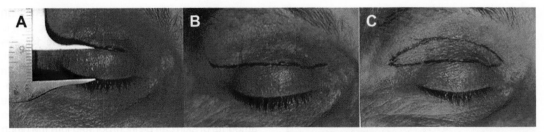

Fig. 4. Eyelid crease marking for a white female. (*A*) A caliper is used to measure the height of her natural lid crease (10 mm). (*B*) Her natural lid crease is marked across the length of the lid, slightly angling the mark superiorly at the puncta medially and canthus laterally. (*C*) The amount of skin to be excised.

Hemorrhage treatment

Preseptal hematoma If hemorrhage does occur after surgery, bleeding may spread diffusely through interstitial tissues or may collect as a focal hematoma (**Fig. 6**). The first step in evaluating a postoperative hematoma is to rule out the presence of a retrobulbar hemorrhage (discussed later) and ensure that vision has not been compromised. Once a retrobulbar hemorrhage has been excluded (no visual compromise), the application of mild, direct, firm pressure with ice to the site of the hematoma is appropriate. Although preseptal hematomas are not usually a threat to vision, the appearance can be a significant source of stress for the patient. In addition, they may lead to varying degrees of cicatrization, eyelid malposition, pigmentary disturbances, and discomfort. Conservative measures such as ice, sleeping with the head of the bed elevated, time, and reassurance are all that is typically needed. On occasion, a focal hematoma may require surgical evacuation, depending on its size, progression, and lack of response to more conservative therapy.

Retrobulbar hematoma Although rare, with an incidence of 0.05%, a retrobulbar hematoma is a potentially serious consequence of blepharoplasty surgery.[13,14] Arterial bleeding, whether deep or superficial, is likely the source of the bleed. The orbital volume is 30 cm^3 and there is little room for tissue expansion. Therefore, as the blood collects in the orbit, the eye becomes proptotic and loss of normal slack in the optic nerve occurs, which can lead to compression of the nerve or its blood supply. This orbital compartment syndrome[15] can lead to significant visual compromise or blindness. The patient typically complains of severe pain and pressure in and around the eye and decreased vision. Clinical signs include (**Fig. 7**):

- Proptosis
- Decreased vision
- A tense orbit

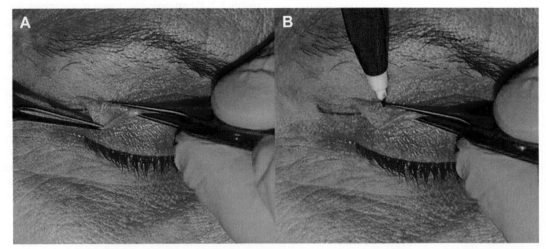

Fig. 5. The pinch technique. (*A*) Using 2 toothless forceps, the excess skin is pinched to remove the redundancy. (*B*) A mark is placed once the desired amount of skin has been incorporated into the tips of the forceps.

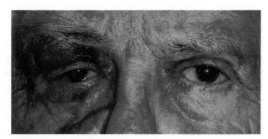

Fig. 6. Severe right eyelid preseptal hematoma following blepharoplasty.

- Increased intraocular pressure
- Limitation of eye movements
- A relative afferent pupillary defect

Because this is a clinical diagnosis, prompt treatment should not be delayed for radiographic studies (eg, computed tomography [CT] scan).

If a retrobulbar hematoma is diagnosed, emergent lateral canthotomy and cantholysis should be performed. The inferior crus of the lateral canthal tendon is lysed first. If improvement does not occur, the superior crus of the tendon can also be lysed. If there is still no improvement, operative control of the bleed, fracture of the orbital floor, and orbital evacuation should be performed. After surgery, serial ophthalmic examinations are performed to ensure that vision is improving, the intraocular pressure is decreasing, and the pupillary response has normalized.

Infection

Infection is another potential serious adverse event after blepharoplasty. The incidence of cellulitis following periorbital surgery is low given the rich blood supply to the eyelids. However, if infection occurs and is left untreated, the consequences can be severe. Cellulitis can be preseptal (isolated to the eyelid) or the more serious orbital cellulitis, in which the infection spreads retroseptally to the orbit proper. Hints of orbital involvement include

reduced vision, pupillary abnormalities, diminished motility, and proptosis. The most common agents causing preseptal and orbital cellulitis are *Staphylococcus* and *Streptococcus*,[16] although rarer pathogens such as atypical mycobacteria have also been reported.[17] The surgeon should maintain a high suspicion for methicillin-resistant *Staphylococcus aureus* (**Fig. 8**) because the incidence is increasing.[18] In addition, rare entities, such as necrotizing fasciitis, have been described following blepharoplasty.[19,20]

Preseptal cellulitis can be managed with oral antibiotics on an outpatient basis. Because infection is anterior to the orbital septum, patients typically manifest a red, tender, and engorged eyelid. However, there are no signs of abnormalities in vision, pupillary reaction, or motility disturbances. Clinical improvement should be seen within 24 to 48 hours. If there is no improvement, hospitalization with intravenous antibiotics should be considered.

In contrast, because of its potential for vision impairment, orbital cellulitis is best managed with hospitalization, imaging, and intravenous antibiotics. Orbital cellulitis results when the infection progresses posterior to the orbital septum into the orbital space.[21] Clinical signs that distinguish orbital cellulitis from preseptal cellulitis include:

- Proptosis
- Chemosis
- Severe pain
- Decreased vision
- Limitation of extraocular movements
- Potentially an afferent pupillary defect

Imaging of the orbits with CT is recommended to identify the presence of an orbital abscess, the extent of the infection, and cavernous sinus involvement.[22] If there is evidence of an abscess with visual impairment, surgical evacuation is warranted. If there is no visual impairment, the patient should be admitted, given intravenous antibiotics, and monitored for improvement.[18] If the abscess persists, it will require surgical drainage.

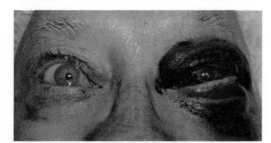

Fig. 7. Retrobulbar hematoma of the left eye. (*Courtesy of* Dr Keith D. Carter.)

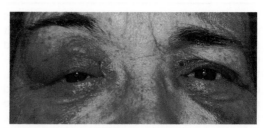

Fig. 8. Postblepharoplasty wound infection of the right upper eyelid. Cultures grew methicillin-resistant *S aureus*.

Corneal Abrasion

Corneal abrasions can occur after surgery from ocular exposure during the procedure. Corneal protectors with ophthalmic ointment should be placed in both eyes before starting surgery to maintain corneal moisture and as another layer of protection to the globe. Although corneal abrasions are painful, they heal quickly. Postoperative lubrication, patching, and occasionally bandage contact lens placement may be necessary. A postoperative abrasion should be managed by an ophthalmologist to prevent potential progression to a corneal ulcer.

Diplopia

When diplopia is present after surgery, it is important to identify whether it is monocular or binocular. Monocular diplopia after surgery results from ointment application, a disrupted tear film, and epithelial injury. Transient binocular diplopia following blepharoplasty often results from infiltration of local anesthetic into the extraocular muscles, and resolves once the anesthetic wears off.[23]

If the diplopia persists in the postoperative period, there are several possibilities. The patient may have a decompensated phoria (latent drift of an eye) or damage to the extraocular muscles, their tendons, or the nerves and blood vessels that supply them. The trochlea is the pulley of the superior oblique muscle tendon and is located just inside the superomedial orbital rim. If aggressive fat removal occurs nasally, damage to the trochlea can occur (iatrogenic Brown syndrome).[24] In lower eyelid blepharoplasty, the inferior oblique separates the nasal and central fat pads and can easily be damaged during fat removal.[25,26] If a patient has new-onset persistent diplopia following blepharoplasty, a complete ophthalmic examination, including an ocular motility evaluation, is warranted. If an ocular deviation is present, strabismus surgery may be necessary for globe realignment.

Lagophthalmos

Lagophthalmos, or the inability to close the eyelids completely, following blepharoplasty may result from varied causes, and is typically temporary and resolves spontaneously. Early and transient lagophthalmos is typically related to postoperative edema, decreased patient effort because of pain, and decreased orbicularis muscle function related to local anesthetic injection or traumatic myopathy. Reassurance is necessary, and temporary use of lubricant eye drops improves patient comfort during this time period, which may last up to 2 to 3 weeks.

Persistent lagophthalmos (more than 3 months) following blepharoplasty is more concerning. Although mild lagophthalmos can be well tolerated, moderate to severe lagophthalmos may require surgical intervention. Symptoms include foreign body sensation, tearing, burning, redness, and decreased visual acuity. On clinical examination, conjunctival injection, superficial punctate keratopathy, or frank abrasion or corneal ulcers may be present. A thorough preoperative assessment should include an inquiry about a history of dry eyes, an assessment of orbicularis function, and a history of laser in situ keratomileusis (LASIK), because these patients are prone to developing symptoms if lagophthalmos develops following surgery.[27]

Persistent lagophthalmos can also have multiple causes. The most common is excessive skin removal from the upper eyelid (**Fig. 9**). Other causes include orbicularis paresis/paralysis from damage to the facial nerve, excessive orbicularis muscle resection, and eyelid retraction. It is generally accepted that at least 20 mm of eyelid skin (brow to lid margin) is required to close the eyelid without force (**Fig. 10**). This distance should be measured from the middle of the eyelid margin to the lower edge of the brow. If a patient has cosmetically altered their brows with tattoo or makeup, the natural brow should still be used as the landmark. During skin excision, care should be taken to preserve the preseptal orbicularis muscle because removal can add to sulcus deformity and lagophthalmos caused by volume deficit and decreased orbicularis function, respectively (**Fig. 11**).

Ptosis

The presence of eyelid ptosis should be identified before blepharoplasty surgery. Patients sometimes have obscuration of the upper eyelid margin from excessive dermatochalasis, giving the false impression of ptosis (**Fig. 12**). Elevating the excess skin gently to measure the margin-to-reflex distance (distance of corneal light reflex to lid margin in primary gaze) allows the surgeon to determine the presence of ptosis. Ptosis is defined by a

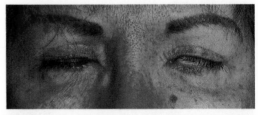

Fig. 9. Patient referred with bilateral lagophthalmos resulting from overzealous skin excision during prior blepharoplasty.

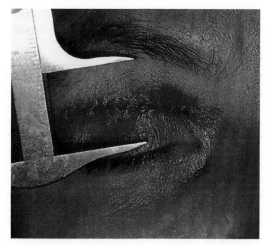

Fig. 10. After blepharoplasty, a minimum of 20 mm of upper eyelid skin should remain from brow to lid margin to allow adequate closure of the eyelid.

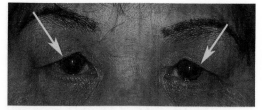

Fig. 12. A patient with pseudoptosis. Excessive dermatochalasis hangs over the upper eyelid margin (*yellow arrows*) giving the appearance that the upper eyelid is lower than it is.

margin-to-reflex distance of 2.5 mm or less. The best way to ensure that ptosis after surgery is not present is to identify its presence before surgery.

In the early postoperative period, ptosis may be caused by the mechanical effects of eyelid edema. However, if ptosis remains after complete resolution of swelling and adequate time for healing, it is possible that the levator muscle/aponeurosis was stretched, damaged, or inadvertently disinserted during surgery. If levator function is reduced after surgery, muscle damage should be suspected. Damage to the levator structures usually occurs during fat removal. Therefore, if fat removal is to be performed, it should be done conservatively and with a sound knowledge of eyelid

anatomy. Ptosis correction after blepharoplasty should be performed only after lid position is stabilized.

Lacrimal Gland Injury

The lacrimal gland is located in the lacrimal gland fossa just posterior to the superolateral orbital rim. Lacrimal gland prolapse can occur for a variety of reasons, with 1 out of every 10 patients having prolapse of the gland on at least 1 side.[28] This often gives a cosmetically unacceptable bulge to the lateral upper eyelid. Sometimes the gland can be seen under the conjunctiva with the eye in adduction (**Fig. 13**). The gland can be mistaken for a lateral fat pad, and therefore is at risk of injury or excision during blepharoplasty (**Fig. 14**), which can significantly increase the risk of permanent symptoms of dry eye, foreign body sensation, corneal damage, and vision loss. Thus it is critical to understand that there is not a third fat pad in the upper lid, and to be familiar with the intraoperative appearance of a prolapsed lacrimal gland. Restoration of the gland to its correct anatomic position via repositioning is the appropriate treatment. A 5-0 nonabsorbable polypropylene suture on a tapered needle (Prolene, Ethicon, Somerville, NJ) is passed through the capsule of the lacrimal gland and periosteum of the anterior tip of the lacrimal gland fossa. A second suture can be applied if necessary. Deep placement of the periosteal fixation suture on the inner aspect of the orbital rim is essential for optimal reposition of the gland.

Asymmetric Eyelid Crease

Despite the eyelid asymmetry that patients may have before blepharoplasty, most expect complete symmetry following surgery. The natural face is not perfectly symmetric.[29] Although eyelid symmetry should be a goal, subtle differences in eyelid crease position are inborn and should be anticipated following surgery. This consideration should be reviewed in the preoperative discussion.

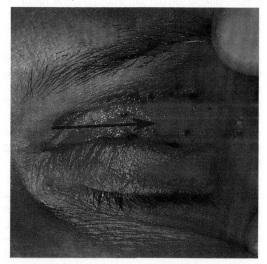

Fig. 11. Preservation of the orbicularis muscle (*black arrow*) during skin excision in blepharoplasty.

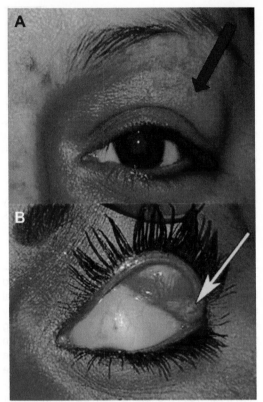

Fig. 13. (*A*) Prolapsed lacrimal gland causing temporal fullness in the left upper eyelid (*black arrow*). (*B*) On eversion of the upper eyelid, the prolapsed gland can be seen beneath the conjunctiva (*yellow arrow*).

Gross crease asymmetry usually results from asymmetric intraoperative markings. Therefore, it is essential to mark the patient precisely before skin incision (**Fig. 15**). Other causes of crease asymmetry include unrecognized preoperative ptosis (with an elevated eyelid crease), differences in globe prominence (crease may ride higher in

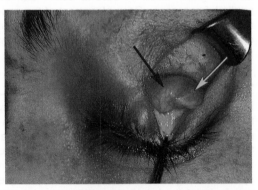

Fig. 14. The prolapsed lacrimal gland (*yellow arrow*) adjacent to the central fat pad (*black arrow*).

a prominent eye), and thyroid-related eyelid disorders (eg, disorders related to globe prominence).

Residual Excess Skin

Regardless of how carefully the eyelid markings are placed, some degree of postoperative eyelid skin asymmetry can occur. This typically occurs in the most lateral and medial portions of the eyelid. Before proceeding to revision, the surgeon must ensure that adequate skin for reexcision remains and that there is not symptomatic dry eye or exposure keratopathy. Furthermore, it is important to reevaluate the position of the eyebrow. If brow ptosis is present, restoration of the brow to its native anatomic position must be considered rather than removing excess skin, which may further accentuate the brow ptosis. Waiting at least 6 months from the initial surgery is recommended.

Sulcus Deformity

Prevention of periocular volume loss is necessary to avoid an aged appearance following blepharoplasty. In the upper eyelid, there are 2 fat pads, nasal and central. The 2 fat pads are distinct in chemical composition and structure. The nasal fat pad is a light yellow, whereas the central is golden in color. The color variance is caused by varying compositions of carotenoids, chemical constituents, and embryologic factors (**Fig. 16**).[30,31] The nasal fat is also denser and admixed with more connective tissue elements. It is a continuation of deeper orbital fat because the levator aponeurosis does not separate it from extraconal and intraconal fat. In contrast, the central fat is preaponeurotic in nature because the levator aponeurosis separates it from deeper orbital fat. With age, the nasal fat pad clinically becomes more prominent, whereas the central fat pad undergoes atrophy.[32] In patients who present for blepharoplasty evaluation with superior sulcus hollowing and a prominent nasal fat pad, it is essential to minimally sculpt only the nasal fat pad, with no removal of the preaponeurotic fat (**Fig. 17**). As an alternative, the excised nasal fat may be placed centrally as a graft, or transposed centrally as a flap.[33] Achieving symmetry of the upper eyelid volume is important to a pleasing aesthetic result.

Canthal Webbing

Canthal webbing following blepharoplasty can occur medially or laterally. Regardless of location, it is often cosmetically unacceptable. Medial canthal webbing occurs when the medial portion of the incision approximates the lid margin to closely, is angled inappropriately, extends too far nasally,

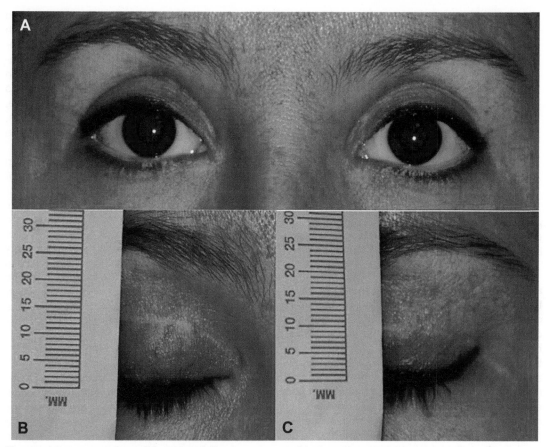

Fig. 15. (*A*) Asymmetric eyelid creases following cosmetic blepharoplasty. (*B*) The right upper eyelid crease measures 14 mm, compared with a 10-mm crease on the left upper eyelid (*C*).

or if too much skin has been excised (**Fig. 18**). Lateral canthal webbing occurs when upper and lower blepharoplasty incisions meet or the upper blepharoplasty incision is angled downward toward the canthus. Canthal webs are difficult to efface and their correction can lead to scarring and a worsened cosmetic appearance. Allow 6 months to 1 year before proceeding with revision, and only proceed after detailed explanation of possible outcomes with the patient.

Fire/Skin Burn/Singed Lashes

Whenever cautery is used there is a risk of intraoperative fire. Combustion requires heat, fuel, and oxygen. Cautery can provide the spark (heat),

Fig. 16. The nasal (*black arrow*) and central (*yellow arrow*) fat pads.

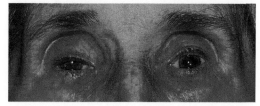

Fig. 17. A patient presenting with bilateral severe superior sulcus hollowing caused by aging. She has no history of previous eyelid surgery.

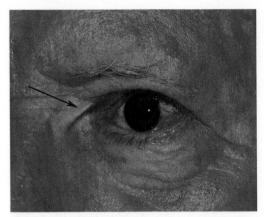

Fig. 18. Left medial canthal webbing (*black arrow*) following excessive skin removal during previous blepharoplasty.

and paper drapes or cilia the fuel. These factors, in the presence of externally supplied oxygen, may create a formula for trouble. If supplemental oxygen is used, the oxygen cannula should always be above the surgical drape to avoid an oxygen trap. In the periocular area, the eyelashes, brows, and skin are most subject to permanent damage (**Fig. 19**). This damage usually occurs when excising nasal fat in the upper eyelid, and the risk of flame initiation is increased by fat saponification from the heat. For this reason, the bovie should be used in short, light, sweeps rather than continuous, heavy, cuts. Avoidance of the fulguration mode of the cautery also minimizes electric arcing of tissues. The use of bipolar cautery may also minimize electric arc discharge.

Wound closure issues and management

A variety of sutures can be used to close blepharoplasty incisions. Surgeon preference dictates

the type of suture, with both absorbable and nonabsorbable variations having been used with good results. Our preference is to avoid inflammatory polyfilament materials, such a silk, because of the possibility of scar and inclusion cysts. We prefer a monofilament suture such as 6-0 nylon or Prolene. The method of closure, whether a running suture, subcuticular technique, or a combination thereof, depends on surgeon preference.

Postoperative wound dehiscence can result from poor wound closure or from accidentally rubbing or picking at the incision. Patients should be counseled on this. Patients with diabetes, hypertension, and poor nutrition may also be predisposed to wound healing issues. In addition, excessive cauterization of the wound edges or the use of cautery or CO_2 laser to perform the skin incision may lead to a poorly healing wound.[34] Appropriate wound closure includes eversion of the upper and lower limb of the wound with each suture pass, to ensure apposition of raw surgical edges rather than epithelialized skin.

Suture Granuloma

Focal inflammation around the suture may occur following surgery. These suture granulomas are usually not painful. However, they are noticeable and often cosmetically unacceptable. Most granulomas resolve with time. If they persist, topical steroid ointment or a steroid injection can be considered. If there is still no resolution, the granuloma can be excised in the office.

Allergy

Postoperative allergic reactions can occur in the lids or the eye. If the eyelids become red and irritated with significant itching, an allergic reaction to the topical ointment or drops is present. Cessation of the medication plus/minus the addition of topical steroid therapy usually allows quick resolution of the problem. If the symptoms are primarily ocular, stopping the medication, with the addition of an intraocular steroid or nonsteroidal antiinflammatory drop, is appropriate.

SUMMARY

Although blepharoplasty remains a safe and effective surgical procedure that is well tolerated by most patients, every surgeon occasionally encounters complications. The prompt recognition and treatment of these complications is important to prevent permanent adverse sequelae. Attaining a detailed patient history, performing a directed and

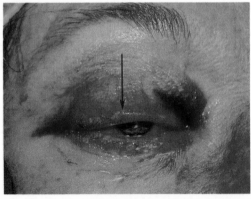

Fig. 19. Singeing of upper eyelid lashes (*arrow*) caused by sudden release of entrapped oxygen from beneath surgical drape during bovie cautery.

through preoperative examination, optimizing the surgical field and technique, being precise with measurements, and monitoring patients closely in the postoperative period will minimize complications and lead to improved outcomes and patient satisfaction.

REFERENCES

1. American Academy of Facial Plastic and Reconstructive Surgery. [Online] 2010 AAFPRS member study. Available at: http://www.aafprs.org/media/stats_polls/aafprsMedia2010.pdf. Accessed January 2011.

2. Battu VK, Meyer DR, Wobig JL. Improvement in subjective visual function and quality of life outcome measures after blepharoptosis surgery. Am J Ophthalmol 1996;121:677–86.

3. Federici TJ, Meyer DR, Lininger LL. Correlation of the vision-related functional impairment associated with blepharoptosis and the impact of blepharoptosis surgery. Ophthalmology 1999;106: 1705–12.

4. Parikh M, Kwon YH. Vision loss after inadvertent corneal perforation during lid anesthesia. Ophthal Plast Reconstr Surg 2011;27(5):e141–2.

5. Tao J, Nunery W, Kresovsky S, et al. Efficacy of fentanyl or alfentanil in suppressing reflex sneezing after propofol sedation and periocular injection. Ophthal Plast Reconstr Surg 2008;24(6):465–7.

6. Price KM, Gupta PK, Wooward JA, et al. Eyebrow and eyelid dimensions: an anthropometric analysis of African Americans and Caucasians. Plast Reconstr Surg 2009;124(2):615–23.

7. Chen WP. Asian blepharoplasty. Update on anatomy and techniques. Ophthal Plast Reconstr Surg 1987; 3(3):135–40.

8. Morris A, Elder MJ. Warfarin therapy and cataract surgery. Clin Experiment Ophthalmol 2001;28(6): 419–22.

9. Heller J, Gabbay JS, Gharjar K, et al. Top-10 list of herbal supplemental medicines used by cosmetic patients: what the plastic surgeon needs to know. Plast Reconstr Surg 2006;117(2):436–45.

10. Dinehart SM, Henry L. Dietary supplements: altered coagulation and effects on bruising. Dermatol Surg 2005;31:819–26.

11. Jaeffer AK, Brotman DJ, Chukwumerije N. When patients on warfarin need surgery. Cleve Clin J Med 2003;70(11):973–84.

12. Kotlus BS, Heringer DM, Dryden RM. Evaluation of homeopathic Arnica montana for ecchymosis after upper eyelid blepharoplasty: a placebo-controlled, randomized, double-blind study. Ophthal Plast Reconstr Surg 2010;26(6):395–7.

13. Hass AN, Penne RB, Stefanyszyn MA, et al. Incidence of postblepharoplasty orbital hemorrhage and associated visual loss. Ophthal Plast Reconstr Surg 2004;20(6):426–32.

14. Teng CC, Reddy S, Wong JJ, et al. Retrobulbar hemorrhage nine days after cosmetic blepharoplasty resulting in permanent vision loss. Ophthal Plast Reconstr Surg 2006;22(5):388–9.

15. Mahaffey PJ, Wallace AF. Blindness following cosmetic blepharoplasty – a review. Br J Plast Surg 1986;39(2): 213–21.

16. Chaudhry IA, Shamsi FA, Elaridi E, et al. Outcome of treated orbital cellulitis in tertiary eye care center in the Middle East. Ophthalmology 2007;114(2): 345–54.

17. Mauriello JA Jr, Atypical Mycobacterial Study Group. Atypical mycobacterial infection of the periocular region after periocular and facial surgery. Ophthal Plast Reconstr Surg 2003;19(3):182–8.

18. Juthani V, Zoumalan CI, Lisman RD, et al. Successful management of methicillin-resistant Staphylococcus aureus orbital cellulitis after blepharoplasty. Plast Reconstr Surg 2010;126(6):305e–7e.

19. Suner IJ, Meldrum ML, Johnson TE, et al. Necrotizing fasciitis after cosmetic blepharoplasty. Am J Ophthalmol 1999;128(3):367–8.

20. Lazzeri D, Agostini T. Eyelid and periorbital necrotizing fasciitis as an early devastating complication of blepharoplasty. Plast Reconstr Surg 2010;126(3): 1112–3.

21. Chiu ES, Capell BC, Press R, et al. Successful management of orbital cellulitis and temporary visual loss after blepharoplasty. Plast Reconstr Surg 2006; 118:67e–72e.

22. Goodwin WJ Jr, Weinshall M, Chandler JR. The role of high resolution computerized tomography and standardized ultrasound in the evaluation of orbital cellulitis. Laryngoscope 1982;92:729–31.

23. Ranin EA, Carlson BM. Postoperative diplopia and ptosis: a clinical hypothesis based on the myotoxicity of local anesthetics. Arch Ophthalmol 1985;103(9): 1337–9.

24. Syniuta LA, Goldberg RA, Thacker NM, et al. Acquired strabismus following cosmetic blepharoplasty. Plast Reconstr Surg 2003;111(6):2053–9.

25. Mowlavi A, Neumeister MW, Wilhelmi BJ. Lower blepharoplasty using bony anatomical landmarks to identify and avoid injury to the inferior oblique muscle. Plast Reconstr Surg 2002;110(5):1218–22.

26. Ghabrial R, Lisman RD, Kane MA, et al. Diplopia following transconjunctival blepharoplasty. Plast Reconstr Surg 1998;102(4):1219–25.

27. Korn BS, Kikkawa DO, Schanzlin DJ. Blepharoplasty in the post-laser in situ keratomileusis patient; preoperative consideration to avoid dry eye syndrome. Plast Reconstr Surg 2007;119(7):2232–9.

28. Smith B, Lisman RD. Dacryoadenopexy as a recognized factor in upper eyelid blepharoplasty. Plast Reconstr Surg 1983;71(5):629–32.

29. Swaddle JP, Cuthill IC. Asymmetry and human facial attractiveness: symmetry may not always be beautiful. Proc Biol Sci 1995;261(1360): 111–6.

30. Sires BS, Saari JC, Garwin GG, et al. The color difference in orbital fat. Arch Ophthalmol 2001;119(6): 868–71.

31. Korn BS, Kikkawa DO, Hicok KC. Identification and characterization of adult stem cells from human orbital adipose tissue. Ophthal Plast Reconstr Surg 2009;25(1):27–32.

32. Oh SR, Chokthaweesak W, Annunziata CA, et al. Analysis of eyelid fat pad changes with aging. Ophthal Plast Reconstr Surg 2011;27(5):348–51.

33. Massry GG. Nasal fat preservation in upper eyelid blepharoplasty. Ophthal Plast Reconstr Surg 2011; 27(5):352–5.

34. Mison MB, Steficek B, Lavagnino M, et al. Comparison of the effects of the CO_2 surgical laser and conventional surgical techniques on healing and wound tensile strength of the skin flaps in the dog. Vet Surg 2003;32(2):153–60.

Adjunctive Skin Care of the Brow and Periorbital Region

Vivian W. Bucay, MD[a,b,*], Doris Day, MD, MA[c,d]

KEYWORDS

- Skin care • Periorbital • Brow • Anti-aging cosmeceuticals • Antioxidants • Retinoids
- Growth factors • Peptides

KEY POINTS

- The unique anatomic characteristics of eyelid skin influence the types of skin care products suited to this area.
- Common concerns, including fine lines and wrinkles, infraorbital dark circles, under-eye puffiness, and thinning lashes and brows, can be treated by specific ingredients.
- Adjunctive skin care to treat the signs of photodamage may include sunscreen, topical antioxidants, retinoids, collagen boosters, and DNA repair enzymes.
- Knowledge of the contributing factors in the development of photodamage, dark circles and under-eye puffiness is needed to make skin care recommendations for these problems.
- It is important to set realistic patient expectations regarding the results of adjunctive skin care therapy.

INTRODUCTION

The periorbital region is often one of the first areas to show signs of aging and patients seek a dermatologist's advice regarding care of the eyelid skin, often starting in their early 20s, well before seeking other antiaging treatments. In the context of a multidisciplinary approach to brow and eyelid rejuvenation, it is the dermatologist's responsibility to be familiar with the many skin care options available for common concerns, including fine lines and wrinkles, infraorbital dark circles, and under-eye puffiness. Eyelid anatomy and aging are addressed in elsewhere in this issue by Lam and colleagues, Fitzgerald, Pepper and Moyer, Lee and Baker, Quatela and Lieberman, Day and Bucay, and Sundaram. They are also discussed in this article as they concern some key concepts relevant to understanding the aforementioned common complaints.

FINE LINES AND WRINKLES

Eyelid skin is the thinnest in the body, at times only 0.2 mm thick, contributing to its susceptibility to actinic and other damage. UV radiation is the primary cause of photodamage resulting in fine lines, mottled pigmentation, and textural changes. Other factors that lead to skin changes include genetic predisposition, smoking, and chronic rubbing due to seasonal allergies, irritants, or contact dermatitis. Components of adjunctive skin care to treat the signs of photodamage may include sunscreen, topical antioxidants, retinoids, collagen boosters, and DNA repair.

Sunscreens

Sunscreens are an indispensable element of adjunctive skin care of the eyelids and periorbital region. Classified as over-the-counter drugs,

[a] Private Practice, University of Texas Health Science Center, 326 W. Craig PL, San Antonio, TX 78212, USA; [b] Department of Physician Assistant Studies, University of Texas Health Science Center, 7703 Floyd Curl Drive, San Antonio, TX 78229, USA; [c] Day Dermatology and Aesthetics, 10 East 70th Street, 1C, New York, NY 10021, USA; [d] The Ronald O. Perelman Department of Dermatology, New York University Langone Medical Center, 550 1st Avenue, New York, NY 10016, USA
* Corresponding author. 326 West Craig Place, San Antonio, TX 78212, USA.
E-mail address: vbucay@aol.com

Clin Plastic Surg 40 (2013) 225–236
http://dx.doi.org/10.1016/j.cps.2012.09.003

sunscreens should offer broad UV protection to include UVA (320–400 nm) and UVB (290–320 nm) and are integral in preventing UV immunosuppression.[1] They should contain only ingredients that have been approved by the US Food and Drug Administration (FDA) as listed in the FDA's Sunscreen Monograph Final Rule.[2] Sunscreens are generally divided into two classes:

1. Chemical—organic
2. Physical—inorganic.

Chemical sunscreens (eg, benzophenone, homosalate, methyl anthranilate, octyl methoxycinnamate, oxybenzone, avobenzone) work by converting UVB radiation into heat, whereas physical sunscreens (eg, zinc oxide, titanium dioxide, kaolin, ichthammol, iron oxide) scatter, reflect and absorb solar radiation across a broad spectrum in the UV and visible ranges. In addition to their greater chemical stability, physical sunscreens have the added benefit of a minimal risk of contact sensitivity, an important consideration for delicate eyelid skin.

Topical Antioxidants

Topical antioxidants scavenge free radicals, which are highly unstable and reactive molecules. Free radicals that are generated from oxygen are known as reactive oxygen species. Capable of damaging cellular membranes, DNA, and cellular proteins, free radicals can be produced by normal cellular metabolism or can be triggered by external factors, including UV radiation and cigarette smoking. Skin aging is generally attributed to a combination of intrinsic and/or chronologic aging and extrinsic and/or environmental aging, and reactive oxygen species play a key role in both types of aging, a concept first published by Harman[3] in 1956. Free radicals can also lead to inflammation, another factor that has been implicated in the aging process.[4]

Vitamin C
Topical vitamin C (ascorbic acid) has been shown to reduce UV-induced erythema, sunburn cell formation,[5,6] and the appearance of wrinkles.[7,8] A combination of topically applied water soluble vitamin C (ascorbic acid), and a lipid soluble form, tetrahexyldecyl ascorbate (THD), has also been shown to reduce wrinkling due to photodamage.[9] Studies have shown that, at the same concentration, THD surpasses the depth of penetration of ascorbic acid by threefold and that its rate of penetration is greater, even when the concentration of ascorbic acid is 25 times that of THD.[10] Vitamin C plays an important role in

collagen production and has been shown to stimulate collagen production when added to cultures of human skin fibroblasts.[11] Vitamin C also restores the antioxidant capacity of vitamin E,[12,13] a much more potent inhibitor of lipid peroxidation.

Vitamin E
Vitamin E is lipid soluble and consists of eight active isomers (tocopherols and tocotrienols), with alpha-tocopherol showing the most biologic activity. Vitamin E reduces the number of sunburn cells, decreases UVB-induced photodamage,[14] and can inhibit UV-induced tumor formation.[15] Alpha-tocopherol, a membrane-bound antioxidant, protects cell membranes from damage caused by phospholipase A, lysophospholipids, and free fatty acids.[14] Vitamin E has been shown to inhibit human macrophage metalloelastase, a matrix metalloproteinase (MMP) that degrades elastin.[15] Furthermore, signs of photoaging were shown to improve in a study comparing the use of a vitamin E cream versus placebo.[16]

Combined vitamins C and E
The combined application of Vitamins E and C that is commercially available in several product lines has been shown to provide more potent photoprotection compared with either agent alone.[6] A limitation to topically applied vitamin E is the potential for contact dermatitis.[17,18]

Green tea
Green tea antioxidants extracted from the leaves and buds of the plant Camellia sinensis include epicatechin, epicatechin-3-gallate, epigallocatechin, and epigallocatechin-3-gallate (EGCG), the latter being the most abundant and potent.[19] Animal studies have shown that topically applied green tea polyphenols can inhibit photocarcinogenesis[20] as well as prevent UV-induced oxidative damage and induction of MMPs.[21] In vivo application of green tea polyphenols to human backs 30 minutes before UV irradiation was shown to reduce erythema, the number of sunburn cells, immunosuppression,[22] and DNA damage.[23] Another study demonstrated the efficacy of topically applied EGCG in reducing UVB-induced inflammation.[24] Although controlled clinical trials are lacking, green tea polyphenols are popular in cosmeceuticals given their ability to multitask. Vivian W. Bucay find them very helpful in mitigating the retinoid-induced irritation.

Vitamin B3
Topically applied niacinamide, the biologically active form of vitamin B3, not only exhibits antioxidant and antiinflammatory properties[25] but also can improve hyperpigmentation by decreasing

transfer of melanosomes to keratinocytes. The effects of topically applied niacinamide include improved skin texture and tone along with a reduction in fine lines and hyperpigmentation.[26]

Side Effects of Topical Antioxidants

Side effects associated with topical antioxidants may include allergic contact dermatitis or irritant dermatitis. Topical vitamin E and niacinamide may induce allergic contact dermatitis, whereas irritant dermatitis may occur with some forms of topical vitamin C, such as the water-soluble forms, because higher concentrations are required for efficacy.

Retinoids

Retinoids are a classification of naturally occurring and synthetic compounds that exhibit the biologic actions of vitamin A. Their inclusion in countless antiaging products was triggered by Kligman and colleagues'[27] groundbreaking research on the effects of tretinoin on photodamaged skin in 1986.

Prescription retinoids

Of the prescription retinoids, only tretinoin and tazarotene have FDA approval for the treatment of photodamage, although nonprescription retinol and retinaldehyde are commonly used for this indication. Wrinkle improvement is the result of retinoid-mediated effects that produce an increase in dermal collagen synthesis by increasing type I procollagen expression[28] mediated by the inhibition of the UV-induction of c-Jun[29] and an alteration of transforming growth factor (TGF)-β expression.[30] Inhibition of dermal collagen degradation is accomplished by inhibition of transcriptional factor activator protein-1 activation of MMP-like collagenase.[31,32]

Retinoids also improve dyschromia by inhibiting tyrosinase activity. This leads to a reduction of melanin synthesis, decrease in melanosome transfer, and increase in shedding of keratinocytes.[33,34] Additionally, retinoids contribute to smoother skin and a reduction in tactile roughness by increasing epidermal proliferation and differentiation, compacting the stratum corneum, and increasing epidermal and dermal intercellular mucin deposition.[35,36]

Over-the-counter retinoids

Over-the-counter alternatives include retinol that, although potentially less irritating than its metabolite retinoic acid (tretinoin), is also 20-fold less potent.[36] Retinaldehyde, a naturally occurring metabolite of retinol and the precursor of retinoic acid, has demonstrated efficacy in treating photodamage[37] but with less irritation than retinoic

acid.[38] Eye skin care products containing hyaluronic acid, ceramides, cholesterol, and dimethylaminoethanol (DMAE) lactate are useful in mitigating dryness and skin irritation, and maintaining an adequate skin barrier.

Side Effects of with Retinoids

The most common side effect associated with retinoid use is an irritant dermatitis, characterized by excessive redness, dryness and flaking. This can be minimized by selecting the appropriate type of retinoid for the patient's skin type, for example, retinoic acid or retinol for someone with thicker, oilier skin and retinaldehyde for those with thinner, drier skin. Additional strategies for mitigating skin irritation include decreasing the amount of product applied and/or the frequency of application. Layering the retinoid over a product containing antiinflammatory ingredients such as green tea polyphenols or coffeeberry also reduces skin irritation. Protective measures regarding sun exposure are strongly recommended and include sunscreen, sunglasses, and hats.

Patients should be counseled against using prescription retinoids during pregnancy and lactation. The authors recommend that each patient consult her obstetrician regarding the use of nonprescription retinoids during pregnancy and lactation.

Collagen Boosters: Peptides and Growth Factors

Peptides

Collagen boosters typically include compounds such as peptides and growth factors. A brief review of the pathogenesis of aging skin will aid in understanding the rationale for the use of these compounds in antiaging products:

- Lines and wrinkles occur both in photoaged and chronologically aged skin
- Coarser lines and wrinkles are characteristic of photoaging, whereas finer lines are more typical of chronologic aging
- The pathogenesis of skin aging is characterized by a decrease in collagen synthesis coupled with an increase in collagen breakdown[39]
- A decrease in procollagen type I mRNA is seen in aging skin,[40] with a greater reduction seen in photodamaged skin compared with nonexposed skin[41]
- UV radiation–induced upregulation of collagenase (MMP-1) leads to damage and degradation of collagen.[42,43]

Mechanisms by which an improvement in lines and wrinkles can be achieved include the upregulation of collagen production coupled with the down-regulation of collagen degradation, with dermal fibroblasts being the target cell in this strategy. To this end, peptides (short chains of amino acid sequences) have been incorporated into cosmeceuticals to stimulate collagen production. Peptides can be subdivided into three categories:

1. Signal peptides
2. Carrier peptides
3. Neurotransmitter-inhibiting peptides.

Perhaps the most studied signal peptide is the five-amino-acid sequence Lys-Thr-Thr-Lys-Ser (KTTKS), which is found on type I procollagen and has been shown to increase the production of extracellular matrix proteins[44] through the feedback regulation of collagen synthesis. Improved delivery of this hydrophilic peptide has been accomplished by adding palmitoyl, a 16-carbon fatty acid fragment, resulting in a compound known as Pal-KTTKS or, its commercial name, Matrixyl and is found in several commercially available products.

An example of a carrier peptide is the tripeptide glycyl-l-histidyl-l-lysine (GHK), which has been shown to facilitate copper uptake by cells[45] and to stimulate fibroblast collagen synthesis.[46] Additional effects of GHK include dermal remodeling by increasing levels of MMP-2 and MMP-2 mRNA and increasing levels of tissue inhibitors of metalloproteinase 1 and 2,[47] increases in type I collagen and glycosaminoglycans,[48] and increases in dermatan sulfate and cell layer-associated heparin sulfate.[49]

In vitro studies have shown that acetyl hexapeptide-3, also known as argireline, functions as a neurotransmitter inhibiting peptide by interfering with sensory nerve action potential-25,[50] thus mimicking the effects of clostridial botulinum neurotoxin. Although there is in vitro evidence of its ability to inhibit acetylcholine release, in vivo studies are limited, probably because of the inability of this compound to penetrate to the muscle. Nonetheless, argireline has been incorporated into several cosmeceutical products.

Additional peptides include tripeptide-1 (Aldenine), which acts by reducing glycation and advanced glycation end products by increasing superoxide dismutase and decreases collagen cross-linking and other peptides, and palmitoyl tetrapetide-7 and palmitoyl oligopeptide (together known as Matrixyl 3000), which act to stimulate type I collagen, fibronectin, and hyaluronic acid.

Additional peptides will be covered under the topic of puffiness and dark circles.

Growth factors

Growth factors are high molecular weight peptides that regulate specific cellular activities, including tissue repair and growth and intercellular signaling. There is evidence to suggest that the following play a role in skin rejuvenation[51]:

- TGF
- Epidermal growth factor
- Platelet-derived growth factor
- Insulin-like growth factor
- Fibroblast growth factor
- Vascular endothelial growth factor (VEGF).

A double-blind study involving 60 subjects examined the safety and efficacy of a proprietary mixture of more than 110 growth factors, cytokines, and soluble matrix proteins secreted by human fibroblasts in the treatment of mild to severe photodamage. Patients were randomized to receive either the active gel or the vehicle and were instructed to apply it twice daily. Both subjective and objective measurements at 3 months showed a greater reduction in fine lines and wrinkles by the active gel when compared with the vehicle, suggesting that a topical gel of growth factors and cytokines can improve the signs of photoaging[52] when used with a sunscreen.

Alternatives to human growth factors are those derived from plants, such as N-furfuryladenine, and animal-derived growth factors, such as snail secretion filtrate, the most biologically active of which is derived from Cryptomphalus aspersa (SCA). This compound has been used successfully in Europe for over 15 years to treat radiation dermatitis.[53,54] SCA is found in commercially available products used to treat the signs of photoaging and at least one published study has demonstrated its efficacy in the treatment of periocular wrinkles.[55]

DNA repair liposomes have been shown to reduce the incidence of UV-induced skin cancer in mice,[56] although to date, there are no controlled clinical studies in humans demonstrating the same. Despite the lack of clinical studies, incorporation of these compounds into antiaging products is becoming increasingly popular, and the author is aware of some ongoing studies involving some of the commercially available products.

DNA repair enzymes include photosomes, which are a plankton-derived form of photolyase and block the transcription of UV-induced pyrimidine dimers, roxisomes or oxoguanine glycosylase-1; a mitochondrial DNA repair enzyme obtained from the Arabidopsis thaliana (mustard) plant, which serves to excise damaged DNA; and ultrasomes, or T4 endonuclease, which is derived from *Micrococcus lysate* and acts by excising UV-induced dimers. Liposomal formulation of these enzymes allows for targeted delivery and enhanced efficacy. Photobiologist and cosmeceutical innovator Daniel Yarosh, PhD, has published more than 100 articles on the subject of DNA repair; his book, *The New Science of Perfect Skin*, is an excellent reference on the science of skin care.[57]

Stem cells are a hot topic in many areas of medicine and their incorporation into skin care is an emerging trend. Plant stem cells, such as apple stem cells, can be found in currently available skin care products; however, the inclusion of autologous human cells in skin care heralds the latest advance in the treatment of photodamage. An additional application of the recent FDA approval of technology involving the injection of an autologous fibroblast suspension for the treatment of fine lines and wrinkles will extend to the use of these same cells to formulate personalized skin care. Controlled clinical trials will be necessary to prove their efficacy.

Complications with Peptides and Growth Factors

A theoretical complication associated with the use of human growth factors is the development of skin cancers or the progression of precancerous lesions to skin cancer in susceptible or predisposed individuals. Vivian W. Bucay emphasize that the potential for skin cancer is theoretical and based on personal experience (the development of actinic keratoses and/or squamous cell skin cancer in one author and four others following use of a cosmeceutical containing VEGF) and that there are no reports in the literature documenting the development of skin cancer associated with cosmeceutical use.

This discussion is limited to VEGF and its effect on skin cancer development because there are ample references in the literature regarding the subject. Research shows that levels of VEGF are at least 10 times higher in patients with melanoma.[58,59] Melanoma cells express receptors for various growth factors, such as VEGF, and increased angiogenesis secondary to excessive VEGF exposure has been shown to be a fundamental step in the transition of dormant tumors to malignancies.[60–62] The role of VEGF in melanoma is discussed because melanoma is the deadliest form of skin cancer, although not the most common. Squamous cell carcinoma is the second most common skin cancer,[63] and important progress regarding the role of VEGF in

tumor initiation and progression has been made. Cancer stem cells have been described in several cancers, including cutaneous squamous cell tumors.[64] Through work on defining the mechanism of action of VEGF-targeted therapies, it is known that VEGF exerts its effects on tumors not only through angiogenesis but also via a direct effect on tumor cells.[65] Using a mouse model for squamous cell tumors (considered ideal for studying skin cancer initiation and growth[66]), Beck and colleagues[67] delineated the dual role of VEGF in regulating the initiation and stemness (the ability of cancer stem cells to renew and differentiate themselves). They showed that VEGF promotes cancer stemness and symmetric cancer stem cell division via neurolipin-1 (Nrp1), a VEGF coreceptor expressed in cutaneous cancer stem cells and the deletion of Nrp1 in normal epidermis prevented skin tumor initiation.

VEGF is upregulated by UVB exposure from sunlight,[68] adding to the susceptibility of unprotected skin. Patients are often reluctant to apply sunscreen to the eyelids and periorbital region, citing such reasons as burning, stinging, and tearing of the eye area. It is the authors' opinion that, although cosmeceutical products containing human growth factors are not subject to the same testing and FDA regulations as prescription drugs are, there is still much to be learned and understood regarding their mechanism of action and caution should be exercised when used in patients with a high risk or history of skin cancer.

INFRAORBITAL DARK CIRCLES AND PUFFINESS

Compared with the extensive research that contributes to our understanding regarding the mechanisms that lead to photoaging, there is a relative paucity of scientific information regarding the causes of under-eye puffiness and dark circles, which cannot be studied via animal models and tissue cultures. For this reason, the underlying causes of these common complaints are discussed here in terms of contributing anatomic and physiologic considerations.

Although not a condition associated with morbidity, dark circles are often a source of cosmetic concern that can have a negative impact on an individual's quality of life[68] because they can convey a sense of sadness or fatigue, even when these are not the case. Causes of dark circles are numerous and usually not limited to a single factor in a given individual and include excessive pigmentation, thin and translucent eyelid skin, shadowing secondary to skin laxity, and anatomic age-related changes leading to hollowing and tear trough deformity.[69,70]

Excessive Pigmentation

Excessive pigmentation may be caused by underlying dermal melanocytosis,[71] which may also be attributed to congenital causes, such as nevus of Ota,[72] sun exposure, drug ingestion,[73] or medical conditions including atopic or contact dermatitis that leads to rubbing or scratching of the periorbital region with the development of postinflammatory hyperpigmentation.[69] Hemosiderin deposition due to "leaky" vasculature or following trauma may also cause pigmentary changes in the lower eyelids. Depending on the underlying cause and the depth of pigmentation, treatment options may include topical prescription medications to treat an underlying medical problem, laser modalities, chemical peels, and/or cosmeceutical agents.

As already mentioned, the eyelids have the thinnest skin of the body, and the orbicularis oculi muscle lies just beneath the eyelid skin with minimal subcutaneous fat found between the muscle and skin. This is a contributing factor to the appearance of dark circles. A prominent subcutaneous and/or muscular vascular plexus will result in a violaceous hue under the eyes that does not blanch but deepens in color with manual stretching of the skin.[74] This maneuver of stretching the skin to produce deepening of the violaceous color may serve as useful diagnostic tool to confirm the vascular cause of the pigmentation.[69] Moreover, in their review on this subject, Roh and Chung[69] state that the successful use of autologous fat transplantation to reduce the appearance of hypervascularity supports the idea that it is the vasculature found within the muscle instead of the combination of thin skin and subcutaneous vascularity that plays a greater role in the appearance of these violaceous infraorbital dark circles.

In addition to autologous fat transplantation, various modalities, including laser and other energy-based devices as well as soft tissue fillers, have been tried with varying success. In keeping with the theme of adjunctive skin care of the eyelids, topical agents that exert effects on the vasculature will be discussed, although, as is the case with many cosmeceuticals, controlled clinical studies to support their use are lacking.

Shadowing

Shadowing due to intrinsic and extrinsic aging of the skin that leads to skin laxity,[75] in combination with age-related changes in the soft tissue and skeleton, is another common cause of dark circles. The appearance of a "tear trough" depression secondary to loss of subcutaneous fat and thinning of the skin over the orbital rim ligament leads to hollowing of the orbital rim,[76] leading to a dark shadow that can be further accentuated by pseudoherniation of the infraorbital fat pad.[77] Short of addressing the issue of photodamaged skin as discussed earlier in this article, adjunctive skin care does not play a role in the treatment of this type of infraorbital dark circle.

Puffiness and bags

Under-eye puffiness and lower eyelid bags are also multifactorial in origin and another common aesthetic complaint, although published studies regarding this topic are scarce. In an analysis of 114 consecutive subjects (67 men and 47 women, mean age 52 years, age range 23–76 years) presenting for aesthetic consultation for lower eyelid bags, Goldman and colleagues[77] conclude that there is not a single anatomic basis for their cause but, instead, identify six anatomic variables. These include

1. Cheek descent and hollow tear trough (52%)
2. Prolapsed of orbital fat (48%)
3. Skin laxity and sun damage (35%)
4. Eyelid fluid (32%)
5. Orbicularis hyperactivity (20%)
6. Triangular cheek festoon (13%).

Not surprising, tear trough depression, skin laxity, and triangular malar mound occurred with greater frequency in those older than 50 years, and linear regression analysis showed that a recommendation for surgery was based on the extent of fat prolapse, skin elasticity, and midface descent.

Surgical intervention, laser resurfacing, soft tissue fillers,[78] neurotoxins, and energy-based skin tightening may be used in varying combinations to address this complaint. Nonetheless, despite the evidence in support of an anatomic basis for under-eye puffiness and bags, patients seek recommendations for cosmeceuticals that can diminish their appearance. Most products used for this indication contain ingredients to reduce fluid retention, strengthen the vasculature, and improve skin laxity.

SKIN CARE INGREDIENTS FOR DARK CIRCLES AND PUFFY EYES

An Internet search for products for "dark circles and puffy eyes" yielded 621,000 results, a testament to the vast array of skin care products devoted to the treatment of these common problems. The lack of controlled trials precludes an evidence-based approach and much of the available information regarding the efficacy of these skin care products is anecdotal and largely dependent on testimonials and marketing campaigns. In preparing this article, several ingredients were noted to be incorporated

Table 1
Physician Dispensed Eye Creams

HydroPeptide Eye (Azure, Issaquah, WA)
Key ingredients: Haloxyl (palmitoyl oligopeptide, palmitoyl tetrapeptide-7, chrysin and N-hydroxysuccinimide), Eyeliss (dipeptide-2), vitamin K, Syn-coll (palmitoyl tripeptide-5), Matrixyl 3000 (palmitoyl tetrapeptide-7, palmitoyl oligopeptide), Dermaxyl (palmitoyl oligopeptide), Aldenine (tripeptide-1), Argireline (acetyl hexapeptide-8), hesperidin methyl chalcone, retinyl palmitate, green tea, sodium hyaluronate
Indications: photoaging, dark circles, puffiness

Gloss Dual-Treatment Eye Area (Young Pharmaceuticals, Hartford, CT)
Key ingredients:
  • STT Eye Area Restorative Eye Cream: 0.5% trichloroacetic acid, vitamin C ester, vitamin E ester, ferulic acid ester, green tea extract, hesperidin methyl chalcone, niacinamide, 18-beta-glycyrrhetinic acid (licorice), Argireline (acetyl-hexapeptide-8), Granactive AGE (palmitoyl hexapeptide-14), Chronoline (caprooyl tetrapaptide-3), B-White *(oligopeptide-68)*
  • MWF Retinol Eye Area: Retinol EmoluGel microsponge
Indications: photoaging, dark circles, puffiness

CELFIX DNA iQuad Infusion Total Eye Complex (PrecisionMD, NY, NY)
Key ingredients: Haloxyl (palmitoyl oligopeptide, palmitoyl tetrapeptide-7, chrysin, N-hydroxysuccinimide), Matrixyl 3000 (palmitoyl tetrapeptide-7, palmitoyl oligopeptide), photolyase liposomes, caffeine, ubiquinone, grape seed oil, green tea extracts, ivy extract, sodium hyaluronate, plankton extract
Indications: photoaging, dark circles, puffiness

Tensage Eye Contour (Biopelle, Ferndale, MI)
Key ingredients: 8% SCA (snail secretion filtrate) derived from *Cryptomphalus aspersa*
Indication: photoaging

NeoStrata SKIN ACTIVE Intensive Eye Therapy (Neostrata Co, Inc., Princeton, NJ)
Key ingredients: NeoGlucosamine™ (melanin production inhibitor), palmitoyl oligopeptide, palmitoyl tetrapeptide-7, tocopheryl acetate (vitamin E), sodium hyaluronate, caffeine, *Malus domestica* fruit cell culture extract (apple stem cell extract)
Indications: photoaging, dark circles, puffiness

RevaléSkin Replenishing Eye Therapy
Key ingredients: 1% CoffeBerry extract
Indications: photoaging, puffiness

Lumière Riche Bio-restorative Eye Balm (NEOCUTIS, Inc. San Francisco, CA)
Key ingredients: PSP® (purified skin proteins- a mixture of human growth factors, cytokines, and interleukins), caffeine, hyaluronic acid
Indications: photoaging, dark circles, puffiness

ELASTIderm™ EYE Complete Complex™ Serum (Obagi Medical Products, Long Beach, CA)
Key ingredients: caffeine, malonic acid, arginine
Indications: photoaging, puffiness

Replenix® Eye Repair Cream (Topix Pharmaceuticals, Inc., N. Amityville, NY)
Key ingredients: all-*trans*-retinol, green tea polyphenols, *Arnica montana*, phytonadione (vitamin K), hesperidin methyl chalcone, sodium hyaluronate, dipeptide-2, N-hydroxysuccinimide, chrysin, palmitoyl oligopeptide, palmitoyl tetrapeptide-7
Indications: photoaging, dark circles, undereye puffiness

Pro+Therapy MD™ Ultimate Lift + Correcting Eye Cream (Valeant Pharmaceuticals, Bridgewater, NJ)
Key ingredients: kinetin (0.1%)-Zeatin (0.1%) Complex; Eye Regener® (a registered trademark of Silab, Brive Cedex, France)- derived from white lupine and alfalfa seed, acts to enhance lymphatic drainage; Intensyl® (a registered trademark of Silab, Brive Cedex, France)- hydrolyzed *Manihot esculenta* tuber extract, 3-D glucan biopolymer acts to smooth and lift skin within 10 minutes
Indications: photoaging, puffiness

(continued on next page)

| **Table 1** |
| *(continued)* |
| MEG 21 EYE TREATMENT (Dynamis Skin Science, Inc., Jenkintown, PA)
Key ingredients: Supplamine®, which is a patented combination of N-Methyl-D-glucamine (meglumine) and arginine. Meglumine inhibits glycation and arginine inactivates glycation byproducts; also contains anti-inflammatory botanical extracts
Indications: photoaging, dark circles, puffiness |

into many of the product lines researched for this topic. This list is by no means exhaustive and, for the sake of simplicity, ingredients are listed under the heading that best describes the underlying cause/targeted problem:

Puffiness

- *Epilobium angustifolium* extract (willow herb): antimicrobial, anti-irritant and antiinflammatory properties
- Dipeptide-2: also known as Eyeliss; improves lymphatic circulation and drainage; inhibits angiotensin-converting enzyme (ACE); strengthens capillaries
- Hesperidin methyl chalcone: improves vascular integrity by strengthening capillaries; decreases capillary permeability
- Caffeine: antioxidant, anti-irritant, purported to decrease fat when applied topically
- Green tea and coffeeberry polyphenols: antioxidant, antiinflammatory, anti-irritant
- Palmitoyl tetrapeptide-7: peptide that improves skin elasticity, firmness, and tone by increasing collagen, hyaluronic acid, and fibronectin
- Palmitoyl oligopeptide: also known as Dermaxyl; boosts cell communication and dermal repair mechanisms
- Palmitoyl tripeptide-5: also known as Syn-Coll; increases collagen 1 production via TGF-β; reportedly 60% more effective than palmitoyl pentapeptide

Hyperpigmentation (Melanin)

- Arbutin: from bearberry; precursor of hydroquinone
- Hydroquinone: decreases melanin synthesis by blocking tyrosinase
- Kojic acid: byproduct of fermentation process in malting rice used in sake production; decreases melanin production; unstable compound so a more stable kojic dipalmitate is often used in skin care products but may not be as effective
- Vitamin C: antioxidant and antiinflammatory; reduces hyperpigmentation and increases collagen production; forms of vitamin C include ascorbic acid, magnesium ascorbyl phosphate, L-ascorbic acid, THD, ascorbyl palmitate, ascorbyl glucosamine, sodium ascorbyl phosphate, ascorbyl glucoside, and ascorbyl tetraisopalmitate.
- Soy: antioxidant and antiinflammatory; inactivates keratinocyte cell receptors that mediate transfer of melanosomes from melanocytes to keratinocytes
- Niacinamide (vitamin B3): antioxidant and antiinflammatory; increases levels of free fatty acids and ceramides in the skin and decreases transepidermal water loss; improves hyperpigmentation by decreasing melanosome transfer from the melanocyte to the keratinocyte.
- Retinol (retinaldehyde, retinyl palmitate): increases cell turnover; inhibits tyrosinase to decrease melanin production
- Azelaic acid: tyrosinase inhibitor
- Lignin peroxidase: enzyme derived from the tree fungus *Phanerochaete chrysosporium* that breaks down lignin (found in tree bark); also breaks down melanin, which is structurally similar to lignin

Vascular Pigmentation

- Chrysin: involved in the clearance of bilirubin, a breakdown product of hemoglobin
- N-hydroxysuccinimide: increases the elimination of hemoglobin breakdown products and increases clearance of iron by rendering it soluble
- Vitamin K: antiinflammatory effects as well as effects on circulation and/or clotting
- Chrysin, N-hydroxysuccinimide, palmitoyl tetrapeptide-3, palmitoyl oligopeptide: this combination is known as Haloxyl. Please refer to **Table 1** for a list of physician dispensed eye creams that contain some of the key ingredients listed below.

EYELASHES AND EYEBROWS

A thorough discussion regarding adjunctive skin care of the periorbital region should include a mention of eyelash and eyebrow enhancing agents. Since its approval by the FDA in December 2008, the only FDA-approved agent for the enhancement of eyelash growth is bimatoprost ophthalmic solution 0.03%, although countless over-the-counter products that claim to enhance eyelashes and eyebrows can be found in a variety or retail outlets ranging from drugstores to high-end department stores. Several skin care companies also manufacture lash-enhancing and brow-enhancing products for office dispensing.

The mechanism of action by which bimatoprost improves lash growth is not completely understood but is thought to involve an increase in the percentage of eyelash follicles in anagen, which may account for increased eyelash length. Bimatoprost also exerts a stimulatory effect on melanogenesis, which may result in darker lashes. Increased lash thickness and fullness may be due to an increase in size of the hair bulb and dermal papilla.[79] Its safety, efficacy, and tolerability are well documented.[80,81]

The successful use of bimatoprost for eyelash enhancement has led to its off-label use to treat eyebrows and, in the experience of the authors, is something often initiated by the patient with successful results. Although not FDA-approved for this purpose, a recent publication seems to support the use of bimatoprost ophthalmic solution 0.03% for eyebrow growth.[82]

Side Effects of Lash Growth Products

Side effects of lash-enhancing products include itchy eyes, redness of the eyes, temporary hyperpigmentation of eyelid skin, and hair growth in other areas that come into contact with the product. Please refer to the Latisse product insert for a complete list of side effects, including the risk of developing brown hyperpigmentation of the iris, which was reported with the use bimatoprost solution used intraocularly for glaucoma.

Patient Expectations Compared with Results of Using Adjunctive Skin Care and Lash Growth Products

In the authors' view, patients want and may even expect surgical results from a topically applied product. It is important to set realistic expectations regarding the role of adjunctive skin care and lash growth products. With the exception of topical prescription retinoids and a prescription lash growth product, there is a paucity of controlled clinical studies that prove the benefits and efficacy of topical cosmeceutical preparations, which is not to say that there is not scientific evidence underlying the rationale for their use.

Signs of early photodamage, such as fine lines and shallow wrinkles, often respond to topically applied products, provided that the patient is compliant regarding sun protection and uses the product consistently. In moderate-to-severe cases of photodamage, resurfacing procedures, such as chemical peels or laser resurfacing, may be more adequate. Treatment of dynamic rhytids is better addressed by neuromodulators. In many cases, a combination approach is the most appropriate approach to treating the signs of photodamage. In this setting, adjunctive skin care is used for maintenance.

Without controlled studies, the use of topical antioxidants, growth factors, peptides, and DNA repair enzymes is based more on their potential benefits and not proof. Monitoring of patients and the reporting of any complications, such as skin cancer, may be indicated, even for cosmeceuticals. Realistically, this may be difficult, given that many of these products are recommended and dispensed by nonmedical personnel, such as an aesthetician, in the setting of the physician's office, a medical spa, or a retail outlet.

Products targeting infraorbital dark circles and puffiness may be effective in mild cases. An understanding of the underlying causative factors is needed to guide treatment. In some instances, fillers or energy-based devices using radiofrequency or high-density focused ultrasound may be a better option; in others, surgery may be the best treatment.

Even in the setting of the initial visit, the authors do not hesitate to refer a patient for surgery when indicated. Patients appreciate candor and honesty and will be happy to return for maintenance, whether it is skin care, botulinum toxin, fillers, chemical peels, laser resurfacing, or energy-based therapies.

SUMMARY

An aging population and the availability and acceptance of surgical procedures to treat the signs of aging of the periorbital area have been accompanied by the development of minimally invasive aesthetic procedures for rejuvenation of this region. A deeper understanding of the contributory anatomic and physiologic factors underlying common cosmetic concerns, such as fine lines and wrinkles, under-eye dark circles, and under-eye puffiness, has allowed us to tailor treatments to the individual's needs.

A parallel explosion in the skin care industry, particularly in the arena of cosmeceuticals, has added to the palette of resources available to address these common cosmetic concerns. UV radiation is the number one cause of photodamage, making sun protection the pillar of any adjunctive skin care regimen. That said, a skin care regimen consisting of topically applied retinoids, antioxidants, collagen boosters, and DNA repair enzymes may be useful as a stand-alone treatment or as maintenance therapy, whether following surgery or one of the many minimally invasive cosmetic procedures.

Most importantly, treating cosmetic concerns does not exempt dermatologists from keeping in mind the patient's medical history. In the context of human growth factors, there is still much to be learned regarding the potency of some of these "hot" compounds found in some skin care products and the theoretical, but possible, complications that may arise from their use in a susceptible individual.

REFERENCES

1. Hanneman KK, Cooper KD, Baron ED. Ultraviolet immunosuppression: mechanisms and consequences. Dermatol Clin 2006;24(1):19–25.
2. Sunscreen drug products for over-the-counter use; final monograph. Food and Drug Administration, HHS. Final rule. Fed Regist 1999;64(98):27666–93.
3. Harman D. Aging: a theory based on free radical and radiation chemistry. J Gerontol 1956;11:298–300.
4. Greenstock CL. Free radicals, aging and degenerative diseases. New York: Alan R. Liss, Inc; 1986.
5. Cohen RM, Pinnell SR. Topical vitamin C in aging. Clin Dermatol 1996;14:227–34.
6. Lin JY, Selim MA, Shea CR, et al. UV Photoprotection by combination topical antioxidants vitamins C and E. J Am Acad Dermatol 2003;48:866–74.
7. Humbert PG, Haftek M, Creidi P, et al. Topical ascorbic acid in photoaged skin. Clinical topographical and ultrastructural evaluation: double-blind study vs. placebo. Exp Dermatol 2003;12(3):237–44.
8. Traikovich SS. Use of topical ascorbic acid and its effects on photodamaged skin topography. Arch Otolaryngol Head Neck Surg 1999;125(10):1091–8.
9. Fitzpatrick RE, Rostan EF. Topical vitamin C for photodamage. Dermatol Surg 2002;28(3):231–6.
10. Barnet Products Corp. Stable forms of vitamin C. Technical bulletin. Englewood Cliffs (NJ): Barnet Products Corp; 2001.
11. Geesin JC, Darr D, Kaufman R, et al. Ascorbic acid specifically increases type I and type III procollagen messenger RNA levels in human skin fibroblast. J Invest Dermatol 1988;90(4):420–4.
12. McCay PB. Vitamin E: interaction with free radicals and ascorbate. Annu Rev Nutr 1985;5:323–40.
13. Chan AC. Partners in defense, vitamin E and vitamin C. Can J Physiol Pharmacol 1993;71:725–31.
14. Trevithick JR, Xiong H, Lee S, et al. Topical tocopherol acetate reduces post-UVB, sunburn-associated erythema, edema, and skin sensitivity in hairless mice. Arch Biochem Biophys 1992; 296(2):575–82.
15. Gensler HL, Magadaleno M. Topical vitamin E inhibition of immunosuppression and tumorigenesis induced by ultraviolet irradiation. Nutr Cancer 1991;15(2):97–106.
16. Kagan VE. Tocopherol stabilizes membrane against phospholipase A, free fatty acids, and lysophospholipids. Ann N Y Acad Sci 1989;570:121–35.
17. Chung JH, Seo JY, Lee MK, et al. Ultraviolet modulation of human macrophage metalloelastase in human skin in vivo. J Invest Dermatol 2002;119(2):507–12.
18. Mayer P. The effects of vitamin E on the skin. Cosmet Toiletries 1993;108:99.
19. Katiyar SK, Ahmad N, Mukhtar H. Green tea and skin. Arch Dermatol 2000;136(8):989–94.
20. Wang ZY, Agarwal R, Bickers DR, et al. Protection against ultraviolet B radiation-induced photocarcinogenesis in hairless mice by green tea polyphenols. Carcinogenesis 1991;12(8):1527–30.
21. Vayalil PK, Mittal A, Hara Y, et al. Green tea polyphenols prevent ultraviolet-induced oxidative damage and matrix metalloproteinases expression in mouse skin. J Invest Dermatol 2004;122(6):1480–7.
22. Elmets CA, Singh D, Tubesing K, et al. Cutaneous photoprotection from ultraviolet injury by green tea polyphenols. J Am Acad Dermatol 2001;44(3): 425–32.
23. Katiyar SK, Afaq F, Perez A, et al. Green tea polyphenol treatment to human skin prevents formation of ultraviolet light B-induced pyrimidine dimers in DNA. Clin Cancer Res 2000;6:3864–9.
24. Katiyar SK, Elmets CA, Agarwal R, et al. Protection against ultraviolet-B radiation-induced local and systemic suppression of contact hypersensitivity and edema responses in C3H/HeN mice by green tea polyphenols. Photochem Photobiol 1995;62: 855–61.
25. Gehring W. Nicotinic acid/niacinamide and the skin. J Cosmet Dermatol 2004;3:88–93.
26. Bissett DL, Oblong JE, Berge CA. Niacinamide: a B vitamin that improves aging facial skin appearance. Dermatol Surg 2005;31(7 Pt 2):860–5.
27. Kligman AM, Grove GL, Hirose R, et al. Topical tretinoin for photoaged skin. J Am Acad Dermatol 1986;15:836–59.
28. Griffiths CE, Russman AN, Majmudar G, et al. Restoration of collagen formation in photodamaged human skin by tretinoin (retinoic acid). N Engl J Med 1993;329:530–5.
29. Fisher GJ, Datta S, Wang Z, et al. c-Jun-dependent inhibition of cutaneous procollagen transcription following ultraviolet irradiation is reversed by all-trans retinoic acid. J Clin Invest 2000;106: 663–70.
30. Fisher GJ, Tavakkol A, Griffiths CE, et al. Differential modulation of transforming growth factor-beta 1 expression and mucin deposition by retinoic acid and sodium lauryl sulfate in human skin. J Invest Dermatol 1992;98:102–8.
31. Fisher GJ, Datta SC, Talwar HS, et al. Molecular basis of sun-induced premature skin aging and retinoid antagonism. Nature 1996;379:335–9.

32. Fisher GJ, Wang ZQ, Datta SC, et al. Pathophysiology of premature skin aging induced by ultraviolet light. N Engl J Med 1997;337:1419–28.

33. Kang S. Photoaging and tretinoin. Dermatol Clin 1998;16:357–64.

34. Orlow SJ, Chakraborty AK, Pawelek JM. Retinoic acid is a potent inhibitor of inducible pigmentation in murine and hamster melanoma cell lines. J Invest Dermatol 1990;16:357–64.

35. Griffiths CE, Finkel LJ, Tranfaglia MG, et al. An in vivo experimental model for effects of topical retinoic acid in human skin. Br J Dermatol 1993;129:389–94.

36. Kang S, Duell EA, Fisher GJ, et al. Application of retinol to human skin in vivo induces epidermal hyperplasia and cellular retinoid binding proteins characteristic of retinoic acid but without measurable retinoic acid levels or irritation. J Invest Dermatol 1995;105:549–56.

37. Diridollou S, Vienne MP, Alibert M, et al. Efficacy of topical 0.05% retinaldehyde in skin aging by ultrasound and rheological techniques. Dermatology 1999;199(Suppl 1):37–41.

38. Saurat JH, Didierjean L, Masgrau E, et al. Topical retinaldehyde on human skin: biologic effects and tolerance. J Invest Dermatol 1994;103:770–4.

39. West MD. The cellular and molecular biology of skin aging. Arch Dermatol 1994;130:87–95.

40. Chung JH, Seo JY, CHoi HR, et al. Modulation of skin collagen metabolism in aged and photoaged human skin in vivo. J Invest Dermatol 2001;117:1218–24.

41. Varoni J, Spearman D, Perone P, et al. Inhibition of type I procollagen synthesis by damaged collagen in photoaged skin and by collagenase-degraded collagen in vitro. Am J Pathol 2001;158:931–42.

42. Ohniski Y, Tajima S, Akiyama M, et al. Expression of elastin-related proteins and matrix metalloproteinases in actinic elastosis of sun-damaged skin. Arch Dermatol Res 2000;292:27–31.

43. Brennan M, Bhotti H, Nerusu KC, et al. Matrix metalloproteinase-1 is the major collagenolytic enzyme responsible for collagen damage in UV-irradiated human skin. Photochem Photobiol 2003; 78:43–8.

44. Katayama K, Armendariz-Borunda J, Raghow R, et al. A pentapeptide from type I procollagen promotes extracellular matrix production. J Biol Chem 1993;268:9941–4.

45. Pickart L, Freedman JH, Loher WJ, et al. Growth-modulating plasma tripeptide may function by facilitating copper uptake into cells. Nature 1980;288: 715–7.

46. Maquart FX, Pickart L, Laurent M, et al. Stimulation of collagen synthesis in fibroblast cultures by the tripeptide-copper complex glycyl-l-histidyl-l-lysine-Cu^{2+}. FEBS Lett 1988;238:343–6.

47. Simeon A, Emonard H, Horneveck W, et al. The tripeptide-copper complex glycyl-l-histidyl-l-glycine-Cu^{2+} stimulates matrix metalloproteinase-2 expression by fibroblast cultures. Life Sci 2000;67:2257–65.

48. Simeon A, Wegrowski Y, Bontemps J, et al. Expression of glycosaminoglycan and small proteoglycans in wounds: modulation of the tripeptide-copper complex glycyl-l-histidyl-l-lysine-Cu^{2+}. J Invest Dermatol 2000;115:962–8.

49. Wegrowski Y, Maquart FX, Borel JP. Stimulation of sulfated glycosaminoglycan synthesis by the tripeptide-copper complex glycyl-l-histidyl-l-lysine-Cu^{2+}. Life Sci 1992;51:1049–56.

50. Blanes-Mira C, Clemente J, Jodas G, et al. A synthetic hexapeptide (argireline) with antiwrinkle activity. Int J Cosmet Sci 2002;24:303–10.

51. Sundaram H, Mehta R, Norine J, et al. Role of physiologically balanced growth factors in skin rejuvenation. J Drugs Dermatol 2009;8(Suppl 5):1–16.

52. Mehta RC, Smith SR, Grove GL, et al. Reduction in facial photodamage by a topical growth factor product. J Drugs Dermatol 2008;7(9):864–71.

53. Abad RF. Treatment of experimental radiodermatitis with a regenerative glucoproteic mucomucopolysaccharide complex. Dermatol Cosmet 1999;9: 53–7.

54. Brieva A, Philips N, Tejedor R, et al. Molecular basis for the regenerative properties of a secretion of the mollusk cryptomphalus aspersa. Skin Pharmacol Physiol 2008;21:15–22.

55. Tribo-Boixareu MJ, Parrado-Romero C, Badr R, et al. Clinical and histological efficacy of a secretion of the mollusk Cryptomphalus aspersa in the treatment of cutaneous photoaging. Cosmetic Dermatol 2009; 22(5):247–52.

56. Yarosh D. Cyclobutane pyrimidine dimer removal enhanced by DNA repair liposomes reduces the incidence of UV skin cancer in mice. Cancer Res 1992;52:4227–37.

57. Yarosh D. The new science of perfect skin. New York: Broadway Books; 2008.

58. Brychtova S, Bezdekova M, Brychta T, et al. The role of vascular endothelial growth factors and their receptors in malignant melanomas. Neoplasma 2008;55(4):273–9.

59. Mehnert JM, McCarthy MM, Jilaveanu L, et al. Quantitative expression of VEGF, VEGF-R1, VEGF-R2, and VEGF-R3 in melanoma tissue microarrays. Hum Pathol 2010;41(3):375–84.

60. Liu B, Earl HM, Baban D, et al. Melanoma cell lines express VEGF receptor and respond to exogenously added VEGF. Biochem Biophys Res Commun 1995; 217:721–7.

61. Benjamin LE, Keshet E. Conditional switching of vascular endothelial growth factor (VEGF) expression in tumors: induction of endothelial cell shedding and regression of hemangioblastoma-like vessels by VEGF withdrawal. Proc Natl Acad Sci U S A 1997; 94:8761–6.

62. McMahon G. VEGF receptor signaling in tumor angiogenesis. Oncologist 2000;5(Suppl 1):3–10.

63. Alam M, Ratner D. Cutaneous squamous cell carcinoma. N Engl J Med 2001;344:975–83.

64. Lobo M, Shimino Y, Qian D, et al. The biology of cancer stem cells. Annu Rev Dev Biol 2007;23:675–99.

65. Ellis LM, Hicklin DJ. VEGF-targeted therapy: mechanisms of anti-tumor activity. Nat Rev Cancer 2008;8:579–91.

66. Perez-Losada J, Balmain A. A stem-cell hierarchy in skin cancer. Nat Rev Cancer 2003;3:434–43.

67. Beck B, Driessens G, Goossens S. A vascular niche and a VEGF-Nrp1 loop regulate the initiation and stemness of skin tumors. Nature 2011;478:399–403. http://dx.doi.org/10.1038/nature10525.

68. Dong W, Yi L, Gao M, et al. IKKα contributes to UVB-induced VEGF expression by regulating AP-1 transactivation. Nucleic Acids Res 2011. http://dx.doi.org/10.1093/nar/gkr1216. [Epub ahead of print].

69. Balkishran R, McMichael AJ, Camacho PT, et al. Development and validation of a health-related quality of life instrument for women with melasma. Br J Dermatol 2003;149:572–7.

70. Roh MR, Chung KY. Infraorbital dark circles: definition, causes, and treatment options. Dermatol Surg 2009;35:1163–71.

71. Lowe NJ, Wieder JM, Shorr N, et al. Infraorbital pigmented skin. Preliminary observations of laser therapy. Dermatol Surg 1995;21:767–70.

72. Hori Y, Takayama O. Circumscribed dermal melanoses. Classification and histologic features. Dermatol Clin 1988;6:315–26.

73. Sun CC, Lu YC, Lee EF, et al. Naevus fusco-caeruleus zygomaticus. Br J Dermatol 1987;117:545–53.

74. Newcomer VD, Lindberg MC, Sternberg TH. A meanosis of the face ("chloasma"). Arch Dermatol 1961;83:284–99.

75. Epstein JS. Management of infraorbital dark circles. A significant cosmetic concern. Arch Facial Plast Surg 1999;1:303–7.

76. Kurban RS, Bhawan J. Histologic changes in the skin associated with aging. J Dermatol Surg Oncol 1990;16:908–14.

77. Goldberg RA, McCann JD, Fiaschetti D, et al. What causes eyelid bags? Analysis of 114 consecutive patients. Plast Reconstr Surg 2005;115:1395–402.

78. Kane MA. Treatment of tear trough deformity and lower lid bowing with injectable hyaluronic acid. Aesthetic Plast Surg 2005;29:363–7.

79. Cohen JL. Enhancing the growth of natural eyelashes. The mechanism of bimatoprost-induced eyelash growth. Dermatol Surg 2010;36:1361–71.

80. Woodward JA, Haggerty CJ, Stinnett SS, et al. Bimatoprost 0.03% gel for cosmetic eyelash growth and enhancement. J Cosmet Dermatol 2010;9:96–102.

81. Yoelin S, Walt TG, Earl M. Safety, effectiveness and subjective experience with topical bimatoprost 0.03% for eyelash growth. Dermatol Surg 2010;36:638–49.

82. Elias MJ, Weiss J, Weiss E. Bimatoprost ophthalmic solution 0.03% for eyebrow growth. Dermatol Surg 2011;37:1057–9.

Index

Note: Page numbers of article titles are in **boldface** type.

http://dx.doi.org/10.1016/S0094-1298(12)00165-4
0094-1298/13/$ – see front matter © 2013 Elsevier Inc. All rights reserved.

Moving?

Make sure your subscription moves with you!

To notify us of your new address, find your **Clinics Account Number** (located on your mailing label above your name), and contact customer service at:

Email: journalscustomerservice-usa@elsevier.com

800-654-2452 (subscribers in the U.S. & Canada)
314-447-8871 (subscribers outside of the U.S. & Canada)

Fax number: 314-447-8029

Elsevier Health Sciences Division
Subscription Customer Service
3251 Riverport Lane
Maryland Heights, MO 63043

*To ensure uninterrupted delivery of your subscription, please notify us at least 4 weeks in advance of move.

Moving?

Make sure your subscription moves with you!

To notify us of your new address, find your Clinics Account Number (located on your mailing label above your name), and contact customer service at:

Email: journalscustomerservice-usa@elsevier.com

800-654-2452 (subscribers in the U.S. & Canada)
314-447-8871 (subscribers outside of the U.S. & Canada)

Fax number: 314-447-8029

Elsevier Health Sciences Division
Subscription Customer Service
3251 Riverport Lane
Maryland Heights, MO 63043

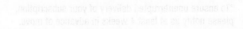

Printed and bound by CPI Group (UK) Ltd, Croydon, CR0 4YY

03/10/2024

01040347-0020